MTP International Review of Science

Physiology
Series One

Consultant Editor
A. C. Guyton

Publisher's Note

The MTP International Review of Science is an important new venture in scientific publishing, which is presented by Butterworths in association with MTP Medical and Technical Publishing Co. Ltd. and University Park Press, Baltimore. The basic concept of the Review is to provide regular authoritative reviews of entire disciplines. Chemistry was taken first as the problems of literature survey are probably more acute in this subject than in any other. Physiology and Biochemistry followed naturally. As a matter of policy, the authorship of the MTP Review of Science is international and distinguished, the subject coverage is extensive, systematic and critical, and most important of all, it is intended that new issues of the Review will be published at regular intervals.

In the MTP Review of Chemistry (Series One), Inorganic, Physical and Organic Chemistry are comprehensively reviewed in 33 text volumes and 3 index volumes. Physiology (Series One) consists of 8 volumes and Biochemistry (Series One) 12 volumes, each volume individually indexed. Details follow. In general, the Chemistry (Series One) reviews cover the period 1967 to 1971, and Physiology and Biochemistry (Series One) reviews up to 1972. It is planned to start in 1974 the MTP International Review of Science (Series Two), consisting of a similar set of volumes covering developments in a two year period.

The MTP International Review of Science has been conceived within a carefully organised editorial framework. The overall plan was drawn up, and the volume editors appointed by seven consultant editors. In turn, each volume editor planned the coverage of his field and appointed authors to write on subjects which were within the area of their own research experience. No geographical restriction was imposed. Hence the 500 or so contributions to the MTP Review of Science come from many countries of the world and provide an authoritative account of progress.

Butterworth & Co. (Publishers) Ltd.

INORGANIC CHEMISTRY SERIES ONE

Consultant Editor
H. J. Eméleus, F.R.S.
Department of Chemistry
University of Cambridge

Volume titles and Editors

1 **MAIN GROUP ELEMENTS—HYDROGEN AND GROUPS I-IV**
Professor M. F. Lappert,
University of Sussex

2 **MAIN GROUP ELEMENTS—GROUPS V AND VI**
Professor C. C. Addison,
F.R.S. and Dr. D. B.
Sowerby, *University of Nottingham*

3 **MAIN GROUP ELEMENTS—GROUP VII AND NOBLE GASES**
Professor Viktor Gutmann,
Technical University of Vienna

4 **ORGANOMETALLIC DERIVATIVES OF THE MAIN GROUP ELEMENTS**
Dr. B. J. Aylett, *Westfield College, University of London*

5 **TRANSITION METALS—PART 1**
Professor D. W. A. Sharp,
University of Glasgow

6 **TRANSITION METALS—PART 2**
Dr. M. J. Mays, *University of Cambridge*

7 **LANTHANIDES AND ACTINIDES**
Professor K. W. Bagnall,
University of Manchester

8 **RADIOCHEMISTRY**
Dr. A. G. Maddock,
University of Cambridge

9 **REACTION MECHANISMS IN INORGANIC CHEMISTRY**
Professor M. L. Tobe,
University College,
University of London

10 **SOLID STATE CHEMISTRY**
Dr. L. E. J. Roberts, *Atomic Energy Research Establishment, Harwell*

INDEX VOLUME

PHYSICAL CHEMISTRY SERIES ONE

Consultant Editor
A. D. Buckingham
Department of Chemistry
University of Cambridge

Volume titles and Editors

1 **THEORETICAL CHEMISTRY**
Professor W. Byers Brown,
University of Manchester

2 **MOLECULAR STRUCTURE AND PROPERTIES**
Professor G. Allen,
University of Manchester

3 **SPECTROSCOPY**
Dr. D. A. Ramsay, F.R.S.C.,
National Research Council of Canada

4 **MAGNETIC RESONANCE**
Professor C. A. McDowell,
F.R.S.C., *University of British Columbia*

5 **MASS SPECTROMETRY**
Professor A. Maccoll,
University College,
University of London

6 **ELECTROCHEMISTRY**
Professor J. O'M Bockris,
University of Pennsylvania

7 **SURFACE CHEMISTRY AND COLLOIDS**
Professor M. Kerker,
Clarkson College of Technology, New York

8 **MACROMOLECULAR SCIENCE**
Professor C. E. H. Bawn,
F.R.S., *University of Liverpool*

9 **CHEMICAL KINETICS**
Professor J. C. Polanyi, F.R.S.,
University of Toronto

10 **THERMOCHEMISTRY AND THERMO-DYNAMICS**
Dr. H. A. Skinner, *University of Manchester*

11 **CHEMICAL CRYSTALLOGRAPHY**
Professor J. Monteath
Robertson, F.R.S., *University of Glasgow*

12 **ANALYTICAL CHEMISTRY —PART 1**
Professor T. S. West,
Imperial College, University of London

13 **ANALYTICAL CHEMISTRY —PART 2**
Professor T. S. West,
Imperial College, University of London

INDEX VOLUME

ORGANIC CHEMISTRY SERIES ONE

Consultant Editor
D. H. Hey, F.R.S.,
Department of Chemistry
King's College, University of London

Volume titles and Editors

1 **STRUCTURE DETERMINATION IN ORGANIC CHEMISTRY**
Professor W. D. Ollis, F.R.S.,
University of Sheffield

2 **ALIPHATIC COMPOUNDS**
Professor N. B. Chapman,
Hull University

3 **AROMATIC COMPOUNDS**
Professor H. Zollinger, *Swiss Federal Institute of Technology*

4 **HETEROCYCLIC COMPOUNDS**
Dr. K. Schofield, *University of Exeter*

5 **ALICYCLIC COMPOUNDS**
Professor W. Parker,
University of Stirling

6 **AMINO ACIDS, PEPTIDES AND RELATED COMPOUNDS**
Professor D. H. Hey, F.R.S.,
and Dr. D. I. John, *King's College, University of London*

7 **CARBOHYDRATES**
Professor G. O. Aspinall,
Trent University, Ontario

8 **STEROIDS**
Dr. W. F. Johns, *G. D. Searle & Co., Chicago*

9 **ALKALOIDS**
Professor K. Wiesner, F.R.S.,
University of New Brunswick

10 **FREE RADICAL REACTIONS**
Professor W. A. Waters,
F.R.S., *University of Oxford*

INDEX VOLUME

MTP International Review of Science

Physiology
Series One

Volume 4
Gastrointestinal Physiology

Edited by **E. D. Jacobson and L. L. Shanbour**
The University of Texas Medical School

Butterworths · London
University Park Press · Baltimore

THE BUTTERWORTH GROUP

ENGLAND
Butterworth & Co (Publishers) Ltd
London: 88 Kingsway, WC2B 6AB

AUSTRALIA
Butterworths Pty Ltd
Sydney: 586 Pacific Highway 2067
Melbourne: 343 Little Collins Street, 3000
Brisbane: 240 Queen Street, 4000

NEW ZEALAND
Butterworths of New Zealand Ltd
Wellington: 26–28 Waring Taylor Street, 1

SOUTH AFRICA
Butterworth & Co (South Africa) (Pty) Ltd
Durban: 152–154 Gale Street

ISBN 0 408 70481 0

UNIVERSITY PARK PRESS

U.S.A. and CANADA
University Park Press
Chamber of Commerce Building
Baltimore, Maryland, 21202

Library of Congress Cataloging in Publication Data

Jacobson, Eugene D.
    Gastrointestinal physiology.

    (Physiology, series one, v. 4)
    1. Alimentary canal. 2. Digestion. I. Shanbour,
L. L., joint author. II. Title. III. Series.
[DNLM: 1. Gastrointestinal system—Physiology.
W1 PH951D ser. 1 v. 4 1974/W1102 G257 1974]
QP156.J3   599′.01′32   73–22455
ISBN 0–8391–1053–7

First Published 1974 and © 1974
MTP MEDICAL AND TECHNICAL PUBLISHING CO LTD
St Leonard's House
St Leonardgate
Lancaster, Lancs
and
BUTTERWORTH & CO (PUBLISHERS) LTD

Typeset and printed in Great Britain by
REDWOOD BURN LIMITED
Trowbridge & Esher
and bound by R. J. Acford Ltd, Chichester, Sussex

Consultant Editor's Note

The International Review of Physiology, a review with a new format, is hopefully also new in concept. But before discussing the new concept, those of us who are joined in making this review a success must admit that we asked ourselves at the outset: Why should we promote a new review of physiology? Not that there is a paucity of reviews already, and not that the present reviews fail to fill important roles, because they do. Therefore, what could be the role of an additional review?

The International Review of Physiology has the same goals as all other reviews for accuracy, timeliness, and completeness, but it has new policies that we hope and believe will engender still other important qualities that are often elusive in reviews, the qualities of critical evaluation and instructiveness. The first decision toward achieving these goals was to design the new format, one that will allow publication of approximately 2500 pages per edition, divided into eight different sub-speciality volumes, each organised by experts in their respective fields. It is clear that this extensiveness of coverage will allow consideration of each subject in far greater depth than has been possible in the past. To make this review as timely as possible, a new edition of all eight volumes will be published every two years giving a cycle time that will keep the articles current. And in addition to the short cycle time, the publishers have arranged to produce each volume within only a few months after the articles themselves have been completed, thus further enhancing the immediate value of each author's contribution.

Yet, perhaps the greatest hope that this new review will achieve its goals of critical evaluation and instructiveness lies in its editorial policies. A simple but firm request has been made to each author that he utilise his expertise and his judgement to sift from the mass of biennial publications those new facts and concepts that are important to the progress of physiology; that he make a conscientious effort not to write a review consisting of annotated lists of references; and that the important material he does choose be presented in thoughtful and logical exposition, complete enough to convey full understanding and also woven into context with previously established physiological principles. Hopefully, these processes will bring to the reader each two years a treatise that he will use not merely as a reference in his own personal field but also as an exercise in refreshing and modernising his whole body of physiological knowledge.

Mississippi   A. C. Guyton

Preface

With this volume we introduce a new look at gastrointestinal physiology. The classical division of the subject into secretion, absorption and motility no longer sustains the complexity, sheer mass of new information and burgeoning concepts which comprise the advances of the past decade. Our emphasis in this book is upon those advances.

Our volume is not intended to serve as intellectual pap for the novice wishing a quick overview of the field. Nor do we claim to have exhausted every aspect and cited every reference; this book is not the department store catalogue of the gastrointestinal field. Lastly, this work is not to become a factual mausoleum, a singular compilation of the state of the art of the early seventies, a repository for future scholars to unearth. The rapid recycling time of two years projected for this book means updating at regular intervals; subsequent editions should reflect the work of tomorrow; this volume is the first of a series.

Much of the task of the editors was done when we selected a body of authors whose writings are both scholarly and lucid. We have attempted in our editing to achieve a more uniform expression which might reduce the stylistic differences of an international group of writers. In this editorial effort we were assisted by Mrs. Barbara G. Cox, Director of Editorial Services, Learning Resources Center of the University of Oklahoma Medical Center.

Houston, Texas

Eugene D. Jacobson
Linda L. Shanbour

Contents

1
Gastrointestinal Hormones
L. R. JOHNSON
University of Texas Medical School, Houston

1.1   INTRODUCTION

During the past decade research dealing with the gastrointestinal hormones has constituted the most exciting and productive area of gastrointestinal physiology. Surprisingly, these hormones are, for the most part, ignored by 'endocrinologists'. In three standard endocrinology textbooks the treatment of the gastrointestinal hormones varied from non-existent[1] to an all inclusive five pages[2]. The third author conceded, as part of his one page treatment, that he had included them 'as a reminder that they are indeed hormones and that they are historically important to endocrinology since gastrin and secretin were the first substances to be called hormones'[3].

There is a sound historical reason why the gastrointestinal hormones have been relegated to the side of the mainstream of endocrinology; the reason is clearly revealed by examining the slow progress made in the study of gastro-intestinal hormones during the years between 1902 and 1964. The science of endocrinology began in 1902 with the discovery of secretin by Bayliss and Starling[4]. Shortly thereafter Hardy introduced the word 'hormone' and the concept of chemical messengers. The first or physiological epoch in the history of the gastrointestinal hormones lasted, from this auspicious beginning, until the early 1960s. In many experiments during these 60 years changes induced in one part of the digestive tract were found to affect secretion and/or motility in another part, and many hormones were implicated to account for these effects. Gastrointestinal endocrinology has never suffered from scarcity of hormones, but there was general failure during those 60 years to isolate and identify those hormones. Mucosal extracts were injected into various animal preparations and effects were attributed to a particular hormone without knowledge of the chemical nature of the extract being injected. Arguments over the existence of individual hormones even retarded the development of gastrointestinal physiology—in one case for as long as 30 years. When the physiological epoch came to an end, we understood what the various con-stituents of a meal did to gastric and pancreatic secretion or to intestinal and gall bladder motility, but we knew little about the hormones supposedly involved in the processes.

In order to establish the existence of a gastrointestinal hormone, four steps are required: first, one must demonstrate—physiologically—that a stimulus applied to one part of the digestive tract changes the activity in another part; second, the effect must persist after all nervous connections between the two parts of the tract have been interrupted; third, from the site of application of the stimulus one must isolate a substance which, when injected into the blood stream, mimics the physiological action caused by the stimulus; and fourth, one must identify the substance chemically and confirm its structure by synthesis. The first 60 years of our history were spent almost exclusively on the first and second of these criteria.

The second or biochemical epoch in the history of gastrointestinal hormones began in 1964 with the isolation, structural determination and synthesis of gastrin by Gregory and his co-workers[5,6]. In the years following, two other gastrointestinal hormones have been isolated and chemically identified, namely, secretin and cholecystokinin; secretin has also been synthesised. The availability of pure hormones has provided the gastrointestinal endocrinologist with the tools to compare responses to endogenous stimuli with those to the pure hormone, examine structure-function relationships, study hormonal interactions, determine active sites and the biochemical and molecular effects of this group of hormones.

1.2 GASTRIN

1.2.1 History

As early as 1879 investigators were aware that gastric secretion could be stimulated by a circulating factor or factors. Edkins cited studies by Heidenhain[7] demonstrating that the presence of food in the main stomach caused the separated pouch to secrete. Heidenhain's conclusion was that the secretagogues were products of digestion and were absorbed from the stomach into the blood to be carried to the pouch. In 1898 Edkins[8] paraphrased this conclusion without committing himself to the nature of the secretagogue, for he wrote of absorbed peptone somehow influencing the epithelium to cause secretion. Following the discovery of secretin and chemical mediators in general, Edkins formulated the gastrin hypothesis in 1905[9]. In his preliminary report to the Royal Society he stated, 'in the process of the absorption of digested food in the stomach a substance may be separated from the cells of the mucous membrane which, passing into the blood or lymph, later stimulates the secretory cells of the stomach to functional activity'[9].

For 43 years following the discovery of gastrin, investigators were occupied by the controversy over the existence of gastrin. The controversy intensified when it was demonstrated that histamine, an ubiquitous substance present in large quantities throughout the body[10] including the gastric mucosa[11], was a powerful stimulant of gastric secretion[12]. Even after histamine and gastrin had been shown to be different substances doubt about the importance of gastrin continued because of the difficulty of demonstrating the endogenous release of gastrin in the absence of nervous influences and absorbed secretagogues.

In 1938 Komarov[13] demonstrated that gastrin was a polypeptide and that it was distinct from histamine. He found gastrin activity in trichloroacetic acid precipitates of antral mucosal extracts and histamine activity in the supernates. It was not until Gregory and Tracy[14] developed their procedures in 1961 that a fully reliable method for extraction of gastrin became available.

The crucial physiological proof for the existence of gastrin was provided in 1948. Grossman et al.[15] demonstrated that a transplanted fundic pouch secreted when the antrum was mechanically distended.

In the mid 1960s the gastrin question was settled definitively. Gregory and his colleagues succeeded in isolating gastrin[5], and Kenner and his group identified the molecular structure[16] and synthesised hog gastrin. The structures of gastrin from man, cat, sheep, cow and dog were identified subsequently. After 60 years all the criteria for establishing the existence of a gastrointestinal hormone had been met.

1.2.2 Structure and chemistry

Gastrin is a 17 amino acid peptide amide having a molecular weight of 2114[17]. The *N*-terminus is a pyroglutamyl residue and the *C*-terminus is phenylalanine amide; thus, gastrin is protected from degradation by both amino- and carboxypeptidases. Gregory and Tracy isolated two types of porcine gastrin having identical amino acid compositions[5]. These differed only in the presence (gastrin II) or absence (gastrin I) of a sulphate group on the ring of the tyrosyl residue at position 12. Sulphation does not appreciably alter the actions or potency of the hormone[5] in dog, cat or man. Way and Durbin[18], however, found that gastrin II was more potent than gastrin I by at least a factor of 10 in eliciting acid secretion from the bullfrog gastric mucosa *in vitro*. Although this result could be attributed to a variation

Human gastrin II

1	2	3	4	5
Pyr —	Gly —	Pro —	Trp —	Leu —

6	7	8	9	10
Glu —	Glu —	Glu —	Glu —	Glu —

11	12		13	14
Ala —	Tyr	HSO₃	Gly —	Trp —

15	16	17	
Met —	Asp —	Phe —	NH₂

Figure 1.1 Amino acid sequence of human gastrin II. The *C*-terminal active tetrapeptide is underlined.

between *in vivo* and *in vitro* conditions, it probably represents a true difference between the orders Mammalia and Amphibia and may constitute an evolutionary change. The evolution of the gastrointestinal hormones is of great interest and bears upon the fact that there are two distinct structural groups of these hormones.

Gastrins have been isolated and chemically identified from 6 mammalian species. Human gastrin was described in 1966 and its complete structure is shown in Figure 1.1[19]. The gastrins differ from human gastrin and each other at the most by two amino acid substitutions (Figure 1.2). All substitutions occur in amino acids 5 through 10 and all those studied to date have a mutation value of 1, meaning that only one nucleotide change in the codon triplet of one of the pairs results in the codon of the other. In unpublished studies (Way, Johnson, and Grossman) the effects of gastrins from man, dog, sheep and cat on feline and canine gastric and pancreatic secretion were qualitatively similar and differed only slightly in potency.

A unique structure activity relationship in the gastrin molecule is that all the biological actions of the whole molecule can be reproduced by the C-terminal tetrapeptide amide (this sequence is underlined in Figure 1.1). Smaller fragments of this peptide or fragments of gastrin not containing the tetrapeptide are devoid of activity. The tetrapeptide itself, however, is

	5	6	7	8	9	10
Man	- Leu -	Glu -	Glu -	Glu -	Glu -	Glu -
Hog	Met					
Cat						Ala
Dog	Met			Ala		
Cow and sheep	Val					Ala

Figure 1.2 Species variations in the structure of gastrin. All variations occur between residues 5 and 10. The remainders of the molecule are identical (see Figure 1.1).

susceptible to some changes without total or even substantial loss of activity[20], especially at the methionine position. Thus, substitutions of nor-leucine or ethionine for methionine yield analogues with high activity. On the other hand, most changes for aspartic acid and removal of the amide group from phenylalanine inactivate the molecule[20].

Although the N-terminal 13 amino acids of gastrin are not needed for activity, they do affect potency. Thus, the cholecystokinin molecule contains the same C-terminal tetrapeptide amide as gastrin, and all differences in activity between these two hormones must be attributed to their remaining structures. The gastrin molecule may be shortened by five amino acids before encountering a loss of potency. Further removal of amino acids from the N-terminus causes loss of activity, and the tetrapeptide itself is about one-twelfth as potent as the whole hormone[6]. A simple acyl derivative of the tetrapeptide, BOC-β-Ala-Trp-Met-Asp-Phe-NH$_2$ (generic name, pentagastrin), is commercially available and is several times more active than the tetrapeptide. Pentagastrin is widely used to study the responses of man and animals to the hormone, gastrin.

1.2.3 Actions

In assessing the effects of gastrointestinal hormones one must be careful to separate physiological actions from pharmacological and to avoid hasty conclusions regarding the effects in one species based upon data obtained from a different species. Two guidelines are usually used in ascertaining whether an effect is physiological. First, the effect should take place in response to a dose of the hormone which does not exceed the maximal dose for the primary action of the hormone, e.g. for gastrin the primary action is stimulation of gastric acid secretion. Second, the effect should be reproduced by endogenous release of the hormone, e.g. endogenous release of gastrin occurs with topical application of acetylcholine to the antrum. The gastrointestinal hormones have a wide spectrum of actions on many organs, including effects on secretion, motility, absorption and metabolism. Before purification and synthesis of the gastrointestinal hormones, some of these actions were attributed to impurities or putative hormones. Since the isolation of CCK and secretin we know that the ability to affect many different targets is a characteristic of gastrointestinal hormones.

1.2.3.1 Digestive

Most of the effects of gastrin concerned with digestion are summarised in Figure 1.3. The primary action, of course, is the stimulation of gastric acid

Stomach

Acid secretion	Strong stimulation
Pepsin secretion	Weak or no stimulation
Motility	Stimulation

Pancreas

Water and HCO_3 secretion	Stimulation
Enzyme secretion	Strong stimulation
Insulin release	Stimulation

Liver

Water and HCO_3 secretion	Stimulation

Intestine

Brunner's glands secretion	Stimulation
Motility	Stimulation
Absorption of H_2O, Na, glucose	Inhibition

Gall bladder

Contraction	Stimulation

Metabolic

Protein synthesis	Stimulation
RNA synthesis	Stimulation
DNA synthesis	Stimulation

Figure 1.3 Effects of gastrin

secretion[9,21]. Gastrin is the most potent gastric secretagogue known, being 1500 times more potent than histamine on a molar basis. In man the ED_{50} is 1.0 ng kg^{-1} min^{-1}. Most investigators consider gastrin to be a weak stimulator of pepsin secretion[21], but recent evidence indicates that the presence of acid itself stimulates pepsin secretion[22], and this may account for the pepsigogic effect of gastrin. In unpublished studies from the author's laboratory, pentagastrin failed to stimulate pepsin secretion from the vagally denervated canine pouch if the pouch contents were kept neutral. In the pancreas gastrin weakly stimulates secretion of fluid and bicarbonate, but evokes a strong increase in enzyme output[23]. It stimulates water and salt secretion from the liver[24] and the glands of Brunner in the duodenal mucosa[25]. Gastrin stimulates gastric motility[26] and affects the motility or contraction of many other organs including the gall bladder[27], uterus[28], oesophagus[29], and intestine[30]. The stimulation of uterine and gall-bladder contraction must be considered pharmacological in that the doses required to observe the effect are considerably higher than the dose which causes maximal gastric acid secretion. Another such effect is the inhibition of gastric acid secretion by high doses of gastrin in the dog[31]. It has recently been demonstrated that gastrin decreases the net absorption of Na^+, K^+, H_2O[32,33] and glucose[33] from the jejunum and ileum. This effect seems due either to an inhibition of active absorption of Na^+ or to a stimulation of Na^+ secretion. These effects on absorption have been demonstrated with endogenous hormone as well as exogenous[33]. It is possible that this mechanism insures the presence of a sufficient volume of fluid in the gut during the time it takes for adequate mixing, digestion, solubilisation and absorption of the more complex components of a meal to occur.

1.2.3.2 Metabolic

Hormones are usually described as regulators of secretion and/or metabolism. The gastrointestinal hormones were originally conceived to account for non-neural effects on secretion and smooth muscle, and it has only been during the past 3 or 4 years that their interesting roles in metabolism have come to light.

There is considerable evidence that gastrin is a trophic hormone for certain tissues of the upper digestive tract, namely, gastric and duodenal mucosa and pancreas. Chronic administration of pentagastrin produces parietal cell hyperplasia in the rat[34]. Johnson et al.[35] demonstrated that pentagastrin stimulated the in vitro incorporation of leucine into protein of gastric and duodenal mucosa; these authors proposed that gastrin was a specific growth regulating hormone for these tissues, since pentagastrin did not increase leucine uptake in liver or skeletal muscle, and effects on the stomach and duodenum were independent of acid secretion. Synthetic human gastrin has also been shown to stimulate the in vivo incorporation of leucine into protein of both duodenal and gastric mucosa[36]. Removal of the major site of gastrin release by antrectomy leads to atrophy of the gastric mucosa and a decrease in the mass of both parietal and chief cells[37].

Mayston and Barrowman[38] reported that repeated injections of penta-gastrin for 2 weeks resulted in hypertrophy of the pancreatic acinar cells accompanied by a decrease in the specific activities of several pancreatic enzymes and a significant increase in the RNA/DNA ratio of the tissue.

They suggested that gastrin may be a trophic hormone for the pancreas[38] in the same manner as had been proposed for the gastric and duodenal mucosa[35].

Evidence has been accumulating that gastrin regulates the growth of some of the most rapidly replicating tissues of the body. It stimulates the incorporation of orotic acid into RNA of duodenal and gastric mucosa[39]. Antrectomy decreases the content of RNA and DNA of rat gastric and duodenal mucosa by about 40% over a period of 4 weeks[40]; this decrease can be reversed significantly by three injections of a physiological dose of pentagastrin during the 24 h before sacrificing the animals[40]. Gastrin (but not histamine) has been shown to stimulate DNA synthesis and mitotic activity in the canine fundic mucosa[41]. These effects of gastrin are probably direct and not due to the release of another hormone, since pentagastrin stimulated proliferation of an epithelial populace from gastric mucosal cells grown in tissue culture[42]. Similarly in cultures of duodenal cells pentagastrin maintained 73% of the cells as proliferative compared to 36% of the controls. Thymidine uptake into nuclear DNA was also stimulated by pentagastrin, and the doubling time of these cultures was 19.5 h compared to 31.5 h for the controls[43].

Obviously, there are many unanswered and exciting questions related to the growth promoting effects of gastrin. While the stimulation of protein, RNA and DNA synthesis are probably involved, where and how does gastrin induce its primary effect? Does it play a role in differentiation of tissue? What about the other gastrointestinal hormones—do they too affect growth?

Gastrin also stimulates insulin secretion and this property is shared by secretin and CCK[44]. The substance, incretin, had been proposed to explain the higher blood insulin levels following an oral glucose load compared to the same amount injected intravenously, but this 'hormone' has now been subsumed under the chemically identified gastrointestinal hormones.

1.2.4 Assay and localisation

Another product of the biochemical epoch has been the development of quantitative assays to measure physiological amounts of gastrin in serum and tissue. These radioimmunoassays have been perfected in several laboratories[45-47] and have essentially replaced the relatively insensitive bioassays which depended on inducing gastric secretion with the unknown sample in a test animal (usually the rat) and comparing it to secretion stimulated by a known amount of histamine or gastrin.

The groundwork for the radioimmunoassay of gastrin was described by McGuigan[48] who was able to produce antibodies to gastrin by repeated injection of the C-terminal tetrapeptide amide coupled to bovine serum albumin. Synthetic human gastrin was then substituted for the tetrapeptide and an antiserum was developed[49]. The tyrosine residue in position 12 is easily labelled with radioactive iodine, measurement of which allowed McGuigan to assay gastrin in the blood with a sensitivity of 10 pg ml^{-1} serum[49]. Similar assays from other laboratories have reported sensitives in the same range[46,47].

Assays employing antibodies to human gastrin I measure gastrin I and II equally well[45]. These antibodies cross-react in an indistinguishable manner with cholecystokinin and with pentagastrin, but the sensitivity is much less than to gastrin itself. In contrast, antibodies prepared to the tetrapeptide cross-react equally well with those compounds which contain the C-terminal 4 amino acids of gastrin, namely gastrins I and II, pentagastrin and cholecystokinin[50].

1.2.4.1 Antrum

The antrum or the pyloric gland region of the stomach is the only normally occurring abundant source of gastrin. Traces of gastrin have also been found in the cardiac region of the stomach[51,54]. The most concentrated gastrin activity is localised in the middle third of the antral mucosa. Using light and electron microscopy Solcia et al.[52,53] identified an antral mucosal endocrine cell, which is found rarely in other parts of the gut; they postulated this cell as the source of gastrin. Subsequently McGuigan[54] used fluorescein-labelled antibodies to human gastrin I to confirm their findings. Gastrin was located in or on abundant cytoplasmic granules of differentiated epithelial cells. Histologically these cells resembled endocrine cells and were structurally similar to 'argentaffin-like' cells[54]. Recently McGuigan and Greider[54] have reported an intensive study correlating the immunochemical localisation of gastrin with light-microscopy and staining techniques. They suggested that a specific name be assigned to the gastrin containing cell for they were unable to classify it on the basis of staining procedures. Bussolati and Pearse[55], on the other hand, were able to stain gastrin containing cells from hog antral mucosa with the Grimelius silver impregnation procedure and classified them in the argyrophilic group. McGuigan and Greider described several endocrine cell types from antral mucosa: the 'gastrin cell' (the name they proposed for the gastrin-containing cell), an autofluorescent cell (previously shown to contain serotonin), and a non-autofluorescent argyrophilic cell[54]. An explanation for the differences between the results of the two groups is not apparent.

The amount of gastrin measured per gram of antral mucosa depends on the methods used in collecting and storing the tissue before assay. Thus, Berson and Yalow[56] measured 11 mg gastrin/g tissue in a specimen which had been quick frozen compared to 2.6 mg in a specimen which had only been iced. Quick-frozen tissue extracted in the frozen condition yielded 25–30 mg gastrin/g compared to 7.0 mg g^{-1} for an adjacent piece kept at 4 °C for 1 h[56]. This emphasises the need for individual laboratories to establish and follow a rigid protocol for both their gastrin assay and for the collection and storage procedures.

Studies of immunoreactive gastrin extracted from human antral tissue yielded two components[56]. On starch gel electrophoresis the major component (approximately 70–90 % of the total) migrated in the same zone as heptadeca-peptide gastrin, moving about twice as far from the origin as serum albumin. The minor component migrated just in advance of serum albumin and, on elution from Sephadex columns, proved to have a molecular weight between

7000 and 7500. Yalow and Berson[57] suggested that the larger component, called 'big gastrin' (BG), contains the heptadecapeptide linked to a more basic peptide with a molecular weight of about 5000.

1.2.4.2 Serum

Normal fasting serum gastrin concentrations vary among laboratories according to different assay methods and standards used. For the most part, human basal gastrin concentrations range between 30 and 120 pg ml^{-1} with a few apparently normal subjects having values in the range of 200–300 pg ml^{-1}[47,58,59].

Gastrin radioimmunoassay has been especially useful in aiding in the diagnosis of gastrinoma, a gastrin-secreting pancreatic islet cell tumour, (the Zollinger–Ellison syndrome) and other conditions coincident with peptic ulcer or gastric secretory abnormalities. Serum gastrin values are frequently higher than 1000 pg ml^{-1} and usually greater than 500 pg ml^{-1} in patients with Zollinger–Ellison syndrome[60,61]. Gastrin values are also usually increased in patients with achlorhydria or hypochlorhydria[61,62]. In cases of pernicious anaemia or achlorhydria without pernicious anaemia serum gastrin values average between 500 and 1000 pg ml^{-1}. Thus the highest serum gastrin concentrations are found in patients having the highest rates of acid secretion (ZE syndrome) on the one hand and no acid secretion on the other. In the case of gastrinoma, tumour secretion of gastrin produces the high values, while in the achlorhydric subject elevated gastrin results from the absence of a normal feed-back inhibition of antral gastrin release by endogenous acid.

Fasting serum gastrin levels in patients with duodenal ulcer disease are not significantly different from those of normal controls in the same studies[58,59,63,64]. The appearance of normal gastrin levels in conjunction with elevated acid secretion raises the question of whether or not the gastrin releasing mechanism in the antrum has become autonomous from the inhibiting mechanism. On the other hand, gastrin values average approximately double control values in patients having gastric ulcer[54,64], and this is no doubt due to a usually decreased acid output.

In contrast to the antrum and other tissues the majority of gastrin present in plasma is the more basic component, BG[57]. The heptadecapeptide-like component (H-L G) and BG are immunoreactively equal and apparently both are physiologically active. BG is not altered by boiling nor is it converted to H-L G by antral extracts[57]. There does not appear to be spontaneous interconversion of the two components in vitro[65]. Whether conversion occurs at the physiological receptor is uncertain. Since BG predominates in plasma independent of whether the sample was taken from a control subject, a patient with ZE syndrome or one with pernicious anaemia[57,65] gastrin may be synthesised and stored in tissues as H-L G and later joined to a second peptide of molecular weight 5000 to form BG. It is even more likely that H-L G and BG are separate gastrin pools and independent of each other. Although BG is preferentially secreted into plasma, feeding releases both components[65]. Obviously, there are a number of interesting and unanswered questions concerning synthesis, storage, release and turnover of gastrin.

The effects following intravenous injection of gastrin in man are of short duration. No increase in acid secretion over baseline values can be detected after 1 h and most of the secretory response has faded by 30 min[66]. Studies in dogs comparing the acid secretory effects of substances given via portal vein infusion with those produced by systemic infusion have shown that the full gastrin heptadecapeptide is relatively immune from biological inactivation by the liver[67]. Pentagastrin and histamine, on the other hand, are markedly inactivated by hepatic passage[67]. Recently Reeder et al.[68] used radioimmunoassay to examine the amount of endogenous gastrin entering and leaving the liver and found no significant decrease caused by hepatic transit. Since all hormones released from the digestive tract must pass through the liver before acting on their normal targets, it is predictable that they might contain structural groups protecting them from hepatic degradation.

Most recent investigations using the radioimmunoassay to estimate the half-life of gastrin in the blood agree and give a value of approximately 5–10 min[47,69,70]. The differences depend primarily on experimental technique, errors due to mixing and the volume of distribution assumed for gastrin. Since gastrin is rapidly inactivated and the liver does not play a significant role in that inactivation, the kidney has become the next candidate for the site of gastrin degradation, because of the large flow of blood through the organ. Recently, Thompson's laboratory reported that renal transit did not appreciably alter basal levels of plasma gastrin as determined by immunoassay[71]. During release of endogenous antral gastrin, however, there was a 30% loss of activity from the blood after a single passage through the kidney. It appears that the major sites of inactivation of elevated levels of endogenous gastrin are probably the kidneys. It also follows from the foregoing that we need to examine the capacities of other tissues (e.g. the lungs) to destroy gastrin and to identify the enzymes involved in its destruction.

1.2.4.3 Intestine

The concentrations of gastrin present in the duodenum and jejunum are significant though considerably less than that present in the antrum[56]. In contrast to the antrum Berson and Yalow[56] found more than half the duodenal gastrin made up of the large component and all jejunal gastrin appeared to be BG. Within the intestine the amount of gastrin decreased from the proximal duodenum to the jejunum. Watson et al.[72], however, determined that 80% of the gastrin activity they measured in the antrum, fundus, and proximal duodenum was H-L G. They found approximately 18,000 μg gastrin/g antrum compared to 200 μg for duodenum and 120 μg g^{-1} for fundus.

Is duodenal gastrin released and is it responsible as such for the well known intestinal phase of gastric secretion? Following gastrectomy in dogs, feeding produced a rise in serum gastrin levels from 47 pg ml^{-1} to 68 pg ml^{-1}, indicating release of extragastric endogenous hormone[73]. Introduction of food into the duodenums of patients with previous gastrectomies and a Bilroth I drainage procedure resulted in a considerable increase in serum gastrin, comparable to that seen in patients with intact stomachs following an identical meal. Serum gastrin did not rise following a meal in patients with a Bilroth II procedure (gastrojejunostomy)[74]. Therefore, it appears that duodenal but not jejunal gastrin may contribute significantly to the response to a meal.

1.2.4.4 Pancreas

The use of bioassay methods measuring stimulation of gastric acid secretion has been ineffectual in establishing the unequivocal presence of gastrin in normal mammalian pancreatic tissue. Immunofluoresence, on the other hand, has localised gastrin within the cytoplasm of certain islet cells in the pancreas. Lomsky et al.[75] found gastrin in the D cells of pancreatic tissue from a variety of species including man. Greider and McGuigan[76] have also localised gastrin in the metachromatic D or delta cells.

The only pathology known to be caused by the overproduction of one of the gastrointestinal hormones is Zollinger–Ellison syndrome. In 1955 Zollinger and Ellison[77] described the association between intractable ulceration of the upper gastrointestinal tract, extremely high levels of gastric acid secretion and non-beta islet cell tumour of the pancreas. At the time they suggested that the tumours might be releasing a gastric secretagogue into the circulation and thus be directly responsible for the development of the ulcers. In 1960 Gregory et al.[78] extracted a gastrin-like substance from one of these tumours and subsequent studies[79,80] on its chemical nature have established its identity. As was true for the antrum and duodenum the majority of tumour gastrin is present as H-L G.

Recognition of the gastrin secreting ability of Zollinger–Ellison tumours focused attention on the pancreas as a site of synthesis and storage of gastrin; however, it is not certain that gastrin normally found in the pancreas is released by physiological stimulation in sufficient quantities to influence the response to a meal.

1.2.5 Release

The release of antral gastrin is normally mediated by neuroendocrine reflexes. These cholinergic reflexes can be divided into two groups: short or local reflexes are intramural and activated by stimuli affecting receptors located in the wall of the stomach; long reflexes involving the extrinsic vagus nerves are initiated by direct vagal stimulation or by stimuli to receptors in the stomach wall which lead to activation of afferent fibres contained in the vagus nerve. Since the efferent path of this latter reflex is also contained in the vagal trunk, it has become known as a vagovagal reflex.

Long reflexes cause small amounts of gastrin to be released, whereas short reflexes may cause the release of sufficient gastrin to produce maximal rates of acid secretion. The small amount of gastrin released by long reflexes is of great importance however, since it occurs in conjunction with direct cholinergic stimulation of the parietal cells. In the dog this combination produces potentiation of the acid response to secretory rates exceeding those which can be attained with either agonist acting alone[81].

Short or local reflexes are stimulated by distension of the stomach and by a few chemical substances. Chemical agents which effectively release gastrin include short chain alcohols such as ethanol and propanol[82]. Methanol is relatively ineffective in releasing gastrin. The amino acids glycine and β-alanine are strong releasers of gastrin[82], indicating that for the most part, only molecules with two or three carbons are highly effective.

Csendes and Grossman[83] recently reported that both D- and L-isomers of alanine and serine are equally effective as releasers of gastrin. This is in contrast to studies of the hormone, cholecystokinin, which can be released only by D-amino acids[84]. Most transport systems distinguish between D- and L-isomers of amino acids. One that does not is the sarcosine carrier which shows equal affinity for D- and L-isomers in the intestinal transport of neutral amino acids. Furthermore, the amino acids having a high affinity for the sarcosine carrier are the same ones which are the most potent releasers of gastrin. This uncovers the interesting possibility of the existence of a similar carrier system in the antral mucosa.

Figure 1.4 summarises the pharmacological evidence that antral gastrin release is mediated by cholinergic nerves, and Grossman[85] has reviewed this area in depth. This rather simple mechanism for gastrin release has been

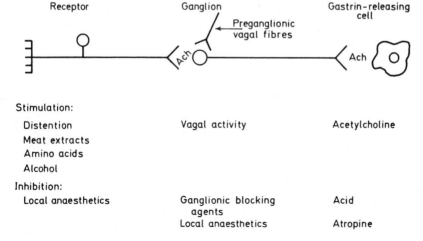

Figure 1.4 Hypothetical local reflex for the release of gastrin by antral stimuli and vagal activation. Agents which inhibit and stimulate at each point are noted. Adapted from Grossman[85].

questioned by the finding in man that systemically injected atropine does not inhibit the release of immunoassayable gastrin in response to a meal[86]. It should be revealing to repeat this experiment in a dog with a Heidenhain pouch so that acid secretion could be monitored simultaneously. This might determine whether or not atropine acts at the parietal cell or the gastrin cell. Perhaps cholinergic release of gastrin is atropine resistant, or non-cholinergic mechanisms may be involved in gastrin release.

Physiological inhibition of gastrin release occurs when the pH of the antral mucosa drops below 3.5[87]. This inhibitory mechanism does not act via a nervous reflex, since acid inhibits gastrin release even after local anaesthesia of the mucosa[87]. The mechanism involved in inhibition of gastrin release by acid is obscure. Most investigators have focused their efforts on either the entrance of H^+ into the mucosa or on the effects of acid on mucosal receptors. A recent study posed a new approach by providing evidence that the crucial point may be reduced penetration into the mucosa of the stimulators of gastrin release[88]. The authors point out that the mucous coat contains glycoproteins with carboxyl groups charged negatively at neutral pH. These groups gain a cation and become neutral at low pH, which reduces membrane osmotic activity with the depletion of counter ions; simultaneously, membrane water is lost and overall membrane permeability decreases. Glycine, on the other hand, is a zwitter ion at pH 7, a cation at pH 1 and would be less permeant at the low pH. This conforms to what Berkowitz et al.[88] found using [^{14}C]glycine. While this idea does not explain all the data on the various releasers of gastrin, it is a new approach to an old problem and is worthy of further testing.

1.2.6 Histamine

No discussion of gastrin is complete without an assessment of the current evidence pertaining to the role of histamine in the stimulation of gastric secretion. As indicated earlier, the historical relationship between histamine and gastrin is a long one involving numerous hypotheses. Only one of these, the so-called final common mediator concept, retains significant support. On the basis of experiments on the histamine content of gastric juice and the gastric mucosa MacIntosh[89] in 1938 proposed that other stimulants released histamine locally within the stomach wall thereby stimulating the parietal cells to secrete acid. This idea has evolved into the statement that 'histamine is the final common local chemostimulator of the parietal cells of the gastric mucosa'[90], which is to say that all other secretagogues, namely gastrin and acetylcholine, act via histamine.

The strongest evidence in favour of the histamine hypothesis comes from experiments with rats. The rat stomach contains histidine decarboxylase, which catalyses the formation of histamine from histidine. The activity of this enzyme increases in response to feeding, gastrin and various means of stimulating the vagus (acetylcholine release)[91]. There is concurrent decrease in the amount of bound histamine within the mucosa[91]. On the basis of these observations Kahlson et al.[91] hypothesised that gastrin, acetylcholine and feeding release mucosal histamine which stimulates the parietal cells; the depletion of histamine stores then triggers a feed-back increase in enzyme activity resulting in the formation of new histamine. Further evidence for the feed-back nature of the system was the observation that injection of histamine itself resulted in a decrease in histidine decarboxylase activity. The salient features of Kahlson's findings and hypothesis are shown in Figure 1.5. This model depends on two unproven and, until recently, untested assumptions:

(1) the release of histamine acts via a feed-back mechanism to increase the activity of histidine decarboxylase; and

(2) mucosal histamine actually stimulates the parietal cell after it is released or formed.

It is well known that vagal stimulation causes gastrin to be released[82]. This suggested the interesting possibility that the increased histidine decarboxylase activity observed in numerous experiments with feeding, insulin, Urecholine , and 2-deoxy-D-glucose was mediated through endogenous gastrin. Johnson *et al.*[92,93] compared histidine decarboxylase activity in

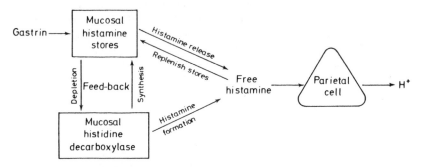

Figure 1.5 Model for involvement of histamine in acid secretion. The only target for gastrin is mucosal histamine. Released histamine stimulates the parietal cells and depletion of the stores stimulates an increase in histidine decarboxylase. (From Johnson and Aures[100], by courtesy of the Society of Experimental Biology and Medicine.)

sham-operated rats and rats in which antral gastrin had been removed by antrectomy. There was no detectable histidine decarboxylase activity in any antrectomised animal while all the sham-operated rats had discernible activity. Re-feeding of fasted animals increased histidine decarboxylase activity in the antrectomised animals, but only to one-third of the levels found in the controls. Pentagastrin itself was equally effective in both groups[92]. Neither insulin, 2-deoxy-D-glucose nor Urecholine increased enzyme activity significantly in the antrectomised rats[93]. Cholecystokinin, which contains the same active *C*-terminal peptide as gastrin, was equally effective in both groups. These observations led to the conclusions that the slight activation seen in the antrectomised rats following feeding was due to the release of cholecystokinin from the small intestine, that gastrin directly stimulated histidine decarboxylase, and that gastrin was responsible for all activation of the enzyme[93]. The fact that enzyme activity decreased following histamine injection[91] can also be explained through gastrin, for histamine stimulates acid secretion leading to antral acidification and decreased gastrin release. Essentially the same results have been reported by Håkanson and Liedberg[94] with the same inherent conclusion that histidine decarboxylase activity is under the control of endogenous gastrin.

Two other types of experiments indicate that histamine does not stimulate the parietal cells in response to gastrin. Adashek and Grossman[95] compared dose response curves to histamine and gastrin in gastric fistula rats. The peak rate for gastrin was twice as high as for histamine. Transformation of these data to obtain Michaelis–Menten constants showed that the V_{max} to gastrin was almost twice that calculated in response to histamine[96]. The different CMRs (calculated maximal responses) or V_{max} for histamine and gastrin mean different efficacies; two agents having different efficacies cannot act through a single agonist. In other words, gastrin does not stimulate the parietal cell via histamine.

Secretin inhibits pentagastrin[97] but not histamine[98] stimulated secretion in the rat. The identical dose of secretin, however, has no effect on induction of histidine decarboxylase activity[99] or histamine release[100] stimulated by gastrin. Therefore, in the presence of secretin, gastrin releases histamine and stimulates histamine formation as it normally does, but acid secretion does not occur. Since secretin does not inhibit histamine stimulated acid secretion, it cannot be assumed that secretin acts on histamine to inhibit gastrin stimulated secretion. Figure 1.6 outlines the actions of gastrin on histamine

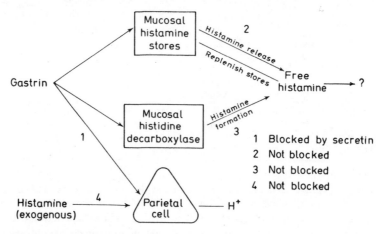

Figure 1.6 Model to correlate stimulation of rat acid secretion by gastrin with the effects of secretin. Gastrin has three targets: histamine stores, histidine decarboxylase, and the parietal cell. (From Johnson and Aures[100], by courtesy of the Society of Experimental Biology and Medicine.)

and the parietal cell according to these findings. On the basis of these experiments, we concluded that histamine is not a physiological mediator of acid secretion[100].

Numerous recent experiments have demonstrated further that under physiological conditions acid secretion occurs without involvement of endogenous histamine. Sewing[101] measured acid secretion, histidine decarboxylase and histamine release in response to a continuous intravenous infusion of pentagastrin. Acid secretion was stimulated and histidine decarboxylase activity increased but there was no release of histamine as is seen with a single bolus injection of gastrin. Sewing concluded that histamine release is actually a pharmacological phenomenon.

Insulin stimulates acid secretion in the antrectomised rat without causing the release of histamine[94]. Since there is no activation of histidine decarboxylase by insulin in the antrectomised rat, acid secretion proceeds independently of both released and newly formed histamine. A more detailed treatment of the work of the past 5 years concerning histamine can be found in a recent review[96].

1.3 CHOLECYSTOKININ

1.3.1 History

Cholecystokinin (CCK) was the last of the three chemically identified gastrointestinal hormones to be discovered. In 1928 Ivy and Oldberg[102] described a humoral mechanism for stimulation of gall-bladder contraction in response to fat in the small intestine. The hormone involved was named cholecystokinin after its primary action. Unlike the history of gastrin, that of CCK is relatively uneventful. The only controversy involving this hormone is a mild one over its name. In 1943 Harper and Raper[103] found that a hormone was released from duodenal mucosa which stimulated pancreatic enzyme secretion and accordingly named it pancreozymin. As the purification of these two hormones proceeded, it became obvious that both properties resided in one substance[104]. For the sake of convenience and because it was the first action described, this hormone is called cholecystokinin. It is, however, still often referred to as pancreozymin or even cholecystokinin-pancreozymin. This is the most noteworthy example of the biochemical epoch resulting in the demise of a classical gastrointestinal hormone.

CCK was purified and its partial structure determined by Jorpes and Mutt[104,105], two Swedish workers who also isolated and purified the third gastrointestinal hormone, secretin. Like gastrin, CCK was isolated from the hog, but in this case the hormone was extracted from the upper small intestine. The full amino acid sequence of CCK has recently been reported, but complete synthesis of the hormone has not taken place.

1.3.2 Structure and chemistry

CCK is a chemical homologue of gastrin, for while it contains 33 amino acids, the 5 C-terminal residues of the two hormones are identical. Thus, CCK contains the minimal active fragment of gastrin, and, as might be expected, the actions of the two agents are qualitatively similar. The differences in the effects of the two compounds are quantitative. This is especially evident with respect to their primary actions. Gastrin stimulates gall-bladder contraction weakly and only at high doses, while CCK is a weak stimulator of gastric secretion and actually inhibits gastric secretion stimulated by gastrin. Since gastrin and CCK both contain the active C-terminal tetrapeptide amide, the differences in the relative potencies of the two hormones must be due to the remainder of the molecules.

Both gastrin II and CCK have sulphated tyrosyl residues near the C-terminus (Figure 1.7). In gastrin the amino acid is in position 6 (counting unconventionally from the C-terminus), whereas in CCK, tyrosine occupies the seventh position. As mentioned earlier, gastrin occurs naturally in both sulphated and non-sulphated forms, and there is no difference in the potency of the two forms in most test systems. CCK, however, occurs naturally only

```
                        7    6    5    4    3    2    1
Gastrin II        - Ala - Tyr - Gly - Trp - Met - Asp - Phe - NH₂
                              |
                            HSO₃


CCK               - Tyr - Met - Gly - Trp - Met - Asp - Phe - NH₂
                         |
                       HSO₃


Caerulein         - Tyr - Thr - Gly - Trp - Met - Asp - Phe - NH₂
                         |
                       HSO₃
```

Figure 1.7 Carboxy-terminal heptapeptide amides numbered unconventionally from the C-terminus.

in the sulphated form and desulphation results in loss of potency[106]. Figure 1.8 illustrates this point with regard to gall-bladder contraction. The natural octapeptide of CCK was 200 times more potent than the desulphated

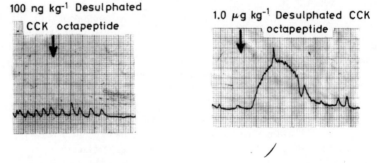

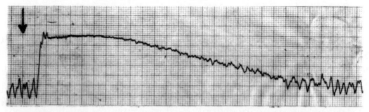

Figure 1.8 Effect of removing the naturally occurring sulphate from the tyrosyl residue in CCK on gallbladder contraction. There is an approximate 200-fold loss in potency. (From Johnson et al.[106], by courtesy of Williams and Wilkins.)

compound[106]. Thus, the tyrosyl residue must be included as part of the active centre of CCK.

Most of the information on the structure-activity relations of the C-terminal portion of CCK has come from the work on caerulein by Erspamer's group in Italy. Caerulein is a decapeptide amide which was isolated from the skin of the Australian frog, *Hyla caerulea*[107,108]. The 5 *C*-terminal amino acids of caerulein are identical to those of gastrin and CCK. Caerulein is more closely related to CCK, for the sulphated tyrosyl residue occurs in position 7 (Figure 1.7). Desulphation of caerulein decreases its stimulatory effect on pancreatic enzyme secretion and gall-bladder contraction to the potency of gastrin in these assay systems[106]. On the other hand, desulphation changes caerulein from a partial to a full agonist like gastrin for gastric acid secretion[109]. As would be expected, desulphated caerulein does not competitively inhibit gastrin stimulated acid secretion, while CCK and natural caerulein do[110]. The gastrin pattern of activity then is elicited when the tyrosyl residue is in position 6 or when it is desulphated in position 7; the CCK pattern predominates when tyrosine is sulphated and in position 7. These data suggest that at one time during phylogenetic development one hormone existed to perform the functions of both CCK and gastrin. A taxonomic investigation of the distribution of these substances would be of interest and would probably uncover other members of the gastrin family similar to caerulein.

1.3.3 Actions

The effects of CCK, in general, resemble those of its structural homologue, gastrin. The most prominent actions of CCK are summarised in Figure 1.9. Given alone, in low doses CCK weakly stimulates gastric acid and pepsin

Stomach		
	Acid secretion	Weak stimulation alone inhibition of gastrin
	Pepsin secretion	Stimulation
	Motility	Stimulation
Pancreas		
	Water and HCO_3 secretion	Stimulation
	Enzyme secretion	Strong stimulation
	Insulin release	Stimulation
Liver		
	Water and HCO_3 secretion	Stimulation
Intestine		
	Brunner's glands secretion	Stimulation
	Motility	Stimulation
	Absorption of H_2O, Na	Inhibition
Gall bladder		
	Contraction	Strong stimulation

Figure 1.9 Effects of cholecystokinin

secretion[105]. It is, however, a potent competitive inhibitor of gastrin stimulated acid secretion in the dog. CCK, however, is a full agonist in the cat. This illustrates one of the clear cut species differences with regard to the action of the gastrointestinal hormones.

CCK is an important physiological stimulator of pancreatic enzyme secretion[105]. In the dog, the ED_{50} for pancreatic flow and enzyme output is about 2.0 μg kg^{-1} h^{-1}. The maximal flow and bicarbonate response is about 20% of that attainable with secretin, while the maximal enzyme output is equal to that of the other strong stimulants of enzyme secretion, gastrin and cholinomimetic drugs[105].

CCK is the strongest of the three known gastrointestinal hormones which cause contraction of the gall bladder[112]. There are no dose-response data for the action of CCK on gall-bladder contraction in man, but in the dog the ED_{50} is about 1.0 μg kg^{-1} h^{-1}. Caerulein is of interest to the clinical gastroenterologist because of its potential use in cholecystography. Bertaccini et al.[113] have reported a successful trial with caerulein in man. Gall-bladder contraction took place within several minutes of injection of caerulein and no side reactions or pain occurred in their patients. The dose of caerulein employed was one-fiftieth (by weight) of the dose of CCK recommended for the same action.

CCK acts on the smooth muscle of the entire digestive tract. Much of this work has been done using the C-terminal octapeptide of CCK which has been synthesised and found to stimulate gall-bladder contraction in all animals tested. Using guinea-pig and dog in vivo gall-bladder contraction to determine relative potency, Rubin et al.[115] found that the octapeptide was 2.5 times more potent than CCK on a molar basis. The octapeptide increases the resting tone of the canine pylorus and the frequency of pyloric squeeze[116]. CCK octapeptide decreases lower oesophageal sphincter pressure in man[117]. It stimulates intestinal motility[118] and inhibits the sphincter of Oddi[114]. The effects of CCK on gastric motility vary depending on the ongoing motility pattern. CCK often inhibits existing motility but stimulates contractions in the quiet stomach[120].

CCK is a mild choleretic[121] and stimulates secretion by the glands of Brunner in the duodenum[122]. Gardner et al.[123] found that CCK inhibited the net transfer of sodium, chloride, and fluid across the everted hamster gut sac. CCK, like gastrin, inhibits absorption from isolated loops of canine jejunum and ileum in situ[124]. In this study, a physiological dose of CCK inhibited absorption of fluid, Na, K, and Cl from both portions of the gut. In the jejunal loop, CCK significantly increased the absorption of glucose. Endogenous CCK released by the presence of fat in the first portion of the gut mimicked the effects of exogenous hormone on ileal absorption. From these results the authors concluded that CCK may insure the presence of sufficient fluid for digestion, solubilisation and absorption of the major foodstuffs.

General metabolic effects of CCK on the gastrointestinal mucosa have not been examined, but in the pancreas the hormone stimulates amino acid uptake and incorporation into protein[125]. Most of the increased protein synthesis measured in these studies is related to the production of pancreatic enzymes[126]. Whether CCK is a trophic hormone for the pancreas, as is the case with gastrin, has not been established. In light of the similar effects of these two agents, however, it is likely that CCK will also be found to regulate pancreatic growth. Like gastrin, CCK stimulates histamine release and the activation of gastric mucosal histidine decarboxylase in the rat[99].

A relatively recent development which has helped move gastrointestinal hormones closer to endocrinology in general, is the realisation that the gastrointestinal hormones release insulin and glucagon[44]. CCK has been reported to increase in plasma following an oral glucose load, but plasma insulin concentration had reached a peak value before CCK[127]. It is unclear whether the carbohydrate content of a normal meal is capable of stimulating CCK release or not. These observations, coupled with the failure of CCK to release insulin from *in vitro* pancreas[128] and isolated islets[129], pose questions concerning the physiological importance of insulin release by CCK. Since digestion products from proteins are potent releasers of CCK, it is possible that glucagon released by CCK may help prevent hypoglycaemia after a high protein intake.

1.3.4 Assay and localisation

Currently there is no reproducible immunoassay in use for measuring CCK. Earlier Young *et al.*[130] had reported a radioimmunoassay for CCK in human serum. Antibodies were obtained from rabbits injected with porcine CCK conjugated by means of carbodiimide to rabbit serum albumin. The antiserum obtained provided for a sensitive radioimmunoassay which could detect 15 μU CCK (comparable to about 12 pg). Healthy adults had undetectable amounts of serum CCK following an overnight fast, but concentrations reached 1280–2400 μU ml^{-1} after a meal composed of 33 g protein and 11 g fat[130]. Other laboratories have reported the development of antibodies to CCK, but much of the difficulty in establishing the assay is due to the instability of I-CCK[131].

Numerous *in vivo* and *in vitro* methods exist for assaying CCK. *In vivo* gall-bladder contraction or pancreatic enzyme secretion are used to monitor CCK release from the upper small intestine. Purified CCK preparations can be assayed using an isolated rabbit gall bladder preparation[132], but the sensitivity of this method (0.05 U) does not approach that obtained with radioimmunoassay. CCK was originally purified from hog duodenum and is generally considered to be confined to the upper small intestine. Specific localisation of CCK in different areas of the intestine and other tissues of the gastrointestinal tract requires development of a standard immunoassay.

1.3.5 Release

CCK is released from the mucosa of the upper small intestine in response to amino acids, fatty acids, and hydrogen ion in the lumen. CCK, like gastrin, is probably synthesised and stored in specialised cells. These cells have not been separated from the other endocrine cells found in the intestinal mucosa. It is not known whether agents which release CCK act directly on the endocrine cells or at another site via a neurohumoral reflex. Unlike gastrin, however, CCK is not released by vagal stimulation. Cholinergic activity either modulates release or plays a permissive role, since vagotomy, atropine and local anaesthetics decrease CCK secretion.

CCK release in response to amino acids and fat has been assessed by studying pancreatic enzyme output in the same animal. Go *et al.*[133] found that phenylalanine, methionine, and valine were active releasers in man, whereas tryptophan was less active. In the dog phenylalanine and tryptophan were potent releasers, valine and leucine were less effective[134], and methionine was ineffective. The discrepancy with methionine probably represents a species difference, for there are numerous species differences regarding the action and interaction of the gastrointestinal hormones. Apparently only the L-isomers of amino acids are effective releasers of CCK, since L-phenylalanine stimulates enzyme secretion in the dog, but D-phenylalanine does not[135]. Proteins do not release CCK when placed in contact with gut mucosa. Whether they must be completely broken down to amino acids or whether intermediate small peptides can release CCK is unknown.

CCK release is related to the rate of entry of amino acid into the gut, i.e. release is dependent on the amount rather than on the concentration of amino acid present. This implies that the rate of absorption of amino acid per length of intestine has a fixed maximum. Therefore, the amount of CCK released depends on the length of intestine exposed to the amino acid.

While the amount of extractable CCK in the mucosa of the small intestine has not been reported as a function of the distance from the pylorus, it appears that it is distributed evenly over the first 90 cm. Meyer and Grossman[134] found that infusion of L-phenylalanine, 45 cm below the pylorus, produced a pancreatic enzyme response equal to that resulting from infusion of the pylorus. In man infusion of amino acids 80 cm beyond the ligament of Treitz produced responses equal to those stimulated by duodenal infusion[136].

According to Meyer (unpublished studies[134]) fatty acids shorter than C_8 do not release CCK. Octanoic acid was found to be a weak releaser, while decanoic was moderately strong; lauric, palmitic, stearic, and oleic acids were equal and strong releasers of CCK. It is likely that fat must be absorbed in order to stimulate CCK release, but this has not been adequately tested for pancreatic enzyme secretion.

Hydrogen ion is a weak releaser of CCK. At low and moderate rates of acid entry into the duodenum, the pancreatic enzyme response can be mimicked by secretin. Moreland and Johnson[137] found that at high rates of entry (24 mequiv. H^+ h^{-1}) the protein output was higher than could be obtained by doses of exogenous secretin producing comparable rates of volume and bicarbonate secretion. Hydrogen ion must, therefore, be considered as a high threshold releaser of CCK. This claim is substantiated by the observation that gall-bladder contraction occurs in response to large acid loads in the duodenum[138]. Secretin alone does not stimulate gall-bladder contraction. Meyer and Grossman[134] have recently calculated that the ratio of secretin to CCK released by acid is about 24 to 1.

1.4 SECRETIN

1.4.1 History

As discussed in Section 1.1 the discipline of endocrinology began in 1902 with the discovery of secretin. Although secretin was the first hormone discovered, its isolation and chemical analysis followed Gregory's comparable work with gastrin. After spending many years on its isolation and purification[139,140], Jorpes and Mutt[141] announced the full amino acid sequence of secretin (Figure 1.10) in 1966. Later that year Bodanszky and co-workers[142]

Porcine secretin

1	2	3	4	5
His -	Ser -	Asp -	Gly -	Thr -

6	7	8	9	10
Phe -	Thr -	Ser -	Glu -	Leu -

11	12	13	14	15
Ser -	Arg -	Leu -	Arg -	Asp -

16	17	18	19	20
Ser -	Ala -	Arg -	Leu -	Gln -

21	22	23	24	25
Arg -	Leu -	Leu -	Gln -	Gly -

26	27	
Leu -	Val -	NH_2

Figure 1.10 Amino acid sequence of porcine secretin

reported the complete synthesis of the hormone. This first attempt at synthesis yielded a product with about half the potency of natural secretin. Elimination of side products derived from rearrangement of the aspartyl residue in position 3 resulted in a material equal in potency to natural secretin, about 4 clinical units μg^{-1}[143].

1.4.2 Structure and chemistry

Secretin is the ranking member of the second family of chemically related hormones and putative hormones isolated from the gastrointestinal mucosa. Secretin is a polypeptide containing 27 amino acid residues and, unlike gastrin and its homologues, contains no active fragment. All 27 amino acids are required for activity; substitution for any one of them renders the molecule inactive. Based on studies of optical rotatory dispersion and circular dichroism of natural and synthetic secretin, Bodanszky et al.[144] concluded that the hormone exists in a preferred tertiary conformation which probably involves a helical structure. It appears that secretin is a miniature protein, the exact primary structure of which is needed to form the bonds yielding the active three dimensional form.

Secretin was isolated from the duodenal mucosa of the hog, and porcine secretin is the only secretin whose structure has been determined. It will be interesting to see whether there will be amino acid substitutions in secretins from other species or whether these will be identical to hog secretin. Presumably any deviations in structure will occur at residues not involved in the active site or in maintaining the active configuration of the hormone.

Secretin is strongly basic since it contains 1 histidyl and 4 arginyl residues, and because two of the three glutamyl residues are amidated at the γ-carboxyl group. This may explain why secretin is released during duodenal acidification, for if it is bound electrostatically to ionised protein carboxyl groups, duodenal acidification may neutralise these negative groups destroying the attractive forces.

1.4.3 Actions

Secretin, like the gastrointestinal hormones in general, has many different target organs (Figure 1.11). Its primary action is the stimulation of pancreatic

Stomach		
	Acid secretion	Strong inhibition of gastrin in dog. Weaker in man
	Pepsin secretion	Strong stimulation
	Motility	Inhibition
	Gastrin release	Inhibition
Pancreas		
	Water and HCO_3 secretion	Strong stimulation
	Enzyme secretion	Stimulation
	Insulin release	Stimulation
	Glucagon release	Inhibition
Liver		
	Water and HCO_3 secretion	Strong stimulation
Intestine		
	Brunner's glands secretion	Stimulation
	Motility	Inhibition
	Absorption of H_2O, Na	Inhibition
Gall bladder		
	Contraction	Stimulation in presence of CCK

Figure 1.11 Actions of secretin

secretion of bicarbonate and fluid, and secretin is the most potent stimulator of this secretion. Volume of pancreatic secretion is proportional to the log dose of secretin, and flow usually begins within 30 s after administration[145,146]. Much of the dose response data on secretin is expressed in various types of clinical units. An explanation of these and their relative potencies can be found in a recent review article by Hubel[147]. In man the ED_{50} is 60 μg kg^{-1} h^{-1}.

The effect of secretin on pancreatic enzyme secretion has been the subject of persistent debate. Enzymes accumulate in the ducts and acini of the unstimulated pancreas. When secretin is administered, the flow of fluid carries these enzymes along in the juice, giving the impression of enzyme secretion. This 'washout' phenomenon has been offered by some as the only explanation for increased enzyme output in response to secretin. Most investigators, however, believe that secretin weakly stimulates pancreatic enzyme secretion. This conclusion is based on finding higher than basal levels of protein persisting in pancreatic juice through long periods of secretin infusion[137] and finding a slight increase in protein output with increasing doses of secretin[148].

Secretin is the most potent pepsigogue of the gastrointestinal hormones, ranking second only to cholinergic stimulation in the ability to evoke pepsin secretion from the chief cells. Unlike some of the other actions of secretin, which vary with animal species, a strong stimulation of pepsin output has been demonstrated in dog[149], cat[149], and man[150].

In the dog, secretin is a potent inhibitor of gastrin stimulated acid secretion. In fact, the response to a near maximal dose of gastrin or pentagastrin is inhibited more than 90% by a submaximal dose of secretin[151]. Secretin exhibits the same inhibitory effect of gastrin stimulated acid secretion in the rat[152]. It is considerably less effective in man[153] and virtually ineffective in the cat[149]. Speculatively, one may relate the effectiveness of secretin as an inhibitor of acid secretion in these various species as a function of its overall action leading to duodenal neutralisation. In the dog, the capacity of the pancreas to secrete bicarbonate in response to secretin falls far short of the maximal acid secretory capacity of the stomach. In man, the difference is smaller and in the cat pancreatic secretion of bicarbonate is approximately equal to gastric secretion of acid. Thus, in each species the combination of secretin stimulated pancreatic secretion of bicarbonate and secretin inhibition of gastric acid secretion approximates neutralisation of the acid output of the stomach.

Most of the effects of secretin on the gastrointestinal tract lead to a decrease in duodenal acidification either by neutralisation, the result of stimulating pancreatic secretion, or by decreasing the amount of acid entering the duodenum, the result of inhibiting gastric secretion. Secretin stimulates bicarbonate flow from the liver and Brunner's glands[122] as well as from the pancreas. In fact, secretin is the most potent choleretic of the gastrointestinal hormones, acting on the cells of the interlobular ducts of the biliary tree to stimulate the flow of water and bicarbonate[154]. Secretin also reduces the amount of acid entering the duodenum by inhibiting gastric motility and emptying[155].

Secretin augments the strength of gall-bladder contraction in dogs in response to CCK[156]. Large amounts of secretin alone, however, appear to have little effect. Secretin reduces the absorption of water by rabbit gall bladder in vitro[157], but there are no adequate studies on in vivo transport.

Secretin inhibits the rise in pressure of the human lower oesophageal sphincter induced by gastrin and reduces the resting pressure[158]. Exogenous secretin in doses about equal to those causing maximal pancreatic secretion reduces small intestinal motility in man. Motility and electrical activity are also reduced in dogs by exogenous secretin[159].

In addition to these direct effects on gastrointestinal function, secretin alters the release of several other hormones. Although secretin is not a powerful inhibitor of gastrin stimulated acid secretion in man, it does inhibit the release of gastrin. Hansky *et al*.[160] have shown that gastrin concentrations fall in fasting patients following the injection of pure natural secretin. The *in vivo* inhibitory effects of secretin on acid secretion must be direct effects at the parietal cell as well as prevention of the release of a normal stimulant of the parietal cells.

Secretin is generally considered to be an effective releaser of insulin[44,161,162]. It will not, however, produce hypoglycaemia in normoglycaemic patients. The physiological significance of the secretin effect on insulin is obscure because of the doses of secretin required, conflicting reports and failure of secretin to release insulin from isolated islets. Furthermore, the secretin-insulin interaction needs to be integrated with the effects of the other gastrointestinal hormones on insulin and glucagon release.

In addition to stimulating insulin release, secretin is a potent inhibitor of glucagon release. Santeusanio *et al*.[163] have recently reported several findings which support this contention. Exogenous secretin decreased the glucagon content of blood from the pancreatico-duodenal vein 60% within 15 min. In combination with modest hyperglycaemia, glucagon release was completely prevented by secretin. Endogenous secretin released by duodenal acidification also significantly suppressed glucagon release. It appears then that secretin is an important antihyperglycaemic agent, both stimulating insulin release and inhibiting the alpha cells.

There has been only one study of the effects of secretin on the growth of the gastrointestinal mucosa. Using rats with chronic gastric fistulas, Stanley *et al*.[164] found that synthetic secretin injected in combination with pentagastrin for a period of 2 weeks prevented the increase in basal and maximal acid output observed in a similar group of rats injected only with pentagastrin. Secretin also reduced the parietal cell hyperplasia and increased mucosal thickness evoked by gastrin. Secretin alone caused a decrease in the parietal cell count when compared to saline injected controls. Secretin may, therefore, antagonise the growth promoting actions of gastrin as well as its effects on secretion and motility.

1.4.4 Assay and localisation

The only reported secretin radioimmunoassay is that of Young *et al*.[165] who studied the release of secretin by duodenal acidification and by a protein meal[166]. Pentagastrin was found to release secretin in an achlorhydric patient and in normal subjects whose gastric secretions were either neutralised or aspirated. They concluded that gastrin directly released secretin and that the effect was not due to acid[166]. Oral glucose was also found to release secretin. These extraordinary observations, some of which were unexpected, stemmed primarily from the success of Young in labelling secretin and in obtaining an antiserum suitable for radioimmunoassay. Unfortunately, it has been impossible to restore the assay and further this work since the untimely and tragic death of Mr. Young in 1970.

Secretin is presently assayed by measuring pancreatic bicarbonate and volume output from a chronic fistula cat or dog. As with all bioassays there are the usual shortcomings of lack of sensitivity and specificity. One cannot measure plasma levels of secretin nor exclude the presence of gastrin and CCK which will weakly stimulate the aqueous component of pancreatic secretion and potentiate the effects of secretin.

In the species so far examined, the amount of secretin which can be extracted per gram of small intestinal mucosa diminishes from the duodenum to ileum[147]. Meyer et al.[167] have shown that the amount of secretin which can be released does not decrease in the first 45 cm from the dog pylorus. Recently these same workers found that introduction of acid 45 cm from the pylorus, while preventing its proximal reflux, stimulated bicarbonate output equal to that obtained by introducing similar amounts of acid at the pylorus[134]. One must conclude from these studies that some secretin which can be extracted from the first 90 cm of gut cannot be released by acid and that there is no gradient for secretin release over the first 90 cm of small intestine.

Secretin (and CCK) are probably synthesised and stored in endocrine cells analogous to the gastrin cell of the antral mucosa. Since secretin can be extracted from cells of the villi and from cells shed into the lumen, the hormone is probably produced by villus epithelial cells. These cells have as yet not been identified among the numerous endocrine-like cells seen in the intestinal mucosa. This will no doubt be of first priority when an immuno-fluorescent antibody is developed for secretin.

1.4.5 Release

The classical studies of Wang and Grossman[168] demonstrated that duodenal installation of fatty acids and amino acids, in addition to hydrochloric acid, stimulated flow and bicarbonate output from the pancreas. The results were interpreted to mean that all of these substances were capable of releasing secretin. Since we now know that CCK can elicit a weak flow of water and bicarbonate from the pancreas, these conclusions must be re-examined. In other words, does the amount of water and bicarbonate secreted from the pancreas in response to amino and fatty acids exceed the response to CCK itself?

Meyer and Grossman[135] examined this question in a series of carefully controlled experiments using L-phenylalanine, a potent CCK releaser. In dogs they found that duodenal infusion of phenylalanine did not augment the bicarbonate response to a high background dose of CCK, whereas a sub-threshold dose of exogenous secretin caused a marked increase in the response. In addition, the bicarbonate response to duodenal infusion of L-phenylalanine was equal to that induced by the dose of exogenous CCK producing a comparable stimulation of protein secretion[135]. Meyer and Grossman concluded that the bicarbonate response to L-phenylalanine depended solely upon the release of CCK. The assumption that this conclusion applies to all amino acids should be tested.

On the other hand, fatty acids given as soap micelles or in bile acid micelles produce a higher ratio of bicarbonate to protein output than does the carboxyterminal octapeptide of CCK[134]. Crude CCK (10% pure) produces a bicarbonate protein ratio like fatty acids. From these results Meyer and Grossman[134] concluded that fatty acids release a second hormone and crude

CCK is an impure material which contains a bicarbonate stimulant in addition to CCK. In both cases, the additional stimulant is assumed to be secretin.

The strongest releaser of secretin is hydrogen ion. While some investigators have reported no threshold below pH 7.0 for secretin release, it has recently been shown that a threshold exists around pH 4.5 above which secretin is not released in amounts sufficient to stimulate pancreatic secretion (Figure 1.12)[169]. Between pH 4.5 and 3.0 there is a rapid rise in pancreatic secretion.

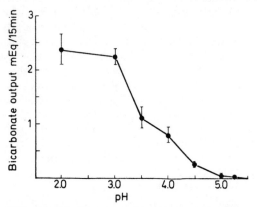

Figure 1.12 Pancreatic bicarbonate response to perfusion of dog duodenum with citrate buffers of different pH. Results demonstrate a threshold for secretin release at pH 4.5. (From Meyer *et al.*[167]), by courtesy of the *American Journal of Physiology*.)

Lowering the pH below 3.0 does not increase secretin release, providing the amount of titratable acid entering the gut is held constant. Below pH 3.0 secretin release and pancreatic bicarbonate secretion are related only to the amount of titratable acid entering the gut per unit time[169]. Thus, at a constant pH the amount of secretin released becomes a function of the length of intestine acidified.

Secretin release is not influenced by the vagus and cholinergic stimulation to the same extent as gastrin release. Vagal stimulation does not release secretin and topical application of acetylcholine to the duodenal mucosa does not stimulate pancreatic secretion[170]. Vagotomy[137] and anticholinergic drugs[171], however, each cause a decrease in the pancreatic response to endogenous secretin without significantly affecting the response to the exogenous hormone. These findings indicate that the cholinergic effect is a permissive one and that cholinergic background facilitates the release of secretin.

1.5 HORMONE INTERACTIONS

The preceding sections dealt with the individual characteristics of the three gastrointestinal hormones whose chemical and physiological identities have been established. It is evident, however, that these hormones have a number of characteristics in common. First, each hormone has a wide spectrum of actions affecting the secretion, motility, absorption and metabolism of many different target organs. Second, many actions overlap: two or three hormones may have the same effect on a given target. Third, a single hormone may stimulate or inhibit depending on what other factors are acting simultaneously. Fourth, there are often substantial species differences in the effects of a hormone on a given target. Finally, pharmacological effects at high doses may differ from physiological effects.

During the response to a meal, the release of the gastrointestinal hormones occurs over a prolonged period of several hours. Therefore, the actual response of a target organ to hormonal stimulation depends on the interaction of the hormones reaching it at any one time. Little is understood of the mechanisms of action of gastrointestinal hormones at the cellular and molecular levels; but analysis of the interactions of gastrin, CCK and secretin on gastric and pancreatic secretion in the dog has provided some insight into the nature of the receptors for these hormones. A theory has been developed which will predict the effects of a given combination on a target if the action of each hormone on the same target is known.

Hormonal interactions are of two general types: augmentation or inhibition. Both augmentation and inhibition may be either competitive or non-competitive (often called potentiation in the case of augmentation). The type of interaction depends upon the efficacies and potencies of the two hormones. The term, 'efficacy', is used to describe the effectiveness of an agonist-receptor combination. The theoretical or calculated maximal response (CMR) to an agent is an index of efficacy. This is analogous to the V_{max} of Michaelis–Menten kinetics and can be determined from various transformations of the Lineweaver–Burke equation, a linear representation for the Michaelis–Menten equation.

Differences in potency arise when the rates of combination between the hormones and receptor system vary. This variation is indicated by a difference in the doses of the two hormones or combination of hormones required for the same effect. Potency is measured by determining the K_m (or the dose needed to produce half the maximal response) from the Michaelis–Menten equation. In secretory studies the K_m is often called the D_{50} and is an index of the affinity of the receptor for the agonist.

If two agents act on the same receptor site, they will produce competitive augmentation if their efficacies are equal or nearly so and competitive inhibition if their efficacies differ. In either case the V_{max} or CMR is unchanged, for it is a property of the receptor site. When the efficacies differ, inhibition occurs because the agent with the lower efficacy will occupy sites which would normally be available to the stronger agonist. This competition decreases the affinity of the sites for the agonist, the D_{50} increases and inhibition results. As one would expect from their similar structures, CCK and gastrin act on the same receptor site. Since the efficacy of CCK on gastric secretion is much lower than that of gastrin, CCK will competitively inhibit gastrin stimulated secretion in the dog[111]. Figure 1.13 demonstrates the dose response relationship to gastrin alone and to gastrin plus CCK. The lines are parallel meaning that increasing the dose of the more effective agent (pentagastrin) overcomes the inhibition. Figure 1.14 is a transformation of the data in Figure 1.13 to yield the Michaelis–Menton constants[111]. The Y-intercepts of the lines, which in this case are nearly equal, are estimates of V_{max}. The negative slopes of the lines, which differ significantly, are

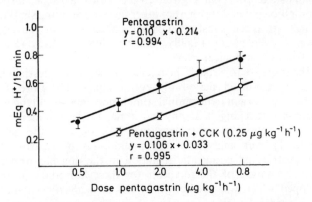

Figure 1.13 Dose response lines for secretion of acid by Heidenhain pouch dogs in response to pentagastrin alone and in combination with CCK. The parallel lines are indicative of competitive inhibition. (From Johnson and Grossman[111], by courtesy of the *American Journal of Physiology*.)

estimates of K_m. It is readily apparent that CCK increased the K_m for pentagastrin, that is, decreased receptor affinity for the agonist.

If two hormones act on different receptor sites they may cause potentiation or non-competitive augmentation if both are stimulatory. This interaction

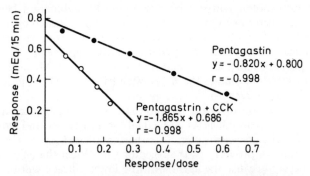

Figure 1.14 Transformation of the data from Figure 1.13 to give Michaelis–Menten constants. The Y-intercepts are estimates of V_{max} and the negative slopes, the K_m. Constant V_{max} and higher K_m indicate competitive inhibition. (From Johnson and Grossman[111], by courtesy of the *American Journal of Physiology*.)

occurs between CCK and secretin in the stimulation of pancreatic secretion of bicarbonate and enzymes. Figure 1.15 shows the CCK, released by perfusing the duodenum with phenylalanine, increases both the bicarbonate

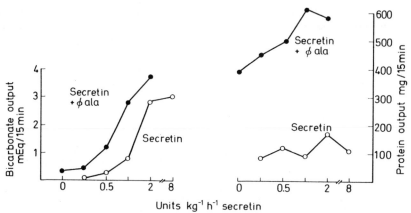

Figure 1.15 Dose response curves for pancreatic bicarbonate and protein output to secretin alone and to secretin plus endogenous CCK released by perfusing the intestine with phenylalanine. This combination illustrates non-competitive augmentation or potentiation. (From Spingola *et al.*[173], by courtesy of the *American Journal of Physiology*.)

and enzyme response to secretin[172]. In each case the maximal response to the combination was higher than the maximal response to either agent alone, indicating that potentiation had occurred[172].

The foregoing results demonstrate that CCK and gastrin act at the same site in the stomach and that secretin and CCK act at different sites in the pancreas. If the receptor sites are similar in the different target organs, one

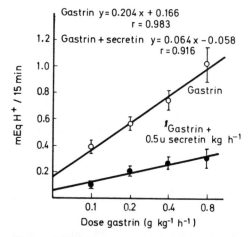

Figure 1.16 Dose response lines for acid secretion from dog Heidenhain pouches stimulated by gastrin and gastrin plus secretin. The non-parallel lines are consistent with non-competitive inhibition. (From Johnson and Grossman[174], by courtesy of F. K. Schattauer Verlag: Stuttgart.)

can predict that secretin and gastrin act at different sites in both the stomach and pancreas. Since secretin inhibits gastrin stimulated acid secretion, it should, therefore, do so non-competitively. Dose response curves for gastrin

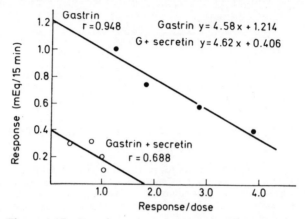

Figure 1.17 Transformation of the data in Figure 1.16 to give Michaelis–Menten constants. The large difference in Y intercepts (V_{max}) and similar slopes (K_m) indicate non-competitive inhibition. (From Johnson and Grossman[174], by courtesy of F. K. Schattauer Verlag: Stuttgart.)

and gastrin plus secretin are shown in Figure 1.16. Secretin causes a relatively constant per cent inhibition, and increasing the dose of gastrin does not decrease the effect of secretin[173]. The transformation of this data is depicted in Figure 1.17, showing that the V_{max} is decreased by secretin and that

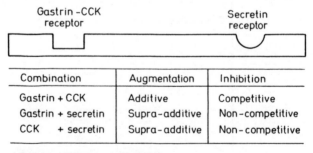

Combination	Augmentation	Inhibition
Gastrin + CCK	Additive	Competitive
Gastrin + secretin	Supra-additive	Non-competitive
CCK + secretin	Supra-additive	Non-competitive

Supra-additive = potentiated

Figure 1.18 Schematic representation of a hypothetical receptor with two sites, one for secretin and one for gastrin and CCK. The model explains interactions of the three gastrointestinal hormones. These are listed below. (From Grossman[175], by courtesy of the Society for Experimental Biology and Medicine.)

secretin is a non-competitive inhibitor[173]. As one would expect, since secretin acts at a different site from that used by gastrin, the affinity of the gastrin receptor site is unchanged and the D_{50}s are equal.

These data indicate that the three gastrointestinal hormones act on two sites which are common to the various target organs. Chemically related gastrin and CCK act on one site and secretin acts on the other. These sites are probably part of the same receptor system, so that combination at one site allosterically affects the other. A model of this receptor developed by Grossman[174] and its predicted interactions are shown in Figure 1.18. Often under physiological conditions only small amounts of hormones are released, therefore, interactions between hormones can account for a large proportion of the response of a particular target. The significance of these effects is fully discussed in the chapters dealing with regulation of function.

1.6 ADDITIONAL HORMONES AND RELATED AGENTS

In addition to gastrin, secretin and CCK there are a number of putative gastrointestinal hormones which were proposed to explain experimental observations. The findings that gastrin, CCK or secretin can account for their actions has eliminated the 'need' for some of these postulated hormones. Cases in point, which have already been discussed, are pancreozymin, incretin and intestinal gastrin. This section deals with other tentative hormones which may prove to have separate physiological roles. In addition, there are a number of other substances found in the gastrointestinal tract which have profound effects on digestive function. These agents may act as local tissue hormones or may be released by physiological stimuli related to a gastrointestinal function.

1.6.1 Enterogastrones

The term, enterogastrone, was coined by Kosaka and Lim[175] in 1930 to identify the hormones involved in the inhibition of gastric secretion which they observed after feeding fat to secreting dogs. Both secretin and CCK are enterogastrones, since they inhibit gastric secretion and are released from the small intestine by fat (enterogastrone literally means a hormone of intestinal origin which inhibits gastric secretion). The remaining question is whether enterogastrone exists as a separate hormone or whether all cases of humorally mediated inhibition arising from the small intestine can be explained by secretin and CCK.

In a study specifically designed to answer this question, it was found that infusion of fat into the canine duodenum caused a 50% inhibition of the Heidenhain pouch response to histamine[176]. Large doses of CCK and secretin did not inhibit the response. These studies were interpreted to mean that fat caused the release of an enterogastrone separate and distinct from CCK and secretin[176].

In 1969 Brown et al.[177] reported the partial purification of a substance from CCK extracts which was also capable of inhibiting gastric secretion. The same group has completed the purification and structural determination of this compound. The polypeptide contains 43 amino acid residues with a molecular weight of 5^{105}. It appears to be more closely related to secretin than gastrin, though it is structurally different from each[178]. The peptide is a potent inhibitor of histamine as well as gastrin stimulated acid secretion[179], indicating that it could be the enterogastrone released by fat which inhibits histamine stimulated secretion[176]. Despite these findings, there is no evidence that this substance is a hormone—that it is actually released from the gut by a physiological stimulus. For these reasons Brown and his colleagues prefer the name 'gastric inhibitory polypeptide' rather than enterogastrone.

Another group of investigators have purified an inhibitory substance from the first part of the hog duodenum which also inhibits histamine stimulated acid secretion[180]. Although referred to as an enterogastrone, there is again no evidence that this particular agent is a hormone. The final resolution of the 'enterogastrone' question obviously depends upon the demonstration of the release of one of these peptides in physiologically active amounts.

1.6.2 Glucagon

Pancreatic glucagon is closely related to secretin chemically as well as physiologically. While secretin contains 27 amino acid residues, glucagon contains 29, and of these, 14 occupy identical positions in the two hormones. Like secretin, glucagon stimulates volume and bicarbonate secretion from the liver[181], inhibits gastric secretion[182] and motility[183], and releases insulin[184]. Unlike secretin, glucagon does not stimulate the resting canine pancreas. In fact, glucagon inhibits pancreatic secretion in response to secretin or secretin plus CCK[185]. There is no question that pancreatic glucagon is a hormone, but whether it can be classified as a gastrointestinal hormone is another matter. Pancreatic glucagon release is stimulated by hypoglycaemia and intravenous amino acids[186].

In 1961 Unger et al.[187] identified immunoassayable glucagon from the gut wall. Gut glucagon-like material (GLI) could be distinguished immunochemically from pancreatic glucagon. GLI has not been characterised or purified, but it is the glucagon released by oral glucose administration[188]. Whether it plays a role as a physiological insulin secretagogue is questionable.

1.6.3 Prostaglandins

The prostaglandins have not been shown to be released into the circulatory system by any physiological stimuli acting within the digestive tract. Nevertheless, these derivatives of prostanoic acid are distributed throughout the gastrointestinal tract and have profound influence on digestive function when administered exogenously. These substances may qualify as 'tissue hormones'; that is, they may regulate cell function at or near their sites of release. The prostaglandins affect motility throughout the digestive tract and can increase or decrease contractions depending on the type of prostaglandin administered and the particular region of the tract under investigation[189]. Prostaglandin E_1 inhibits gastric secretion in rats and dogs[190,191] and has created some interest as a possible antisecretory drug[190].

1.7 A LOOK AHEAD

In the few years since the beginning of the biochemical epoch of gastro-intestinal hormone investigation, knowledge in the field has progressed by leaps and bounds. Building on the foundation of that knowledge, future work should progress at an even faster pace. While it is difficult to predict the precise direction these efforts will take, some courses stand out as the most likely.

There will continue to be intense interest in the area of isolation and identification of gastrointestinal hormones. It is a safe prediction that the number of hormones will not remain at 3. In addition, we will no doubt learn the structure of so-called big gastrin and the significance of the different forms of this hormone.

Development of reproducible radioimmunoassays for secretin and CCK will be accomplished in the near future. This will make possible a plethora of studies defining precisely the conditions for release of these hormones. As with gastrin, the cells of origin and the distribution of these hormones will also become apparent.

It is becoming increasingly obvious that the gastrointestinal hormones do more than turn faucets on and off. They all appear to regulate metabolism of the gastrointestinal tract, gastrin being an important growth factor for the gastric and duodenal mucosa. Therefore, interest has been stimulated in the mechanisms by which the gastrointestinal hormones produce these effects and studies pertaining to DNA, RNA and protein synthesis are being reported. In addition, much effort has been expended to ascertain the relation-ships between these hormones and the cyclic nucleotides. The end of these efforts to integrate hormone physiology with biochemical processes is not in sight.

One area totally ignored until recently concerns the nature of the receptor(s) for the gastrointestinal hormones. This should be of intense interest for basic scientists and clinicians alike, since endocrine malfunction can be caused by a receptor defect as well as over or under production of the hormone.

Optimistically, I predict that the primary causes of peptic ulcer will be elucidated and a medical control for the disease developed. Whether this therapy will involve one of the gastrointestinal hormones directly or only the knowledge obtained from studying them remains to be seen. Our infor-mation is expanding too rapidly in this area to miss a significant breakthrough.

In any event, if we use the knowledge obtained during the past decade vigorously and effectively, the gastrointestinal hormones will resume their position in the mainstream of endocrinology.

References

1. Tapperman, J. (1962). *Metabolic and Endocrine Physiology* (Chicago: Year Book Medical Publishers)
2. Turner, C. D. and Bagnara, J. T. (1971). *General Endocrinology*, 578 (Philadelphia: W. B. Saunders)
3. Sawin, C. T. (1969). *The Hormones Endocrine Physiology*, 19 (Boston: Little, Brown)

4. Bayliss, W. M. and Starling, E. H. (1902). The mechanism of pancreatic secretion. *J. Physiol.*, **28**, 325

5. Gregory, R. A. and Tracy, H. J. (1964). The constitution and properties of two gastrins extracted from hog antral mucosa. *Gut*, **5**, 103

6. Gregory, R. A. and Tracy, H. J. (1964). Physiological properties of a series of synthetic peptides structurally related to gastrin I. *Nature (London)*, **204**, 935

7. Heidenhain, R. (1879). Über der Absonderung der Fundusdrüsen des Magens. *Pflüg. Arch. Physiol.*, **19**, 148

8. Edkins, J. S. (1898). *Text-Book of Physiology*, Vol. I, 531 (E. A. Schäfer, editor) (Edinburgh: Pentland)

9. Edkins, J. S. (1905). On the chemical mechanism of gastric secretion. *Proc. Roy. Soc. London B*, **76**, 376

10. Dale, H. H. and Laidlow, P. P. (1910). The physiological action of B-iminazolylethylamine. *J. Physiol.*, **41**, 318

11. Sacks, J., Ivy, A. C. and Vandolah, J. E. (1932). Histamine as the hormone for gastric secretion. *Amer. J. Physiol.*, **101**, 331

12. Popielski, L. (1920). β-imidazolyläthylamin und die Organ extrakte; B-imieläzolylathylamin als machtiger Erreger der Magendrusen. *Pflüg. Arch. Physiol.*, **178**, 214

13. Komarov, S. A. (1938). Gastrin. *Proc. Soc. Exp. Biol. Med.*, **38**, 514

14. Gregory, R. A. and Tracy, H. J. (1961). The preparation and properties of gastrin. *J. Physiol.*, **156**, 523

15. Grossman, M. I., Robertson, C. R. and Ivy, A. C. (1948). Proof of a hormonal mechanism for gastric secretion—the humoral transmission of the distention stimulus. *Amer. J. Physiol.*, **153**, 1

16. Gregory, H., Hardy, P. M., Jones, D. S., Kenner, G. W. and Sheppard, R. C. (1964). The antral hormone gastrin. I. Structure of gastrin. *Nature (London)*, **204**, 931

17. Anderson, J. D., Barton, M. A., Gregory, R. A., Hardy, P. M., Kenner, G. W., MacLeod, J. K., Preston, J., Sheppard, R. D. and Morley, J. S. (1964). The antral hormone gastrin. II. Synthesis of gastrin. *Nature (London)*, **204**, 933

18. Way, L. W. and Durbin, R. P. (1969). Response of the bullfrog gastric mucosa to gastrin I and gastrin II. *Gastroenterology*, **56**, 1266

19. Bentley, P. H., Kenner, G. W. and Sheppard, R. C. (1966). Human gastrin: isolation, structure and synthesis. Structures of human gastrins I and II. *Nature (London)*, **209**, 583

20. Morley, J. S., Tracy, H. J. and Gregory, R. A. (1965). Structure-function relationships in active C-terminal tetrapeptide sequence of gastrin. *Nature (London)*, **207**, 1356

21. Emas, S. and Grossman, M. I. (1967). Effect of truncal vagotomy on acid and pepsin responses to histamine and gastrin in dogs. *Amer. J. Physiol.*, **212**, 1007

22. Johnson, L. R. (1972). Regulation of pepsin secretion by topical acid in the stomach. *Gastroenterology*, **62**, 766

23. Stening, G. F. and Grossman, M. I. (1969). Gastrin-related peptides as stimulants of pancreatic and gastric secretion. *Amer. J. Physiol.*, **217**, 262

24. Jones, R. S. and Grossman, M. I. (1970). Choleretic effects of cholecystokinin, gastrin II and caerulein in dog. *Amer. J. Physiol.*, **219**, 1014

25. Stening, G. F. and Grossman, M. I. (1969). The hormonal control of Brunner's glands. *Gastroenterology*, **56**, 1047

26. Isenberg, J. and Grossman, M. I. (1969). Effect of gastrin and SC 15396 on gastric motility in dogs. *Gastroenterology*, **56**, 450

27. Vagne, M. and Grossman, M. I. (1968). Cholecystokinetic potency of gastrointestinal hormones and related peptides. *Amer. J. Physiol.*, **215**, 881

28. Easley, R. B., Thompson, G. H., Erdos, E. G., Kaul, P. N. and Jacobson, E. D. (1970). Effects of a gastrin-like peptide on uterine smooth muscle. *Proc. Soc. Exp. Biol. Med.*, **133**, 870

29. Castell, D. O. and Harris, L. D. (1970). Hormonal control of gastroesophageal sphincter strength. *N. Eng. J. Med.*, **282**, 886

30. Benne, H. A. and Misiewicz, J. J. (1967). The role of gastrin in gastrointestinal motility. *Gastroenterology*, **53**, 680

31. Gillespie, I. E. and Grossman, M. I. (1963). Inhibition of gastric secretion by extracts containing gastrin. *Gastroenterology*, **44**, 301
32. Gingell, J. C., Davies, M. W. and Shields, R. (1968). Effect of synthetic gastrin-like pentapeptide upon the intestinal transport of sodium, potassium and water. *Gut*, **9**, 111
33. Bynum, T. E., Jacobson, E. D. and Johnson, L. R. (1971). Gastrin inhibition of intestinal absorption in dogs. *Gastroenterology*, **61**, 858
34. Crean, G. P., Marshall, M. W. and Rumsey, R. D. E. (1969). Parietal cell hyperplasia induced by the administration of pentagastrin (ICI 50, 123) to rats. *Gastroenterology*, **57**, 147
35. Johnson, L. R., Aures, D. and Yuen, L. (1969). Pentagastrin induced stimulation of the *in vitro* incorporation of ^{14}C-leucine into protein of the gastrointestinal tract. *Amer. J. Physiol.*, **217**, 251
36. Johnson, L. R., Aures, D. and Hakanson, R. (1969). Effect of gastrin on the *in vivo* incorporation of ^{14}C-leucine into protein of the digestive tract. *Proc. Soc. Exp. Biol. Med.*, **132**, 996
37. Martin, F., Macleod, I. B. and Sircus, W. (1970). Effect of antrectomy on the fundic mucosa of the rat. *Gastroenterology*, **59**, 437
38. Mayston, P. D. and Barrowman, L. A. (1971). The influence of chronic administration of pentagastrin on the rat pancreas. *Quart. J. Exp. Physiol.*, **56**, 113
39. Chandler, A. M. and Johnson, L. R. (1972). Pentagastrin stimulated incorporation of ^{14}C-orotic acid into RNA of gastric and duodenal mucosa. *Proc. Soc. Exp. Biol. Med.* (in press)
40. Johnson, L. R. and Chandler, A. M. (1972). RNA and DNA content of gastric and duodenal mucosa from antrectomized and pentagastrin treated rats. *Amer. J. Physiol.* (in press)
41. Willems, G., Vansteenkiste, Y. and Limbosch, J. M. (1972). Stimulating effect of gastrin on cell proliferation kinetics in canine fundic mucosa. *Gastroenterology*, **62**, 583
42. Miller, L. R., Jacobson, E. D. and Johnson, L. R. (1972). Long-term cultivation of gastric epithelium *in vitro*. *Gastroenterology*, **62**, 784
43. Lichtenberger, L., Miller, L. R., Erwin, D. N. and Johnson, L. R. (1973). The effect of pentagastrin on adult rat duodenal cells in culture. *J. Cell Biol.* (in press)
44. Unger, R. H., Ketterner, H., Dupre, J. and Eisentrant, A. M. (1967). The effects of secretin, pancreozymin and gastrin on insulin and glucagon secretion in anesthetized dogs. *J. Clin. Invest.*, **46**, 630
45. McGuigan, J. E. (1969). Studies of the immunochemical specificity of some antibodies to human gastrin. *Gastroenterology*, **56**, 429
46. Charters, A. C., Odell, W. D., Davidson, W. D. and Thompson, J. C. (1969). Gastrin: immunochemical properties and measurement by radioimmunoassay. *Surgery*, **66**, 104
47. Yalow, R. S. and Berson, S. A. (1970). Radioimmunoassay of gastrin. *Gastroenterology*, **58**, 1
48. McGuigan, J. E. (1967). Antibodies to the carboxyl-terminal tetrapeptide of gastrin. *Gastroenterology*, **53**, 697
49. McGuigan, J. E. (1968). Immunochemical studies with synthetic human gastrin. *Gastroenterology*, **54**, 1005
50. McGuigan, J. E. (1968). Antibodies to the C-terminal tetrapeptide amide of gastrin: assessment of antibody binding to cholecystokinin-pancreozymin. *Gastroenterology*, **54**, 1012
51. Edkins, J. S. (1906). The chemical mechanism of gastric secretion. *J. Physiol.*, **34**, 133
52. Solcia, E., Vassallo, G. and Sampietro, R. (1967). Endocrine cells in the antropyloric mucosa of the stomach. *Z. Zellforsch. Mikrosk. Anat.*, **81**, 474
53. Solcia, E., Vassallo, G. and Capella, C. (1969). Studies on the G cells of the pyloric mucosa, the probable site of gastrin secretion. *Gut*, **10**, 379
54. McGuigan, J. E. and Greider, M. H. (1971). Correlative immunochemical and light microscopic studies of the gastrin cell of the antral mucosa. *Gastroenterology*, **60**, 223
55. Bussolati, G. and Pearse, A. G. E. (1970). Immunofluorescent localization of the gastrin-secreting G cells in the pyloric antrum of the pig. *Histochemie*, **21**, 1

56. Berson, S. A. and Yalow, R. S. (1971). Nature of immunoreactive gastrin extracted from tissues of gastrointestinal tract. *Gastroenterology*, **60**, 215
57. Yalow, R. S. and Berson, S. A. (1970). Size and charge distinctions between endogenous human plasma gastrin in peripheral blood and heptadecapeptide gastrins. *Gastroenterology*, **58**, 609
58. Hansky, J. and Cain, M. D. (1969). Radioimmunoassay of gastrin in human serum. *Lancet*, **2**, 1388
59. Ganguli, P. C. and Hunter, W. M. (1972). Radioimmunoassay of gastrin in human plasma. *J. Physiol.*, **220**, 499
60. McGuigan, J. E. and Trudeau, W. L. (1968). Immunochemical measurement of elevated levels of gastrin in the serum of patients with pancreatic tumors of the Zollinger–Ellison variety. *New Eng. J. Med.*, **278**, 1308
61. Ganguli, P. C., Cullen, D. R. and Irvine, W. J. (1971). Radioimmunoassay of plasmagastrin in pernicious anemia, achlorhydria without pernicious anemia, hypochlorhydria, and in controls. *Lancet*, **1**, 155
62. McGuigan, J. E. and Trudeau, W. L. (1970). Serum gastrin concentrations in pernicious anemia. *New Eng. J. Med.*, **282**, 358
63. Reeder, D. D., Jackson, B. M., Ban, J. L., Davidson, W. D. and Thompson, J. C. (1970). Effect of food on serum gastrin concentrations in duodenal ulcer and control patients. *Surg. Forum*, **21**, 290
64. Trudeau, W. L. and McGuigan, J. E. (1971). Relations between serum gastrin levels and rates of gastric hydrochloric acid secretion. *New Eng. J. Med.*, **284**, 408
65. Yalow, R. S. and Berson, S. A. (1971). Further studies on the nature of immunoreactive gastrin in human plasma. *Gastroenterology*, **60**, 203
66. Makhlouf, G. M., McManus, J. P. A. and Card, W. I. (1964). Dose-response curves for the effect of gastrin II on acid gastric secretion in man. *Gut*, **5**, 379
67. Thompson, J. C., Reeder, D. D., Davidson, W. D., Chargers, A. C., Bruckner, W. L., Lemmi, C. A. E. and Miller, J. H. (1969). Effect of hepatic transit of gastrin pentagastrin and histamine measured by gastric secretion and by assay of hepatic vein blood. *Ann. Surg.*, **170**, 493
68. Reeder, D. D., Brandt, E. N. Jr, Watson, L. C., Hjelmquist, U. B. E. and Thompson, J. C. (1972). Pre- and post-hepatic measurements of mass of endogenous gastrin. *Surgery* (in press)
69. Ganguli, P. C., Elder, J. B., Smith, I. S. and Hunter, W. M. (1970). The half-life ($T\frac{1}{2}$) of synthetic human gastrin I in man. *Brit. J. Surg.*, **57**, 848
70. Reeder, D. D., Jackson, B. M., Brandt, E. N. Jr, and Thompson, J. C. (1972). Rate and pattern of disappearance of exogenous gastrin in dogs. *Amer. J. Physiol.*, **222**, 1571
71. Hjelmquist, U. B. E., Reeder, D. D., Brandt, E. N. Jr and Thompson, J. C. (1972). Effect of the kidney on endogenous gastrin. *Surg. Forum* (in press)
72. Watson, L. C., Reeder, D. D. and Thompson, J. C. (1970). Total gastrin in canine fundus, antrum and proximal duodenum. *Clin. Res.*, **20**, 468
73. Miller, J. H., Jackson, B. M. and Thompson, J. C. (1970). Effect of total gastrectomy and partial evisceration on circulating gastrin concentration. *Surg. Forum*, **21**, 153
74. Stern, D. H. and Walsh, J. H. (1972). Release of duodenal gastrin in man. *Clin. Res.*, **20**, 223
75. Lomsky, R., Langr, F. and Vortel, V. (1969). Immunochemical demonstration of gastrin in mammalian islets of Langerhans. *Nature* (*London*), **223**, 618
76. Greider, M. and McGuigan, J. E. (1971). Cellular localization of gastrin in human pancreas. *Diabetes*, **20**, 389
77. Zollinger, R. M. and Ellison, E. H. (1955). Primary peptic ulcerations of jejunum associated with islet cell tumors or pancreas. *Ann. Surg.*, **142**, 709
78. Gregory, R. A., Tracy, H. J., French, J. M. and Sircus, W. (1960). Extraction of gastrin-like substance from pancreatic tumour in case of Zollinger–Ellison-syndrome. *Lancet*, **1**, 1045
79. Grossman, M. I., Tracy, H. J. and Gregory, R. A. (1961). Zollinger–Ellison syndrome in a Bantu woman, with isolation of a gastrin-like substance from the primary and secondary tumors. II. Extraction of gastrin-like activity from tumors. *Gastroenterology*, **41**, 87

80. Gregory, R. A., Tracy, H. F., Agarwal, K. L. and Grossman, M. I. (1969). Amino acid constitution of the two gastrins isolated from Zollinger–Ellison tumour tissue. *Gut*, **10**, 6003
81. Johnson, L. R. and Grossman, M. I. (1969). Potentiation of the gastric acid response in dog. *Gastroenterology*, **56**, 687
82. Elwin, C. E. and Uvnas, B. (1966). Distribution and local release of gastrin. 69 *Gastrin, Proceedings of a Conference* (M. I. Grossman, editor) (Los Angeles: University of California Press)
83. Csendes, A. and Grossman, M. I. (1972). D- and L-isomers of serine and alanine equally effective as releasers of gastrin (in press)
84. Meyer, J. H. and Grossman, M. I. (1970). Comparison of D- and L-phenylalanine as pancreatic stimulants. *Gastroenterology*, **58**, 1046
85. Grossman, M. I. (1967). Neural and hormonal stimulation of gastric secretion of acid. *Handbook of Physiology*. Section 6, Vol. II, 835 (C. F. Code, editor) (Washington, D.C.: American Physiological Society)
86. Walsh, J. H., Yalow, R. S. and Berson, S. A. (1970). Effect of feeding and atropinization of plasma gastrin concentrations. *Gastroenterology*, **58**, 1005
87. Schofield, B. (1966). Inhibition by acid of gastrin release. *Gastrin, Proceedings of a Conference*,171 (M.I. Grossman, editor) (Los Angeles: University of California Press)
88. Berkowitz, J. M., Buetow, G., Walden, M. and Praissman, M. (1971). Molecular factors in antral permeation: their proposed role in gastrin release. *Amer. J. Physiol.*, **221**, 259
89. MacIntosh, F. C. (1938). Histamine as a normal stimulant of gastric secretion. *Quart. J. Exp. Physiol.*, **28**, 87
90. Code, C. F. (1965). Histamine and gastric secretion: a later look, 1955–1965. *Federation Proc.*, **24**, 1311
91. Kahlson, G., Rowengren, E., Svahn, D. and Thunberg, R. (1964). Mobilization anf formation of histamine in the gastric mucosa as related to acid secretion. *J. Physiol.*, **174**, 400
92. Johnson, L. R., Jones, R. S., Aures, D. and Häkanson, R. (1969). The effect of antrectomy on gastric histidine decarboxylase activity in the rat. *Amer. J. Physiol.*, **216**, 1051
93. Aures, D., Johnson, L. R. and Way, L. W. (1970). Gastrin: obligatory intermediate for activation of gastric histidine decarboxylase activity in the rat. *Amer. J. Physiol.*, **219**, 214
94. Häkanson, R. and Liedberg, G. (1970). The role of endogenous gastrin in the activation of histidine decarboxylase activity in the rat. Effect of antrectomy and vagal denervation. *Europ. J. Pharmacol.*, **12**, 94
95. Adashek, D. and Grossman, M. I. (1963). Response of rats with gastric fistulas to injection of gastrin. *Proc. Sec. Exp. Biol. Med.*, **112**, 629
96. Johnson, L. R. (1971). Control of gastric secretion: no room for histamine? *Gastroenterology*, **61**, 106
97. Tumpson, D. B. and Johnson, L. R. (1969). Effect of secretin and cholecystokinin on the response of the gastric fistula rat to pentagastrin. *Proc. Soc. Exp. Biol. Med.*, **131**, 186
98. Johnson, L. R. and Tumpson, D. B. (1970). Effect of secretin on histamine stimulated secretion in the gastric fistula rat. *Proc. Soc. Exp. Biol. Med.*, **133**, 125
99. Caren, J. F., Aures, D. and Johnson, L. R. (1969). Effect of secretin and cholecystokinin on histidine decarboxylase activity in the rat stomach. *Proc. Soc. Exp. Biol. Med.*, **131**, 1194
100. Johnson, L. R. and Aures, D. (1970). Evidence that histamine is not the mediator of acid secretion in the rat. *Proc. Soc. Exp. Biol. Med.*, **134**, 880
101. Sewing, K.-Fr. (1972). Is there a feedback relationship between histamine content and histidine decarboxylase activity in the gastric mucosa? (in press)
102. Ivy, A. C. and Oldberg, E. (1928). A hormone mechanism for gallbladder contraction and evacuation. *Amer. J. Physiol.*, **86**, 599
103. Harper, A. A. and Raper, H. S. (1943). Pancreozymin, a stimulant of the secretion of pancreatic enzymes in extracts of the small intestine. *J. Physiol.*, **102**, 115
104. Jorpes, J. E. (1968). The isolation and chemistry of secretin and cholecystokinin. *Gastroenterology*, **55**, 157

105. Stening, G. F. and Grossman, M. I. (1969). Gastrin-related peptides as stimulants of pancreatic and gastric secretion. *Amer. J. Physiol.*, **217**, 262

106. Johnson, L. R., Stening, G. F. and Grossman, M. I. (1970). Effect of sulfation on the gastrointestinal actions of caerulein. *Gastroenterology*, **58**, 208

107. Anastasi, A., Erspamer, V. and Endean, R. (1967). Isolation and structure of caerulein, and active decapeptide from the skin of Hyla caerulea. *Experientia*, **23**, 699

108. DeCaro, G., Endean, R., Erspamer, V. and Roseghini, M. (1968). Occurence of caerulein in extracts of the skin of *Hyla caerulea* and other Australian hylids, *Brit. J. Pharmacol.*, **33**, 48

109. Gadacz, T. R. and Way, L. W. (1972). Comparison of the effect of several gastrin-related compounds on acid secretion in dogs. *Amer. J. Surg.*, **123**, 143

110. Brooks, A. M., Johnson, L. R., Spencer, J. and Grossman, M. I. (1970). Failure of desulfated caerulein to inhibit pentagastrin-stimulated acid secretion. *Amer. J. Physiol.*, **219**, 794

111. Johnson, L. R. and Grossman, M. I. (1970). Analysis of inhibition of acid secretion by cholecystokinin in dogs. *Amer. J. Physiol.*, **218**, 550

112. Amer, M. S. (1969). Studies with cholecystokinin II. Cholecystokinetic potency of porcine gastrins I and II and related peptides in three systems. *Endocrinology*, **84**, 1277

113. Bertaccini, G., Braibanti, T. and Uva, F. (1969). Cholecystokinetic activity of the new peptide caerulein in man. *Gastroenterology*, **56**, 862

114. Onde Hi, M. A., Rubin, B. and Engel, S. L. (1970). Cholecystokinin-pancreozymin: Recent developments. *Amer. J. Dig. Dis.*, **15**, 149

115. Rubin, B., Engel, S. L. and Drung, A. M. (1969). Cholecystokinin-like activities in guinea pigs and in dogs of the C-terminal octapeptide (SQ 19,844) of cholecystokinin, *J. Pharm. Sci.*, **18**, 955

116. Isenberg, J. I. and Csendes, A. (1971). The effect of the octapeptide of cholecystokinin on canine pyloric squeeze. *Gastroenterology*, **60**, 778

117. Resin, H., Stern, D. H., Sturdevant, R. Z. and Isenberg, J. I. (1972). Effect of octapeptide of cholecystokinin on lower esophageal pressure in man, *Gastroenterology*, **62**, 797

118. Hedner, P., Persson, H. and Rorsman, G. (1967). Effect of cholecystokinin on the small intestine. *Acta Physiol. Scand.*, **70**, 250

119. Lin, T. M. and Spray, G. F. (1969). Effect of pentagastrin, cholecystokinin, caerulein, and glucagon on the choledochal resistance and bile flow of conscious dog. *Gastroenterology*, **56**, 1178

120. Cameron, A. J., Phillips, S. F. and Summerskill, W. H. J. (1967). Effect of cholecystokinin on motility of human stomach and gallbladder muscle *in vitro*. *Clin. Res.*, **15**, 416

121. Jones, R. S. and Grossman, M. I. (1970). Choleretic effects of cholecystokinin, gastrin II and caerulein in dog. *Amer. J. Physiol.*, **219**, 1014

122. Stening, G. F. and Grossman, M. I. (1969). The hormonal control of Brunner's glands. *Gastroenterology*, **56**, 1047

123. Gardner, J. D., Peskin, G. W., Cerda, J. J. and Brooks, F. P. (1967). Alterations of *in vitro* fluid and electrolyte absorption by gastrointestinal hormones. *Amer. J. Surg.*, **113**, 57

124. Bussjaeger, L. J. and Johnson, L. R. (1972). Evidence for the hormonal regulation of intestinal absorption (in press)

125. Webster, P. D. (1969). Comparison of metabolic and secretory effects of methacholine and pancreozymin on the pancreas. *Gastroenterology*, **56**, 1267

126. Sahba, M. M., Morissett, J. A. and Webster, P. D. (1970). Synthetic and secretory effects of cholecystokinin-pancreozymin on the pigeon pancreas. *Proc. Soc. Exp. Biol. Med.*, **134**, 728

127. Young, J. D., Lazarus, L. and Chisholm, D. J. (1968). Secretin and pancreozymin after glucose. *Lancet*, **2**, 914

128. Turner, D. S. (1969). Intestinal hormones and insulin release: *In vitro* studies using rabbit pancreas. *Hormone Metab. Res.*, **1**, 168

129. Buchanan, K. D., Vance, J. E. and Williams, R. H. (1969). Insulin and glucagon release from isolated islets of Langerhans. *Diabetes*, **18**, 381

130. Young, J. D., Lazarus, L., Chisholm, D. J. (1969). Radioimmunoassay of cholecystokinin-pancreozymin in human serum *J. Nucl. Med.*, **10**, 743
131. Berson, S. A. and Yalow, R. S. (1972). Radioimmunoassay in gastroenterology. *Gastroenterology*, **62**, 1061
132. Amer, M. S. and Becvar, W. E. (1969), A sensitive *in vitro* method for the assay of cholecystokinin. *J. Endocrinol.*, **43**, 1
133. Go, V. L. W., Hofmann, A. F. and Summerskill, W. H. J. (1970). Pancreozymin bioassay in man based on pancreatic enzyme secretion: potency of specific amino acids and other digestive products. *J. Clin. Invest.*, **49**, 1558
134. Meyer, J. H. and Grossman, M. I. (0000). Release of secretin and cholecystokinin. *Symposium on Gastrointestinal Hormones*, Erlangen, Germany (in press)
135. Meyer, J. H. and Grossman, M. I. (1970). Comparison of D- and L-phenylalanine as pancreatic stimulants. *Gastroenterology*, **58**, 1046
136. Go, V. L. W., Hofmann, A. F. and Summerskill, W. H. J. (1969). Pancreozymin: sites of secretion and effects on pancreatic enzyme output in man. *J. Clin. Invest.*, **48**, 29a
137. Moreland, H. J. and Johnson, L. R. (1971). Effect of vagotomy on pancreatic secretion stimulated by endogenous and exogenous secretin. *Gastroenterology*, **60**, 425
138. Ivy, A. C. (1934). Physiology of gallbladder. *Physiol. Rev.*, **14**, 1
139. Jorpes, J. E. and Mutt, V. (1961). On the biological activity and amino acid composition of secretin. *Acta Chem. Scand.*, **15**, 1790
140. Jorpes, J. E., Mutt, V. and Magnusson, S. (1962). Amino acid composition and N-terminal amino acid sequence of porcine secretin. *Biochem. Biophys. Res. Commun.*, **9**, 275
141. Mutt, V. and Jorpes, J. E. (1966). Secretin: Isolation and determination of structure. *Proceedings of the Fourth International Symposium on the Chemistry of Natural Products*. (Stockholm, Sweden)
142. Bodanszky, M., Ondetti, M. A. and Levine, S. D. (1966). Synthesis of a heptacosa peptide amide with the hormonal activity of secretin. *Chem. Industr.*, **42**, 1757
143. Grossman, M. I. (1968). Gastrointestinal hormones. *Med. Clin. N. Amer.* **52**, 1297
144. Bodanszky, A., Ondetti, M. A., Mutt, V. and Bodanszky, M. (1969). Synthesis of secretin. IV. Secondary structure in a miniature protein. *J. Amer. Chem. Soc.*, **91**, 944
145. Gregory, R. A. (1962). *Secretory Mechanisms of the Digestive Tract*, 159 (London: Edward Arnold Ltd.)
146. Hickson, J. C. D. (1970). The secretory and vascular response to nervous and hormonal stimulation in the pancreas of the pig. *J. Physiol.*, **206**, 299
147. Hubel, K. A. (1972). Secretin: A long progress note. *Gastroenterology*, **62**, 318
148. Spingola, L. J., Meyer, J. H. and Grossman, M. I. (1970). Potentiated pancreatic response to secretin and endogenous cholecystokinin (CCK). *Clin. Res.*, **18**, 175
149. Stening, G. F., Johnson, L. R. and Grossman, M. I. (1969). The effect of secretin on acid and pepsin secretion in cat and dog. *Gastroenterology*, **56**, 468
150. Brooks, A. M., Isenberg, J. and Grossman, M. I. (1969). The effect of secretin, glucagon and duodenal acidification on pepsin secretion in man. *Gastroenterology*, **57**, 159
151. Johnson, L. R. and Grossman, M. I. (1968). Secretin: The enterogastrone release: by acid in the duodenum. *Amer. J. Physiol.*, **215**, 885
152. Tumpson, D. B. and Johnson, L. R. (1969). Effect of secretin and cholecystokinin on the response of the gastric fistula rat to pentagastrin. *Proc. Soc. Exp. Biol. Med.*, **131**, 186
153. Brooks, A. M. and Grossman, M. I. (1970). Effect of secretin and cholecystokinin on pentagastrin-stimulated gastric secretion in man. *Gastroenterology*, **59**, 114
154. Wheeler, H. O. and Mancusi-Ungaro, P. L. (1966). Role of bile ducts during secretion choleresis in dogs. *Amer. J. Physiol.*, **210**, 1153
155. Dinoso, V., Chey, W. Y. and Lorber, S. H. (1966). Effect of secretin on gastric secretion and motor function of the upper gastro-intestinal tract in man. *Clin. Res.*, **14**, 295
156. Stening, G. F. and Grossman, M. I. (1969). Potentiation of cholecystokinetic action of cholecystokinin (CCK) by secretin. *Clin. Res.*, **17**, 528

157. Kraft, A. V., Tompkins, R. K. and Emdahl, G. L. (1969). Alterations in membrane transport produced by diarrheogenic non-beta islet cell tumors of the pancreas. *Surg. Forum*, **20**, 338

158. Cohen, S. and Lipshutz, W. (1971). Hormonal regulation of lower esophageal sphincter competence: Interaction of gastrin and secretin. *J. Clin. Invest.*, **50**, 449

159. Kelly, K. A., Woodward, E. R. and Code, C. F. (1969). Effect of secretin and cholecystokinin on canine gastric electrical activity. *Proc. Soc. Exp. Biol. Med.*, **130**, 1060

160. Hansky, J., Soveny, J. and Korman, M. G. (1971). Effect of secretin on serum gastrin measured by immunoassay. *Gastroenterology*, **61**, 62

161. Jorpes, E. and Mutt, V. (1967). Secretin and glucagon as insulin releasing factors. *Nord. Med.*, **77**, 30

162. Deckert, T. (1968). Stimulation of insulin secretion by glucagon and secretin. *Acta Endocrinol.*, **57**, 578

163. Santensaulo, F., Faloona, G. R. and Unger, R. H. (1972). Suppressive effect of secretin upon alpha cell function. *J. Clin. Invest.*, **51**, 1743

164. Stanley, M. S., Coalson, R. E., Grossman, M. I. and Johnson, L. R. (1972). Influence of secretin and pentagastrin on acid secretion and parietal cell number in rats. *Gastroenterology*, **63**, 264

165. Young, J. D., Lazarus, L. and Chisholm, D. J. (1968). Radioimmunoassay of secretin in human serum. *J. Nucl. Med.*, **9**, 641

166. Chisholm, D. J., Young, J. D. and Lazarus, L. (1969). The gastrointestinal stimulus to insulin release I. Secretin. *J. Clin. Invest.*, **48**, 1453

167. Meyer, J. H., Way, L. W. and Grossman, M. I. (1970). Pancreatic response to acidification of various lengths of proximal intestine in the dog. *Amer. J. Physiol.*, **219**, 971

168. Wang, C. C. and Grossman, M. I. (1961). Physiological determination of release of secretin and pancreozymin from intestine of dogs with transplanted pancreas. *Amer. J. Physiol.*, **164**, 527

169. Meyer, J. H. and Grossman, M. I. (1970). Pancreatic bicarbonate response to various acids in the duodenum of dogs. *Amer. J. Physiol.*, **219**, 964

170. Sum, P. T., Schipper, H. L. and Preshaw, R. M. (1969). Canine gastric and pancreatic secretion during intestinal distention and intestinal perfusion with choline derivatives. *Canad. J. Physiol. Pharmacol.*, **47**, 115

171. Thomas, J. E. (1964). Mechanism of the action of pancreatic stimuli studied by means of atropine-like drugs. *Amer. J. Physiol.*, **206**, 124

172. Spingola, L. J., Meyer, J. H. and Grossman, M. I. (1970). Potentiated pancreatic response to secretin and endogenous cholecystokinin (CCK). *Clin. Res.*, **18**, 175

173. Johnson, L. R. and Grossman, M. I. (1969). Characteristics of inhibition of gastric secretion by secretin. *Amer. J. Physiol.*, **217**, 1401

174. Grossman, M. I. (1970). Effect of gastrin, cholecystokinin and secretin on gastric and pancreatic secretion: A theory of interaction of hormones. *Origin, Chemistry, Physiology and Pathophysiology of the Gastrointestinal Hormones*, 129 (W. Creutzfeldt, editor) (F. K. Schattauer Verlag: Stuttgart)

175. Kosaka, T. and Lim, R. K. S. (1930). Demonstration of the humoral agent in fat inhibition of gastric secretion. *Proc. Soc. Exp. Biol. Med.*, **27**, 890

176. Johnson, L. R. and Grossman, M. I. (1969). Effects of fat, secretin and cholecystokinin on histamine-stimulated gastric secretion. *Amer. J. Physiol.*, **216**, 1176

177. Brown, J. C., Pederson, R. A., Jorpes, J. E. and Mutt, V. (1969). Preparation of highly active enterogastrone. *Com. J. Physiol. Pharmacol.*, **47**, 113

178. Brown, J. C. and Dryburgh, J. R. (000). A gastric inhibitory polypeptide. II. The complete amino acid sequence. *Can. J. Biochem.* (in press)

179. Pederson, R. A. and Brown, J. C. (1972). Inhibition of histamine-, pentagastrin-, and insulin-stimulated canine gastric secretion by pure 'gastric inhibitory polypeptide'. *Gastroenterology*, **62**, 393

180. Lucien, H. W., Itoh, Z. and Schally, A. V. (1970). Inhibitory effects of a purified enterogastrone, secretin, and cholecystokinin on histamine-stimulated gastric acid secretion. *Gastroenterology*, **59**, 707

181. Morris, T. Q., Sardi, G. and Bradley, S. E. (1967). Character of glucagon induced choleresis. *Fed. Proc.*, **26**, 774

182. Lin, T. M. and Spray, G. F. (1968). Effect of glucagon on gastric HCl secretion. *Gastroenterology*, **54**, 1254
183. Stunkard, A. J., Van Itallie, T. B. and Reiss, B. B. (1955). Mechanism of satiety: Effect of glucagon on gastric hunger contractions in man. *Proc. Soc. Exp. Biol. Med.*, **89**, 258
184. Samols, E., Marri, G. and Marks, V. (1965). Promotion of insulin secretion by glucagon. *Lancet*, **2**, 415
185. Dyck, W. P., Rudick, J., Hoexter, B. and Janowitz, H. D. (1969). Influence of glucagon on pancreatic exocrine secretion. *Gastroenterology*, **56**, 531
186. Rocha, D. M., Faloona, G. R. and Unger, R. H. (1972). Glucagon-stimulating activity of 20 amino acids in dogs. *J. Clin. Invest.*, **51**, 2346
187. Unger, R. H., Eisentraut, A. M. and McColl, M. S. (1961). Glucagon antibodies and an immunoassay for glucagon. *J. Clin. Invest.*, **40**, 1280
188. Samols, E., Tyler, J. and Marri, G. (1965). Stimulation of glucagon secretion by oral glucose. *Lancet*, **2**, 1257
189. Bennett, A. and Flesher, B. (1970). Prostaglandins and the gastrointestinal tract. *Gastroenterology*, **59**, 790
190. Robert, A., Nezamis, J. E. and Phillips, J. P. (1968). Effect of prostaglandin E_1 on gastric secretion and ulcer formation in the rat. *Gastroenterology*, **54**, 481
191. Robert, A., Phillips, J. P. and Nezamis, J. E. (1968). Inhibition by prostaglandin E_1 of gastric secretion in the dog. *Gastroenterology*, **54**, 1263

2
Gastrointestinal Mucosal Metabolism

University of Texas Medical School, Houston

2.1 INTRODUCTION

Although the subject of gastrointestinal metabolism spans innumerable sub-topics, the primary emphasis in this chapter will be placed on topics of current research interest. These selected topics will be related to discussions in other chapters, especially gastrointestinal hormones and gastrointestinal electrophysiology. Unfortunately, this approach excludes consideration of research currently in a quiescent phase. Historical material, however, has already been well documented elsewhere.

To begin this chapter where the previous chapter ended, the possible hormonal mediation of gastric and intestinal ion transport by adenosine 3′,5′-monophosphate (cyclic AMP) will be discussed. Then the role of the brush border and its associated glycocalyx in intestinal absorption will be considered. To complete the chapter and prepare for the next, the final topic involves the proposed enzymatic mechanisms for gastrointestinal ion transport. In particular, the presumed relations between ion-specific adenosine triphosphatases (ATPases) and gastric secretion or intestinal absorption will be examined in the light of recent investigations.

2.2 MUCOSAL HORMONE MEDIATION

The recent research of Sutherland and many others has revolutionised our concept of hormonal action by providing us with a connecting link between the extracellular hormone and the intracellular site of action[1]. This connecting link is a membrane-bound enzyme, adenylate cyclase (AC), which catalyses the transformation of intracellular ATP to cyclic AMP, upon activation by the conjugate hormone[2]. The intracellular cyclic AMP, in turn, activates an appropriate enzyme system that completes the hormonal expression until the nucleotide has been hydrolysed by phosphodiesterase (PDE) to form an inactive metabolite, adenosine 5′-monophosphate (5′AMP)[3].

This general scheme describes the mediation of hormones like epinephrine which affect the intermediary metabolism of target organs[4]. In addition, however, Orloff and Handler discovered that cyclic AMP could mimic the action of the hormone vasopressin in stimulating ion transport through an epithelium[5]. These two potential sites of action are depicted in Figure 2.1.

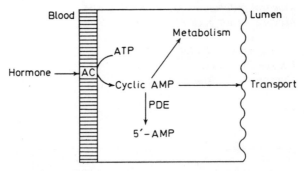

Figure 2.1 Two potential modes of cyclic AMP mediation in a gastrointestinal mucosal cell. (Modified from Robison and Sutherland[2] by permission of the American Heart Association Inc.)

The metabolic and transport reactions of cyclic AMP will be discussed relative to two gastointestinal functions that have received great attention, namely gastric and intestinal secretions. Although cyclic AMP may also be implicated in other gastrointestinal secretions (e.g. salivary and pancreatic secretions[6]), the general principles can be adequately grasped by examining the two best-studied examples.

2.2.1 Cyclic AMP and gastric acid secretion

In appraising the evidence for or against the mediation of cyclic AMP in gastric acid secretion, one must appreciate that the gastric mucosa performs functions other than acid secretion, that the response of the parietal cell secreting acid differs from that of the intact mucosa and that only stimulation of acid secretion by gastrin unequivocally reflects the action of a hormone, compared with stimulation by other secretagogues. Finally, criteria must be established to relate cyclic AMP mediation to the secretory process[1].

Harris *et al.* proposed one such set of criteria to determine whether the stimulation of acid secretion by the methylxanthines was mediated by cyclic AMP[7]. The methylxanthines are pharmacological compounds known to inhibit the degradative enzyme of cyclic AMP, PDE[3], which would raise the level of mucosal cyclic AMP. The deduced criteria for cyclic AMP mediation of acid secretion were (a) the response to methylxanthine should mimic that to exogenous cyclic AMP; (b) exogenous cyclic AMP should initiate acid secretion; (c) methylxanthines should increase mucosal cyclic AMP; (d) the increase in mucosal cyclic AMP should precede or parallel the increase in acid secretion; (e) the dose response to methylxanthines should parallel that to mucosal cyclic AMP; and (f) theophylline should increase mucosal cyclic AMP more than caffeine, since the former drug more effectively inhibits PDE. Although these criteria refer to pharmacologic stimulation of acid secretion, criteria (b) and (d) are general and have influenced the approach that others have taken to establish mediation by cyclic AMP.

Alonso and Harris noted that methylxanthines stimulated acid secretion in the isolated bullfrog gastric mucosa and that theophylline was a more potent stimulant than caffeine[8]. Caffeine also stimulated mucosal oxygen consumption in ordinary Ringer's solution, but not when the impermeant anion glucuronate was substituted for chloride. Since Hogbèn had previously demonstrated the active transport of chloride through the isolated bullfrog gastric mucosa[9], the failure of caffeine to stimulate oxygen consumption in glucuronate Ringer's solution was interpreted to mean that the principal action of caffeine, and hence cyclic AMP, related to ion transport rather than to intermediary metabolism.

Harris and Alonso later showed that exogenous cyclic AMP increased both acid secretion and oxygen consumption[10]. In these studies, the increase in mucosal oxygen consumption was reproducible in glucuronate Ringer's solution. This observation shifted the presumed site of action to cell metabolism. An intermediate response was obtained in another species, the isolated leopard frog gastric mucosa (Figure 2.2). The partial reproducibility here probably reflects the situation in which cyclic AMP affects two interdependent phenomena, metabolism and transport. In these experiments, cyclic AMP did increase both acid secretion and the short-circuit current (Isc) in parallel. Acid secretion (H^+) is related to the Isc through Hogben's equation[9]:

$$Isc = Cl^- \text{ (net } S \rightarrow M) - H^+$$

where Cl^- (net $S \rightarrow M$) is the net flux of chloride under a condition of zero electrochemical potential difference. The simultaneous and equivalent increase in Isc and H^+ led Harris and Alonso to postulate that cyclic AMP stimulated active chloride transport in addition to active hydrogen transport.

In isolated mucosae, the dual effect of cyclic AMP on metabolism and transport may be explained in terms of a tissue whose secretory function is limited by the available supply of endogenous and exogenous substrate. This possibility was supported by the finding of Alonso et al. that exogenous fatty acids stimulated acid secretion[11].

Since methylxanthines and histamine are structurally similar in possessing an imidazole ring, the possibility was explored that methylxanthines stimulated acid secretion and oxygen consumption as analogues of histamine rather than as inhibitors of PDE[12]. The common base of imidazole as well as N-methylimidazole, however, reduced rather than increased acid secretion. The Isc rose equivalently, indicating inhibition of hydrogen but not chloride transport according to Hogben's equation.

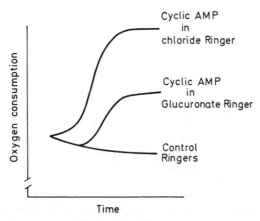

Figure 2.2 Effects of cyclic AMP on oxygen consumption of gastric mucosa from the leopard frog in chloride and glucuronate media. (Modified from Harris and Alonso[10])

Having concluded that methylxanthines act by means of a metabolic action of cyclic AMP, Harris and his collaborators studied some probable metabolic sites of action. The earlier work of Sutherland's group had established the complex activation of muscle and liver phosphorylase by cyclic AMP[1]. Since phosphorylase catalysed the mobilisation of glycogen to glucose and the amphibian gastric mucosa contains large stores of glycogen[11], this site of action was attractive, particularly in an energy-limited, isolated mucosa. Incubation with cyclic AMP did elevate both active and total phosphorylase activity in the gastric mucosa of the leopard frog, but the increase was not dramatic[13]. The small rise was explained as a consequence of a prevalent active phosphorylase in gastric mucosa as compared to skeletal muscle.

In their culminating studies, Alonso et al. demonstrated that cyclic AMP simultaneously accelerated glycogenolysis, oxygen consumption and lactate formation[14]. Expected oxygen consumption was calculated from glycogen utilisation and lactate production. The expected oxygen consumption was about one-half that actually measured, indicating that the other half must have derived from mucosal triglyceride oxidation. The ratio of expected to measured oxygen consumption remained unchanged after cyclic AMP administration, so it was deduced that cyclic AMP-stimulated lipolysis as well as glycogenolysis. The site of action was presumed to be some integrative step like the citric acid cycle or oxidative phosphorylation.

In general, Harris and his associates amply satisfied their criteria implicating cyclic AMP in the stimulation of acid secretion by methylxathines in the isolated anuran gastric mucosa. Nakajima et al. have confirmed and extended these results on the urodelan gastric mucosa of another amphibian, the mudpuppy[15]. Later studies indicated that histamine and pentagastrin could approximately double the mucosal cyclic AMP, an effect that these authors attributed to the activation of AC by secretagogues[16]. PDE was localised in the acid-secreting cells[17].

Intriguing as the results on isolated amphibian gastric mucosae were, their physiological relevance needed to be studied in isolated and intact mammalian gastric mucosae. In a preliminary report, Perrier and Laster observed that mucosal AC from the guinea-pig could be stimulated several-fold by histamine but not by gastrin[18]. This stimulation could be competitively inhibited by the antihistaminic chlorpheniramine, even though antihistaminies are known to have no effect on gastric acid secretion stimulated by histamine. Domschke et al. also reported that intravenous infusion of histamine in rats caused dose-dependent increases in acid secretion and mucosal cyclic AMP[19]. These attempts to correlate the levels of cyclic AMP and acid secretion in rodents must be tempered by the observations that the isolated gastric mucosae of rats[20] and guinea-pigs[21] are refractory to histamine stimulation. Furthermore, Tague and Shanbour found no differences between the levels of cyclic AMP from intact rat gastric mucosae exposed either to saline or 20% ethanol saline[22]. This ethanol concentration inhibits histamine-stimulated acid secretion in the dog chambered gastric segment[23] and presumably also in the rat stomach.

The cyclic AMP hypothesis has recently been examined critically by Mao et al.[24]. In experiments on anaesthetised dogs, they simultaneously tested the effects of stimulants or inhibitors of acid secretion and prospective stimulants or inhibitors of AC and PDE, both in vivo or in vitro. These studies effectively dissociated changes in acid secretion from cyclic AMP in the dog stomach. First, histamine initiates acid secretion in vivo but fails to stimulate AC in vivo or in vitro (Figure 2.3). Second, theophylline and papaverine fail to initiate acid secretion in vivo but do inhibit mucosal PDE in vitro. Finally, the more permeable dibutyryl derivative of cyclic AMP fails to evoke acid secretion, although total blood flow to the chambered gastric segment rises. Whereas any one set of these observations might be criticised on the basis of a manifold causality for a negative result, the argument in toto leaves little to be debated.

In a later study, Mao et al. demonstrated that gastrin as well as histamine stimulated acid secretion while failing to increase cyclic AMP content in mucosal biopsies[25]. Conversely, the intra-arterial infusion of papaverine increases mucosal cyclic AMP while failing to stimulate acid secretion.

Mao et al. criticised the evidence in favour of cyclic AMP mediation of acid secretion because it was obtained from in vitro mucosae that spontaneously secrete acid[25]. Amphibians and rodents do secrete acid spontaneously, and the underlying biochemical processes may well differ from those involved in stimulated acid secretion[26]. They also pointed out that *in vitro* gastric function may be limited by the available metabolic energy and that stimulants of AC and inhibitors of PDE may energetically reinforce the mucosa, thereby increasing acid secretion. Unlike the situation *in vivo*, the isolated frog gastric mucosa secretes in response to exogenous fatty acids[11] and the isolated rat gastric mucosa in response to exogenous glucose[27].

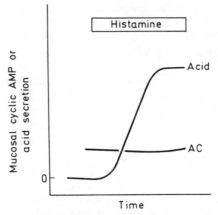

Figure 2.3 Effects of intravenous infusion of histamine on acid secretion and adenylate cyclase (AC) activity of gastric mucosa from the dog. (Modified from Mao *et al.*[24].)

One should also note the limitation of studies which measure gastric mucosal cyclic AMP, AC and PDE. The parietal cell mass constitutes a fraction of the total mucosa; changes or absence of changes in mucosal cyclic AMP content or enzymatic activity may reflect events in other cell types in the tissue. For example, splanchnic vascular smooth muscle has been shown to dilate upon stimulation by agents that raise the level of cyclic AMP[28], and contractions of the muscularis mucosae of the stomach cease after administration of cyclic AMP[29].

At present, the case favouring cyclic AMP mediation in the isolated amphibian gastric mucosa and the case against mediation in the intact canine gastric mucosa seem equally convincing. The physiologist can only hope that the final resolution will be more general than the *in vitro–in vivo* and species differences would suggest.

2.2.2 Cyclic AMP and intestinal secretion

In contrast to gastric secretion, choleraic secretion appears to be remarkably free of *in vivo–in vitro* and species differences. Not only is choleraic secretion independent of the host species, but the diarrhoeal state may be elicited by several bacterial vectors dwelling within the intestinal lumen. *Vibrio cholerae* produces the cholera toxin, and *Clostridium welchii* and *Escherichia coli* release other toxins which evoke diarrhoea[30]. Although only the mediation of choleraic secretion will be considered, the process may be representative of many interactions that frequently occur between the intestinal mucosa and its microflora. Normally, however, the predominant intestinal function must be absorptive rather than secretory.

In their studies of the isolated rabbit ileum, Schultz and Zalusky identified the Isc with the active transport of sodium from mucosa to serosa[31,32]. Both could be increased by mucosal glucose through coupled sodium and glucose transport[33]. Thus, the driving forces for normal absorption of isotonic fluid appeared to be independent and coupled transport of sodium from lumen to blood. Although entirely satisfactory for the intestinal absorptive state, this scheme cannot adequately explain intestinal secretion.

The virtual identity of Isc with active sodium transport in the rabbit ileal wall neither suggests nor precludes the simultaneous transport of other ion species. A similar situation prevails in the isolated rat stomach. In the undissected rat stomach wall, sodium transport accounts for most of the Isc. The dissected rat gastric mucosa, however, transports chloride even in excess of sodium transport[20].

Field *et al.* also found that removal of the attached muscle coat uncovered a chloride transport process in the rabbit ileal mucosa[34]. Unlike the gastric mucosa, the ileal mucosa transported chloride from mucosa to serosa. Although the discovery of an absorptive chloride transport would appear somewhat irrelevant to choleraic secretion, the opposite is true. When cholera toxin was added to the mucosal solution, the net absorptive transport of sodium was abolished and a net secretory transport of chloride was produced[35]. The latter effect was overwhelming as shown by increased Isc and PD. Furthermore, Field *et al.*[34] confirmed the earlier findings of Carpenter *et al.*[36] in dog jejunal loops; i.e. cholera toxin does not affect the fraction of sodium transport that is coupled to glucose absorption. In rabbit ileal mucosa, this fraction is about four-fifths the total sodium transport[34]. Thus, the principal action of cholera toxin in inducing intestinal secretion consists of unmasking a secretory chloride transport rather than inhibiting an absorptive sodium transport.

Although cholera toxin is hardly a hormone[4], much evidence has been developed to show that cyclic AMP mediates its action on the gut. In this modern sense, cholera toxin may partly resemble a 'first messenger'. If one judges solely from the biochemical effects of cholera toxin, such quasi 'first messengers' may play a similar role in pathophysiological non-steady states as the classical hormones play in the physiological steady state.

Field and his associates have shown that the hormone vasopressin increases the Isc of rabbit ileal mucosa, albeit transiently[37]. Furthermore, cyclic AMP or theophylline elicits an equal and sustained increase. Whether the elevated Isc results from a rise in absorptive sodium transport or an induction of secretory chloride transport has not been determined.

In subsequent and more elaborate studies, Field described the effects of exogenous cyclic AMP on rabbit ileal mucosa more completely[38]. First he determined that cyclic AMP, its dibutyryl derivative and theophylline are equally effective but not additive in raising the Isc. As for the mucosal administration of cholera toxin, the serosal administration of these agents abolishes absorptive sodium transport and reverses absorptive chloride transport. As with cholera toxin, they have no effect on coupled sodium and glucose transport. These parallel actions of cholera toxin and cyclic AMP suggest a common mechanism (Figure 2.4). Other workers have found that theophylline increases the normal secretory chloride transport of isolated guinea-pig ileal mucosa[39].

This general picture also seems to reflect the action of cholera toxin *in vivo*. For example, cholera toxin significantly augments the trans-mural PD across rabbit jejunal loops[40] and more than doubles the mucosal concentration of cyclic AMP in canine intestinal mucosa[41]. Infusion of theophylline induces net secretion from dog jejunal loops[42].

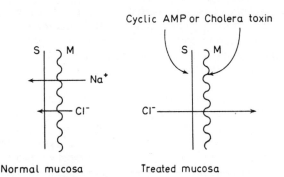

Figure 2.4 Effects of cylic AMP and cholera toxin on ion transport through ileal mucosa from the rabbit. (Modified from Field[38].)

Definitive proof for the cyclic AMP mediation of choleraic secretion awaited the demonstration by Kimberg *et al.* that cholera toxin could increase AC activity in guinea-pig and rabbit ileal mucosa both *in vitro* and *in vivo*[43]. Cholera toxin has no effect on mucosal PDE activity. A similar stimulation of AC activity has been observed in mucosal biopsy specimens from patients in the diarrhoeal phase of cholera compared with those in the convalescent phase (Figure 2.5)[30].

Cholera toxin acts from the mucosal side of the gut, whereas cyclic AMP is effective from the serosal side. This observation permits the establishment of criteria that can put the proposed cyclic AMP mediation of choleraic secretion to test. First, the side effects of the intravenous administration of cholera toxin should be explicable in terms of cyclic AMP changes in non-intestinal tissues. Second, the time for cholera toxin to diffuse from the mucosal surface to the serosal AC should entail a necessary lag that precedes choleraic secretion. Finally, the biochemical localisation of a serosal AC for cholera toxin should be feasible.

One prominent effect of the intravenous administration of cholera toxin is sustained hyperglycemia[44]. Apparently, it results from stimulation of glycogenolysis in the liver, because the AC activity of mouse liver cells increases several-fold after inoculation with cholera toxin[45]. The AC activity stimulated by cholera toxin equals that stimulated by epinephrine, and the effects are not additive. Intravenous inoculation with cholera toxin has been reported to reduce liver glycogen[46]. Thus, cholera toxin mimics epinephrine in stimulating glycogenolysis by means of a cyclic AMP-sensitive phosphorylase system.

A delay of 1–3 h normally separates the inoculation of cholera toxin and its first effects[43]. This is true both *in vitro* and *in vivo*. Although a few minutes delay might imply the postulated diffusion time, a delay of hours seems more characteristic of intermediate and perhaps synthetic reactions. Serebro *et al.* have demonstrated that pre-treatment with cycloheximide, an inhibitor of protein synthesis, prevents the copious secretion of choleraic fluid in rabbits[47]. Whatever its cause, a delay does appear to characterise the action of cholera.

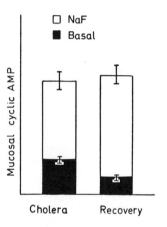

Figure 2.5 Adenylate cyclase activity (as measured by cyclic AMP levels) of jejunal mucosa from paired human patients during cholera and after recovery (Modified from Chen *et al.*[30])

Although AC has been found in preparations of intestinal plasma membranes, it is absent from isolated brush borders, both before and after treatment with cholera toxin *in vivo*[48]. From these observations, Parkinson *et al.* concluded that the membrane-bound AC, which is stimulated by cholera toxin, must be localised in the lateral and basal membranes of mucosal cells.

The cyclic AMP mediation of choleraic secretion appears a sufficient if not necessary explanation on the basis of the test criteria. Other less predictable observations are also consistent with the cyclic AMP hypothesis. We cannot predict whether a hormonal effect on ion movement through epithelial tissue involves active transport or changes in membrane permeability. For example, the action of vasopressin (mediated by cyclic AMP) involves both an increase in sodium transport and an increase in membrane permeability[5]. Conceivably, heightened permeability could reverse fluid absorption to fluid secretion, as during cholera. However, Lifson *et al.* showed that cholera toxin did not affect the movement of small non-electrolytes through the intestinal epithelium of dog jejunal loops in response to a hydrostatic or osmotic gradient[49]. That choleraic fluid is not a filtrate may also be surmised from the failure of a large reduction in mesenteric arterial pressure to reduce choleraic fluid production[44].

Active ion transport generally depends on aerobic metabolism and its derivative oxidative phosphorylation. For this reason, the observation that cholera toxin failed to alter either the oxygen consumption or the ATPase activity of everted rabbit jejunum is initially surprising[50]. However, one should recall that cholera toxin simultaneously inhibits absorptive transport and stimulates secretory transport.

Finally, one should note that the common element in gastric and choleraic secretion is the active transport of chloride from serosa to mucosa. The evidence favouring cyclic AMP mediation of this transport process is scanty and inferential for gastric secretion but well documented and direct for choleriac secretion. The simultaneous hydrogen transport in gastric secretion and sodium transport in intestinal absorption obscure the potential relation between cyclic AMP and chloride transport in the gastrointestinal tract. The issue is further obscured by the observation that cholera toxin may inhibit rather than stimulate gastric acid secretion[44]. Clearly, a need exists to re-evaluate the role that cyclic AMP plays in mediating chloride transport through the isolated, short-circuited gastric mucosa.

2.3 MUCOSAL CELL KINETICS

The susceptibility of the gastrointestinal mucosa to radiation damage emphasises the importance of mitotic activity in the alimentary tract. Without constant and rapid cell renewal, normal cell desquamation would soon be fatal. On the other hand, with uncontrolled cellular division a malignant carcinoma would ensue. Not only is mitotic activity essential to the constitution of the mucosa, it underlies the development of unspecialised crypt cells into the villous cells that accomplish digestion and transport. The brush border of the villous cells contains the binding proteins for substances that are absorbed in the intestine. Turnover of the brush border and its components occurs even more rapidly than that of the over-all mucosal ontogeny.

2.3.1 Mucosal mitosis

Mitotic activity of the mucosa is measured in turnover time, the time required to replace a number of cells equal to that initially present in the epithelium.[51] The mitotic index is the percentage of cells in mitosis histochemically; the labelling index is the percentage of cells in the DNA synthetic phase. The labelling index gained prominence after autoradiographic labelling with tritiated thymidine was introduced as a technique for determining mitotic activity[52]. This technique assumes that all cells synthesising DNA incorporate tritiated thymidine and divide mitotically[53]. Because non-incorporated thymidine is rapidly metabolised and cleared from the body, the uptake technique has found clinical application[51].

In the fundic gastric mucosa, the uptake of tritiated thymidine is first observed in the deep part of the foveolae and the mucous neck area[51]. Starting from this area of proliferation, most of the newly synthesised cells migrate upward to the surface. Parietal cells do not synthesise DNA or divide but originate from other cells. The turnover time in the rat fundus is 1.5 days, and the labelling index is 5.6%. The turnover time declines after ingestion of food. (This postprandial proliferation is discussed in the chapter on gastro-intestinal hormones.)

In the intestinal mucosa, the uptake of tritiated thymidine is first observed in the lower two-thirds of the crypts of Lieberkuhn[53] (Figure 2.6). From the

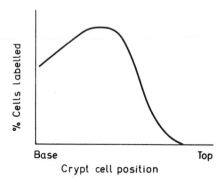

Figure 2.6 Distribution in cell positions of labelled cells in intestinal mucosa from the rat after administration of tritiated thymidine. (Modified from Cairnie *et al.*[53])

crypts, the newly synthesised cells migrate upward to the villi, the tips of which are reached in 2–3 days in the rat. As they migrate to the villi, the crypt cells proliferate but do not differentiate. In the crypt, the undifferentiated cell is rich in the enzymes necessary for cell division but lacks many of the specialised digestive enzymes[54]. The full complement of digestive enzymes is acquired at the junction of the crypt and villus. The ratio of protein to DNA is smaller in the crypts than in the villi, a consequence of the smaller size of the crypt cells[55].

In celiac sprue, the mature epithelial cells are apparently attacked selectively, resulting in a compensatory increase in mitotic activity[56]. The lower crypt cells appear normal and give rise to structurally differentiated cells near the luminal surface of the crypts. When the cells emerge on to the epithelial surface, however, the microvilli become abnormal and undergo lysosomal autodigestion. Celiac sprue is thought to result from a deficiency of a peptide hydrolase needed to digest a toxic fraction of dietary wheat gluten[57].

2.3.2 Mucosal brush border

The brush border of the differentiated mucosal cell consists of the surface microvilli, intercellular tight junctions and the terminal web that underlies the surface[58]. The portion external to the plasma membrane of the brush border is the glycocalyx. The brush border and its associated glycocalyx constitute the organelle for intestinal absorption.

Brush borders were first isolated by Miller and Crane, who demonstrated that this cell fraction contained almost all the sucrase and maltase activities of the unfractionated homogenate[59]. In addition, brush borders were found to contain the other disaccharidases, isomaltase and lactase[58]. The turnover time of disaccharidases (11.5 h) has been shown to be shorter than that of brush borders (18 h) or that of whole rat mucosa (31 h)[60]. These observations indicate that cell migration alone cannot account for enzyme turnover.

The activity of lactase declines rapidly after infancy in mammals, except for certain human ethnic groups[61] (Figure 2.7). The virtual absence of lactase

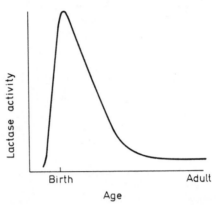

Figure 2.7 Lactase activity of rat intestinal mucosa from foetal stage to adulthood. (Modified from Kretchmer[62] *Lactase and Lactase.* Copyright © 1972, by courtesy of *Scientific American Inc.* All rights reserved.)

in the brush border adequately explains the intolerance to milk lactose in most human adults, the major symptom being diarrhoea[62].

Beside disaccharidases, the brush border contains alkaline phosphatase, leucine aminopeptidase and $(Na^+ + K^+)$-ATPase[58]. Together with the disaccharidases, these comprise the intrinsic enzymes of the brush border. The glycocalyx of the brush border can additionally absorb extrinsic enzymes, such as pancreatic amylase.

Although one would expect absorbed substances to react with some component of the brush border, convincing evidence for such a binding protein is rare. The concentration of calcium-binding protein increases during calcium absorption and in response to vitamin D administration[63]. In contrast, the glucose-binding protein of the brush border does not respond physiologically[64]. Its binding to glucose requires no sodium (as does glucose transport), is inhibited by non-transported sugars like 2-deoxyglucose and is not inhibited by transported sugars like 3-O-methylglucose. Similarly, a leucine-binding protein of the brush border is not inhibited by valine, as is leucine transport[65]. Even though these properties of binding proteins for monosaccharides and amino acids differ from the respective transport processes in the mucosa, binding proteins have nevertheless been regarded as (altered) carrier proteins for intestinal transport.

The glycocalyx consists of fine filaments radiating from the microvilli of the brush border[66]. It is prominent on absorptive cells but not on crypt or goblet cells. Although it stains for acid mucopolysaccharides, the glycocalyx does not derive from the mucus of goblet cells[67]. The glycoprotein of the glycocalyx may be labelled with radioisotopic glucosamine, and the resultant distribution of label in cell fractions is identical to that of sucrase, a plasma membrane marker[68]. These observations indicate the intimate relation between the microvillous membrane and its surface coat. This intimacy may affect the absorption of weak electrolytes, including many drugs. In the apparent absence of specific transport processes, these weak electrolytes permeate the mucosal membrane in their undissociated state[69]. The degree to which they are un-ionised governs their absorption, and the pH of the mucosal unstirred layer regulates their association according to the Henderson–Hasselbach equation. In the rat intestine, the local pH required to explain the absorption of weak electrolytes is 5.3, whereas the luminal contents are neutral or alkaline[69]. This suggests a role for the acid-staining glycocalyx in the mucosal unstirred layer. In contrast, the rat gastric mucosa envinces no such microclimate affecting permeation of weak electrolytes[70]. In the dog stomach, the rapid transport of weak electrolytes, such as aminopyrine, permits measurement of mucosal clearance as an estimate of blood flow, in accordance with the Fick principle[71].

This brief sketch of cellular kinetics emphasises the dynamic state of the gastrointestinal mucosa. Mucosal cells are constantly sloughed and replaced, and often their intrinsic digestive enzymes are renewed even more rapidly. Despite their rapid turnover, the absorptive mucosal cell achieves exquisite differentiation in the brush border and its beguiling glycocalyx. Through the expansive area of its microvilli and the distinctive microclimate of its glyco-calyx, the brush border governs the relative rate of passive absorption. More important, however, the brush border contains the carrier proteins and the transport enzymes for active aborption.

2.4 MUCOSAL TRANSPORT ENERGETICS

Documented explanations of ion transport across unit membranes of nerve axon and erythrocyte[72] have influenced the approach to bioenergetics of trans-epithelial ion transport across gastrointenstinal membranes. Of critical importance is the role of an ATPase that may be activated by the ions it transports. In the case of nerve axon and erythrocyte, a membranous ATPase does respond to the transported ions (sodium and potassium). Our concern, however, is with the physiological importance of ion-specific ATPases that reside in gastrointestinal mucosa. Although the cation-specific ATPase of the intestinal mucosa and the anion-specific ATPase of the gastric mucosa suggest mechanisms for intestinal absorption and gastric secretion, the dis-crepancies and contradictions inherent in this approach must be scrutinised and alternative approaches explored.

2.4.1 Ion-specific ATPases

Guinea-pig intestinal mucosa contains a magnesium-dependent ATPase whose activity is stimulated by the combined action of sodium and potassium;

this stimulation is inhibited by ouabain[73]. In the intestinal mucosa of the rat, most of the ATPase that responds to sodium and potassium[74] and to ouabain[75] resides in the basolateral membrane of the epithelium. Addition of exogenous ATP to isolated bullfrog intestine stimulates sodium transport; ouabain inhibits it[76]. Although drawn from different species, this is evidence for an adequate mechanism for the intestinal absorption of sodium. The apparent absence, under steady-state conditions, of an equivalent intestinal secretion of potassium eludes explanation by this mechanism.

Since absorptive transport of sodium is coupled to that of certain organic solutes[33], one might expect the postulated ATPase to be activated not only by sodium but also by the transported organic solute. Such evidence has not been forthcoming. The addition of the transported amino acids, glycine or lysine, which do not further activate the $(Na^+ + K^+)$-APTase from rat intestinal mucosa[77]. A concentration of ouabain that completely inhibits $(Na^+ + K^+)$-ATPase has no effect on the uptake of phenylalanine (another transported amino acid) by rat intestinal rings[78]. At a concentration comparable to that of the cytoplasm, exogenous ATP strongly inhibits the uptake by isolated rat intestinal mucosal cells of transported leucine, isoleucine, lysine, alanine and valine[79].

Similarly, transported hexoses such as glucose, 3-O-methylglucose, galactose and mannose inhibit the $(Na^+ + K^+)$-ATPase from rat intestinal mucosa[80]. Inhibition is considerable at glucose concentrations above 10 mmol l^{-1} in the presence of sodium and potassium (Figure 2.8). When the

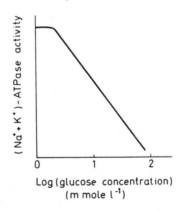

Figure 2.8 Inhibition of intestinal $(Na^+ + K^+)$-ATPase by glucose in intestinal mucosa from the rat. (Modified from Dettmer et al.[80])

major part of sodium transport may be coupled to glucose transport[34], such inhibition renders untenable a single ATPase for the transport of these coupled species. In fact, the ATPase of the basolateral membranes from rat intestinal mucosa is more sensitive to ouabain inhibition and the ATPase of the brush border is more sensitive to phlorhizin inhibition[81].

These studies, however, seem to support the sodium-gradient hypothesis of Crane[82] because the transport of amino acids and hexoses is dissociated from that of sodium with respect to the activity of $(Na^+ + K^+)$-ATPase. According to the sodium-gradient hypothesis (*discussed in the chapter on gastrointestinal electrophysiology*), only sodium transport need be energised to account for the apparent active transport of other coupled solutes[83].

In contrast to the intestinal ATPase that is stimulated by cations and inhibited by ouabain, gastric mucosal ATPase is stimulated by anions and inhibited by thiocyanate. Durbin and Kasbekar showed that the microsomal ATPase from bullfrog gastric mucosa is most sensitive to bicarbonate; chloride is not essential to its activity[84]. The relative insensitivity of this HCO_3^--ATPase to chloride raises a question regarding its physiological importance. Not only is chloride actively transported during gastric secretion[9], it also participates in an exchange with bicarbonate at the serosal surface[85]. In either case, one would expect the carrier involved to respond to chloride. Although active hydrogen secretion is not easily distinguished from active bicarbonate absorption in the process of acidification, the rising pCO_2 of the mucosal solution during gastric acid secretion indicates active hydrogen secretion rather than active bicarbonate absorption[86]. Thus, the HCO_3^--ATPase of the gastric mucosa seems disconnected from the process of gastric acid secretion; its anionic specificity and susceptibility to thiocyanate, however, have continued to attract attention.

When a non-secreting tadpole stomach develops into a secreting bullfrog stomach, a specific increase occurs in the fraction of gastric mucosal ATPase that is sensitive to thiocyanate and insensitive to ouabain[87]. Although the sensitivity to thiocyanate associates this ATPase with gastric secretion, the insensitivity to ouabain does not. In the isolated gastric mucosae of both the bullfrog[88] and the rat[20] ouabain specifically inhibits active hydrogen and chloride transport.

The thiocyanate-sensitive HCO_3^--ATPase from the oxyntic cells of the mudpuppy has been localised in the smooth microsomal cell fraction[89]. The activity of this enzyme in the stomach, however, is much less than that in the gills or brain of this species. Its ubiquity raises question about the specificity of HCO_3^--ATPase for gastric acid secretion.

Most of the ATPase in lizard gastric mucosa is sensitive to anions rather that to cations[90]. The anionic character of thiocyanate may well underlie its inhibition of HCO_3^--ATPase. In fact, the affinity of thiocyanate for this enzyme exceeds that of several other anions tested (Figure 2.9).

To complete this comparative review, a HCO_3^--ATPase has been identified in the vesicular membrane fraction of dog gastric mucosa[91]. A similar thiocyanate-sensitive HCO_3^--ATPase has been found in dog pancreas[92].

The available evidence does not support a close connection between HCO_3^--ATPase and gastric acid secretion. First, this enzyme is active in organs that do not secrete acid. Second, the insensitivity of this enzyme to chloride effectively dissociates its activity from the known anionic transport process contributing to gastric acid secretion.

Although sodium transport from mucosa to serosa has been well established for isolated mammalian mucosae[93], a sodium-gradient hypothesis seems an unlikely explanation for active secretion of acid. The isolated amphibian gastric mucosa for instance, can secrete acid in the absence of any sodium transport[9]. The inhibitory effect of ouabain on acid secretion does, however, suggest some role for sodium transport in this secretion.

Dinitrophenol, an uncoupler of oxidative phosphorylation, reduces acid secretion by the frog mucosa in a dose-dependent fashion[94]. This inhibition, however, is not reversed by exogenous ATP (ATP further inhibits acid

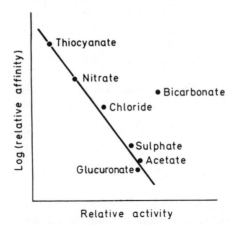

Figure 2.9 Relation of binding to activation of HCO_3^--ATPase by anions in the gastric mucosa from the lizard. (Modified from DePont et al.[90])

secretion). Inhibition by dinitrophenol differs from that by thiocyanate in that the former enhances mucosal resistance while the latter diminishes it. Since inhibition of ion transport should be accompanied by an increase in mucosal resistance[23], thiocyanate inhibition requires further explanation. Perhaps related to its affinity for HCO_3^--ATPase, thiocyanate is actively transported by the gastric mucosa[95]. This transport occurs at the expense of chloride transport[96]. But to account for the overall decline in resistance, thiocyanate transport must predominate over its inhibition of hydrogen and chloride transport. The decrease in resistance induced by thiocyanate is not invariable[97].

Thiocyanate inhibition is not localised to the gastric mucosa because oxygen consumption and ATP binding of rat liver mitochondria can be reduced by thiocyanate[98]. Still, in the *in vivo* dog stomach, thiocyanate inhibits acid secretion while leaving oxygen consumption unchanged[99]. The problem of distinguishing the principal action from the side effects of an inhibitor like thiocyanate becomes even more complicated when one considers the redox change that thiocyanate may induce in gastric mucosal extramitochondrial cytochrome c.

2.4.2 Extramitochondrial processes

In its capacity as an energy-limited tissue, the isolated gastric mucosa has presented a unique opportunity for the biochemical resolution of transport processes. Davenport and Chavré showed that the isolated mouse stomach wall oxidises acetoacetate as well as glucose in support of acid secretion, although the acetoacetate requires a cholinergic stimulant for its action[100]. In the spontaneously secreting bullfrog mucosa under endogenous stimulation fatty acids appear to energise acid secretion even in preference to glycolytic products whose oxidation is limited by a co-factor of pyruvate dehydrogenase lipoate[11]. These results emphasise the role of mitochondrial oxidation in support of stimulated acid secretion. Such mitochondrial oxidation could, by oxidative phosphorylation, be converted to the cellular chemical energy, ATP.

Some difficulties in adopting this approach to acid secretion have already been broached. First, exogenous ATP inhibits rather than stimulates acid secretion and, second, the HCO_3 -ATPase of the gastric mucosa is not highly specific with respect to either transported ions or acid-secreting tissues. The inhibitory effect of exogenous ATP has been studied in detail by Kidder in isolated bullfrog gastric mucosa[101]. Not only does exogenous ATP inhibit aerobic acid secretion, it fails to stimulate acid secretion in the anoxic mucosa. The anoxic musosa should be relatively depleted of endogenous ATP. The inhibition of aerobic acid secretion is accompanied by the apparent oxidation of cytochrome c in gastric mucosa. Cytochrome c is present in relative excess in the gastric mucosa, and apparently the excess is extramitochondrial[102].

The addition of thiocyanate to isolated bullfrog mucosa also leads to an apparent oxidation of this extramitochondrial cytochrome c[103]. In this action, thiocyanate resembles an entire class of secretory inhibitors characterised by inclusion of a nitrogen atom with an unshared pair of electrons; e.g., ammonium, nitrite, cyanate and thiocyanate[104]. These ions cause an oxidative shift in the spectrum of gastric mucosal cytochrome c. In contrast, the secretagogue histamine evokes a reductive shift in this spectrum[102]. The oxidative shift is thought to reflect the inhibitory complexing of thiocyanate with cytochrome c[103].

These results can be partly explained in terms of the chemiosmotic hypothesis proposed by Mitchell[105], i.e., that membranes may actively transport ions *in lieu of* oxidative phosphorylation. In the case of the gastric mucosa, the ion transport of acid secretion would not necessarily be limited by the supply of ATP or by the mitochondrial oxidation that produces ATP. The reciprocal relation between ion transport and oxidative phosphorylation, according to this hypothesis, may explain an inhibitory effect with excess exogenous ATP.

The isolated rat gastric mucosal preparation has been used to gain unique insight into the extramitochondrial support of acid secretion[27]. Of the substrates tested, only glucose and ribose maintained spontaneous acid secretion; pyruvate and butyrate did not (Figure 2.10). Pyruvate and butyrate were

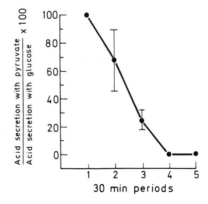

Figure 2.10 Acid secretion by rat gastric mucosa exposed to pyruvate relative to that by paired mucosa exposed to glucose. (Modified from Sernka and Harris[27].)

selected as prime candidates for mitochondrial oxidation through the citric acid cycle and they did stimulate mucosal oxygen consumption. Thus, their failure to support acid secretion cannot be attributed to mucosal imper-meability. Instead, it appears that mitochondrial oxidation does not support spontaneous acid secretion by this mucosa. In contrast, glucose and ribose support acid secretion by oxidation through an extramitochondrial pathway, the pentose phosphate shunt.

The pentose phosphate shunt has been detected in rat gastric mucosa by incubating paired tissue slices with either $(1\text{-}^{14}C)$glucose or $(6\text{-}^{14}C)$glucose and comparing the relative amounts of $^{14}CO_2$ evolved. Since the C-1 carbon atom of glucose is preferentially oxidised through the pentose phosphate shunt but not through the citric acid cycle, a ratio of evolved $^{14}CO_2$ greater than unity implies the presence of the pentose phosphate shunt. The measured ratio for rat gastric mucosa exceeds both unity and the ratio obtained for rat dia-phragm (Figure 2.11). The relative magnitude of this ratio, however, does not necessarily provide a measure of shunt activity.

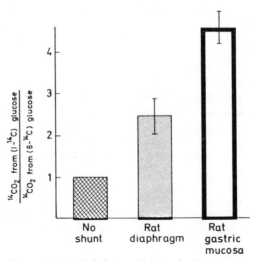

Figure 2.11 Relative activity of the pentose phosphate shunt. (Modified from Sernka and Harris[27] also, unpublished observations.)

The activity of the pentose phosphate shunt has been determined in the supernatant fraction of homogenised rat gastric mucosa. All enzymes of the shunt reside in the soluble cytoplasm, so that only the necessary substrate, co-enzyme and electron coupler need be added. Although the glucose 6-phosphate substrate is common to both the shunt and the glycolytic pathway, the co-enzymes for these two pathways differ. Whereas oxidation of glucose 6-phosphate through the glycolytic pathway requires NAD^+ as co-enzyme, the pentose phosphate shunt uniquely requires $NADP^+$ as its oxidising agent. The rapid oxidation of glucose 6-phosphate by $NADP^+$, but not by NAD^+, indicates the high activity of the pentose phosphate shunt in rat gastric mucosa (Figure 2.12).

These results on isolated rat gastric mucosa emphasise the importance of an extramitochondrial process in the ion transport that comprises acid secretion.

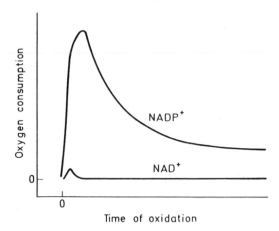

Figure 2.12   Co-enzyme oxidation of glucose 6-phosphate in the supernatant fraction from rat gastric mucosa. (Modified from Sernka and Harris[27]; also, unpublished observations.)

They do not additionally exclude an essential role for mitochondrial oxidation and oxidative phosphorylation. The isolated rat gastric mucosa secretes acid spontaneously, but does not respond to secretagogues like histamine[20]. Acid secretion stimulated by secretagogues in other species or preparations may well depend on mitochondrial processes[106]. Secretagogues do not stimulate the activity of shunt enzymes in rat gastric mucosa[26]. To resolve the underlying oxidative support for stimulated acid secretion, a more responsive preparation like the isolated dog gastric mucosa[93] must be investigated.

Finally, the insight into the bioenergetics of gastrointestinal active transport gained through application of the sodium-gradient and chemiosmotic hypotheses derives from an essential relation in irreversible thermodynamics, Onsager's law, which predicates that the various forces acting on a membrane may be coupled to one another[107]. This coupling allows intestinal sodium transport to determine the transport of many organic solutes. A more abstruse coupling may allow oxidations within gastric membranes either to generate ATP or to transport ions directly.

2.5 CONCLUSIONS

With respect to the mediation of gastrointestinal ion transport by cyclic AMP, some critical experiments conducted on the mammalian gastric mucosa have challenged the established view that cyclic AMP mediates gastric acid secretion. Equally definitive experiments performed on the mammalian ileal mucosa have established that cyclic AMP does mediate the intestinal secretion of cholera. With regard to the functional significance of the brush border to intestinal absorption, the identity of binding proteins with transport carriers has been questioned and the emerging importance of the glycocalyx has been underscored. Finally, recent data conflicts with a simple enzymatic interpretation of gastric acid secretion or intestinal fluid absorption. The intestinal cation-specific ATPase responds to transported organic solutes unexpectedly, and the gastric anion-specific ATPase is specific neither to the gastric mucosa nor the transported anion. Current debate centres about the conceivable role of extramitochondrial processes in gastric acid secretion[108-110].

References

1. Robison, G. A., Butcher, R. W. and Sutherland, E. W. (1971). *Cyclic AMP* (New York: Academic Press)
2. Robison, G. A. and Sutherland, E. W. (1970). Sympathin E, sympathin I, and the intracellular level of cyclic AMP, *Circulation Research*, **26–27[I]**, 147
3. Butcher, R. W. and Sutherland, E. W. (1962). Adenosine 3',5'-phosphate in biological materials. I. Purification and properties of cyclic 3',5'-nucleotide phosphodiesterase and use of this enzyme to characterise adenosine 3',5'-phosphate in human urine, *J. Biol. Chem.*, **237**, 1244
4. Robison, G. A. (1972). Cyclic AMP and hormone action, *Amer. J. Pharm. Educ.*, **36**, 723
5. Orloff, J. and Handler, J. S. (1962). The similarity of effects of vasopressin, adenosine-3',5'-monophosphate (cyclic AMP) and theophylline on the toad bladder, *J. Clin. Invest.*, **41**, 702
6. Scratcherd, R. and Case, R. M. (1969). The role of cyclic adenosine-3'5'-monophosphate (AMP) in gastrointestinal secretion, *Gut*, **10**, 957
7. Harris, J. B., Nigon, K. and Alonso, D. (1969). Adenosine-3',5'- monophosphate: intracellular mediator for methyl xanthine stimulation of gastric secretion. *Gastroenterology*, **57**, 377
8. Alonso, D. and Harris, J. B. (1965). Effect of xanthines and histamine on ion transport and respiration by frog gastric mucosa, *Amer. J. Physiol.*, **208**, 18
9. Hogben, C. A. M. (1955). Active transport of chloride by isolated frog gastric epithelium: origin of the gastric mucosal potential, *Amer. J. Physiol.*, **180**, 641
10. Harris, J. B. and Alonso, D. (1965). Stimulation of the gastric mucosa by adenosine-3',5'-monophosphate, *Fed. Proc.*, **24**, 1368
11. Alonso, D., Nigon, K., Dorr, I. and Harris, J. B. (1967). Energy sources for gastric secretion: substrates, *Amer. J. Physiol.*, **212**, 992
12. Alonso, D., Rynes, R. and Harris, J. B. (1965). Effect of imidazoles on active transport by gastric mucosa and urinary bladder, *Amer. J. Physiol.*, **208**, 1183
13. Nigon, K. and Harris, J. B. (1968). Adenosine monophosphates and phosphorylase activity in frog stomachs, *Amer. J. Physiol.*, **215**, 1299
14. Alonso, D., Park, O. H. and Harris, J. B. (1968). Adenosine monophosphates and glycogenolysis in frog gastric mucosa, *Amer. J. Physiol.*, **215**, 1305
15. Nakajima, S., Shoemaker, R. L., Hirschowitz, B. I. and Sachs, G. (1970). Comparison of actions of aminophylline and pentagastrin on *Necturus* gastric mucosa, *Amer. J. Physiol.*, **219**, 1259
16. Nakajima, S., Hirschowitz, B. I. and Sachs, G. (1971). Studies on adenyl cyclase in *Necturus* gastric mucosa, *Arch. Biochem. Biophys.*, **143**, 123
17. Sung, C. P., Wiebelhaus, V. D., Jenkins, B. C., Adlercreutz, P., Hirschowitz, B. I. and Sachs, G. (1972). Heterogeneity of 3',5'-phosphodiesterase of gastric mucosa, *Amer. J. Physiol.*, **223**, 648
18. Perrier, C. V. and Laster, L. (1969). Adenyl cyclase activity of guinea pig gastric mucosa, *Clin. Res.*, **17**, 596

19. Domschke, W., Domschke, S., Classen, M. and Demling, L. (1972). Cyclic AMP and the stimulation of gastric secretion by histamine in rats, *Gastroenterology*, **62**, 744

20. Sernka, T. J. and Hogben, C. A. M. (1969). Active ion transport by isolated gastric mucosae of rat and guinea pig, *Amer. J. Physiol.*, **217**, 1419

21. Shoemaker, R. L., Sachs, G. and Hirschowitz, B. I. (1966). Secretion by guinea pig gastric mucosa *in vitro*, *Proc. Soc. Exp. Biol. Med.*, **123**, 824

22. Tague, L. L. and Shanbour, L. L. Effects of ethanol on gastric mucosal cAMP, *Clin. Res.*, **20** [4], 736

23. Sernka, T. J., Gilleland, C. W. and Shanbour, L. L. (1973). Effects of ethanol on active transport in the dog stomach, *Amer. J. Physiol.*, in press

24. Mao, C. C., Shanbour, L. L., Hodgins, D. S. and Jacobson, E. D. (1972). Cyclic adenosine 3',5'-monophosphate (cyclic AMP) and secretion in the canine stomach, *Gastroenterology*, **63**, 427

25. Mao, C. C., Jacobson, E. D. and Shanbour, L. L., Mucosal cyclic AMP and secretion in the dog stomach, *Amer. J. Physiol.*, **225**, 893

26. Sernka, T. J. (1972). Response of the pentose phosphate shunt in rat gastric mucosa to stimulants and inhibitors of acid secretion, *Gastroenterology*, **62**, 808

27. Sernka, T. J. and Harris, J. B. (1972). Pentose phosphate shunt and gastric acid secretion in the rat, *Amer. J. Physiol.*, **222**, 25

28. Shepherd, A. P., Solomon, N., Shanbour, L. L. and Jacobson, E. D. (1972). The role of cyclic AMP in mesenteric vasodilation, *Gastroenterology*, **62**, 811

29. Rehm, W. S., White, A. S., Sanders, S. S. and Feagin, F. F. (1970). Adenine compounds on changes in optical density and motility of frog gastric mucosa, *Amer. J. Physiol.*, **218**, 1010

30. Chen, L. C., Rohde, J. E. and Sharp, G. W. G. (1972). Properties of adenyl cyclase from human jejunal mucosa during naturally acquired cholera and convalescence, *J. Clin. Invest.*, **51**, 731

31. Schultz, S. S. and Zalusky, R. (1964). Ion transport in isolated rabbit ileum. I. Short-circuit current and sodium fluxes, *J. Gen. Physiol.*, **47**, 567

32. Schultz, S. S. and Zalusky, R. (1964). Ion transport in isolated rabbit ileum. II. The interaction between active sodium and active sugar transport, *J. Gen. Physiol.*, **47**, 1043

33. Schultz, S. S. and Curran, P. F. (1970). Coupled transport of sodium and organic solutes, *Physiol. Rev.*, **50**, 637

34. Field, M., Fromm, D. and McColl, I. (1971). Ion transport in rabbit ileal mucosa. I. Na and Cl fluxes and short-circuit current, *Amer. J. Physiol.*, **220**, 1388

35. Field, M., Fromm, D., Al-Awqati, Q. and Greenough, W. B. III (1972). Effect of cholera enterotoxin on ion transport across ileal mucosa, *J. Clin. Invest.*, **51**, 796

36. Carpenter, C. C. J., Sack, R. B., Feeley, J. C. and Steenberg, R. W. (1968). Site and characteristics of electrolyte loss and effect of intraluminal glucose in experimental canine cholera, *J. Clin. Invest.*, **47**, 1210

37. Field, M., Plotkin, G. R. and Silen, W. (1968). Effects of vasopressin, theophylline and cyclic adenosine monophosphate on short-circuit current across isolated rabbit ileal mucosa, *Nature (London)*, **217**, 469

38. Field, M. (1971). Ion transport in rabbit ileal mucosa. II. Effect of cyclic 3',5'-AMP, *Amer. J. Physiol.*, **221**, 992

39. Powell, D. W., Binder, H. J. and Curran, P. F. (1972). Electrolyte secretion by the guinea pig ileum *in vitro*, *Amer. J. Physiol.*, **223**, 531

40. Moritz, M., Iber, F. L. and Moore, E. W. (1971). Rabbit cholera: relation of transmural potentials to water and electrolyte fluxes, *Amer. J. Physiol.*, **221**, 19

41. Schafer, D. E., Lust, W. D., Sircar, B. and Goldberg, N. D. (1970). Elevated concentration of adenosine 3',5'-cyclic monophosphate in intestinal mucosa after treatment with cholera toxin, *Proc. Nat. Acad. Sci., USA*, **67**, 851

42. Pierce, N. F., Carpenter, C. C. J. Jr., Elliott, H. L. and Greenough, W. B. III (1971). Effects of prostaglandins, theophylline, and cholera exotoxin upon transmucosal water and electrolyte movement in the canine jejunum, *Gastroenterology*, **60**, 22

43. Kimberg, D. V., Field, M., Johnson, J., Henderson, A. and Gershon, E. (1971). Stimulation of intestinal mucosal adenyl cyclase by cholera enterotoxin and prostaglandins, *J. Clin. Invest.*, **50**, 1218

44. Carpenter, C. C. J. (1971). Cholera enterotoxin—recent investigations yield insights into transport processes, *Amer. J. Med.*, **50**, 1
45. Gorman, R. E. and Bitensky, M. W. (1972). Selective effects of cholera toxin on the adrenaline responsive component of hepatic adenyl cyclase, *Nature (London)*, **235**, 439
46. Zieve, P. D., Pierce, N. F. and Greenough, W. B. III (1970). Stimulation of glycogenolysis by purified cholera enterotoxin in disrupted cells, *Clin. Res.*, **18**, 690
47. Serebro, H. A., Iber, F. L., Yardley, J. H. and Hendrix, T. R. (1969). Inhibition of cholera toxin action in the rabbit by cycloheximide, *Gastroenterology*, **56**, 506
48. Parkinson, D. K., Ebel, H., Dibona, D. R. and Sharp, G. W. (1972). Localization of the action of cholera toxin on adenyl cyclase in mucosal epithelial cells of rabbit intestine, *J. Clin. Invest.*, **51**, 2292
49. Lifson, N., Hakim, A. A. and Lender, E. J. (1972). Effects of cholera toxin on intestinal permeability and transport interactions, *Amer. J. Physiol.*, **222**, 1479
50. Keusch, G. T., Rahal, J. J. Jr., Weinstein, L. and Grady, G. F. (1970). Biochemical effects of cholera enterotoxin: oxidative metabolism in the infant rabbit, *Amer. J. Physiol.*, **218**, 703
51. Willems, G. (1972). Cell renewal in the gastric mucosa, *Digestion*, **6**, 46
52. Taylor, J. H., Woods, P. S. and Hughes, W. L. (1957). The organization and duplication of chromosomes as revealed by autoradiographic studies using tritium-labelled thymidine, *Proc. Nat. Acad. Sci., USA*, **43**, 122
53. Cairnie, A. B., Lamerton, L. F. and Steel, G. C. (1965). Cell proliferation studies in the intestinal epithelium of the rat. I. Determination of the kinetic parameters, *Exp. Cell Res.*, **39**, 528
54. Gardner, J. D., Brown, M. S. and Laster, L. (1970). The columnar epithelial cell of the small intestine: digestion and transport (first of three parts), *New Eng. J. Med.*, **283**, 1196
55. Koldovský, O., Herbst, J. J., Burke, J. and Sunshine, P. (1970). RNA and DNA in intestinal mucosa during development of normal and cortisone-treated rats, *Growth*, **34**, 359
56. Trier, J. S. and Browning, T. H. (1970). Epithelial-cell renewal in cultured duodenal biopsies in celiac sprue, *New Eng. J. Med.*, **283**, 1245
57. Gardner, J. D., Brown, M. S. and Laster, L. (1970). The columnar epithelial cell of the small intestine: digestion and transport (third of three parts), *New Eng. J. Med.*, **283**, 1317
58. Crane, R. K. (1968). Digestive-absorptive surface of the small bowel mucosa, *Ann. Rev. Med.*, **19**, 57
59. Miller, D. and Crane, R. K. (1961). The digestive function of the epithelium of the small intestine. II. Localization of disaccharide hydrolysis in the isolated brush border portion of intestinal epithelial cells, *Biochim. Biophys. Acta*, **52**, 293
60. James, W. P. T., Alpers, D. H., Gerber, J. E. and Isselbacher, K. J. (1971). The turnover of disaccharidases and brush border proteins in rat intestine, *Biochim. Biophys. Acta*, **230**, 194
61. Alpers, D. H. and Isselbacher, K. J. (1970). Disaccharidase deficiency, *Adv. Met. Disorders*, **4**, 75
62. Kretchmer, N. (1972). Lactose and lactase, *Sci. Amer.*, **227**, [4], 70
63. Wasserman, R. H., Corradino, R. A. and Taylor, A. N. (1968). Vitamin D-dependent calcium-binding protein. Purification and some properties. *J. Biol. Chem.*, **243**, 3978
64. Eichholz, A., Howell, K. E. and Crane, R. K. (1969). Studies on the organization of the brush border in intestinal epithelial cells. IV. Glucose binding to isolated intestinal brush borders and their subfractions, *Biochim. Biophys. Acta*, **193**, 179
65. Reiser, S. and Christiansen, P. A. (1971). The properties of the preferential uptake of L-leucine by isolated intestinal epithelial cells, *Biochim. Biophys. Acta*, **225**, 123
66. Ito, S. (1965). The enteric surface coat on cat intestinal microvilli, *J. Cell Biol.*, **27**, 475
67. Forstner, G. G. (1970). (1-^{14}C)glucosamine incorporation by subcellular fractions of small intestinal mucosa. Identification by precursor labelling of three functionally distinct glycoprotein classes, *J. Biol. Chem.*, **245**, 3584
68. Forstner, G. G. (1971). Release of intestinal surface-membrane glycoproteins associated with enzyme activity by brief digestion with papain, *Biochem J.*, **121**, 781
69. Hogben, C. A. M., Tocco, D. J., Brodie, B. B. and Schanker, L. S. (1959). On the mechanism of intestinal absorption of drugs, *J. Pharmac. Exp. Therap.*, **125**, 275

70. Sernka, T. J. (1969). *Ion transport through gastric mucosa*, 62 (Ann Arbor: University Microfilms)
71. Jacobson, E. D. (1968). Clearances of the gastric mucosa, *Gastroenterology*, **54**, 434
72. Glynn, I. M. (1968). Membrane adenosine triphosphatase and cation transport, *Brit. Med. Bull.*, **24**, 165
73. Taylor, C. B. (1962). Cation-stimulation of an ATPase system from the intestinal mucosa of the guinea-pig, *Biochim. Biophys. Acta*, **60**, 437
74. Quigley, J. P. and Gotterer, G. S. (1969). Distribution of $(Na^+ - K^+)$-stimulated ATPase activity in rat intestinal mucosa, *Biochim. Biophys. Acta*, **173**, 456
75. Fujita, M., Matsui, H., Nagano, K. and Nakao, M. (1971). Asymmetric distribution of ouabain-sensitive ATPase activity in rat intestinal mucosa, *Biochim. Biophys. Acta*, **233**, 404
76. Gerencser, G. A. and Armstrong, W. McD. (1972). Sodium transfer in bullfrog small intestine. Stimulation by exogenous ATP, *Biochim. Biophys. Acta*, **255**, 663
77. Quigley, J. P. and Gotterer, G. S. (1969). Properties of a high specific activity, $(Na^+ - K^+)$-stimulated ATPase from rat intestinal mucosa, *Biochim. Biophys. Acta*, **173**, 469
78. Robinson, J. W. L. (1970). The difference in sensitivity to cardiac steroids of $(Na^+ - K^+)$-stimulated ATPase and amino acid transport in the intestinal mucosa of the rat and other species, *J. Physiol. (London)*, **206**, 41
79. Reiser, S. and Christiansen, P. A. (1971). Inhibition of amino acid uptake by ATP in isolated intestinal epithelial cells, *Biochim. Biophys. Acta*, **233**, 480
80. Dettmer, D., Glander, H. J. and Müller, F. (1972). Effects of monosaccharides on the sodium activation curve of the intestinal $(Na^+ - K^+)$-ATPase, *Biochim. Biophys. Acta*, **266**, 128
81. Quigley, J. P. and Gotterer, G. S. (1972). A comparison of the $(Na^+ - K^+)$-ATPase activities found in isolated brush border and plasma membrane of the rat intestinal mucosa, *Biochim. Biophys. Acta*, **255**, 107
82. Crane, R. K. (1962). Hypothesis for mechanism of intestinal active transport of sugars, *Fed. Proc.*, **21**, 891
83. Crane, R. K. (1965). Na^+-dependent transport in the intestine and other animal tissues, *Fed. Proc.*, **24**, 1000
84. Durbin, R. P. and Kasbekar, D. K. (1965). Adenosine triphosphate and active transport by the stomach, *Fed. Proc.*, **24**, 1377
85. Hogben, C. A. M. (1952). Gastric anion exchange: its relation to the immediate mechanism of hydrochloric acid secretion, *Proc. Nat. Acad. Sci. USA*, **38**, 13
86. Schilb, T. P. and Brodsky, W. A. (1966). Acidification of mucosal fluid by transport of bicarbonate ion in turtle bladders, *Amer. J. Physiol.*, **210**, 997
87. Limlomwongse, L. and Forte, J. G. (1970). Developmental changes in ATPase and K^+-stimulated phosphatase of tadpole gastric microsomes, *Amer. J. Physiol.*, **219**, 1717
88. Cooperstein, I. L. (1959). The inhibitory effect of strophanthidin on secretion by the isolated gastric mucosa, *J. Gen. Physiol.*, **42**, 1233
89. Wiebelhaus, V. D., Sung, C. P., Helander, H. F., Shah, G., Blum, A. L. and Sachs, G. (1971). Solubilization of anions ATPase from *Necturus* oxyntic cells. *Biochim. Biophys. Acta*, **241**, 49
90. DePont, J. J. H. H. M., Hansen, T. and Bonting, S. L. (1972). An anion-sensitive ATPase in lizard gastric mucosa, *Biochim. Biophys. Acta*, **274**, 189
91. Sachs, G., Shah, G., Strych, A., Cline, G. and Hirschowitz, B. I. (1972). Properties of ATPase of gastric mucosa. III. Distribution of HCO_3^--stimulated ATPase in gastric mucosa, *Biochim. Biophys. Acta*, **266**, 625
92. Simon, B., Kinne, R. and Sachs, G. (1972). The presence of a HCO_3^--ATPase in pancreatic tissue, *Biochim. Biophys. Acta*, **282**, 293
93. Kitahara, S., Fox, K. R. and Hogben, C. A. M. (1969). Acid secretion, Na^+ absorption, and the origin of the potential difference across isolated mammalian stomachs, *Amer. J. Digest. Diseases*, **14**, 221
94. Rehm, W. S. and LeFevre, M. E. (1965). Effect of dinitrophenol on potential resistance and H^+ rate of frog stomach, *Amer. J. Physiol.*, **208**, 992
95. Hogben, C. A. M. and Green, N. D. (1958). Active transport of bromide, iodide and thiocyanate by isolated gastric mucosa, *Fed. Proc.*, **17**, 72

96. Imamura, A. (1967). Effect of carbon dioxide upon the thiocyanate inhibition of hydrochloric acid secretion in frog gastric mucosa, *Biochim. Biophys. Acta*, **135**, 155
97. Sachs, G., Collier, R. H., Pacifico, A., Shoemaker, R. L., Zweig, R. A. and Hirschowitz, B. I. (1969). Action of thiocyanate on gastric mucosa *in vitro*, *Biochim. Biophys. Acta*, **173**, 509
98. Sachs, G., Collier, R. H. and Hirschowitz, B. I. (1970). Action of SCN⁻ on rat liver mitochondria, *Proc. Soc. Exp. Med. Biol.*, **133**, 456
99. Moody, F. G. (1968). Oxygen consumption during thiocyanate inhibition of gastric acid secretion in dogs, *Amer. J. Physiol.*, **215**, 127
100. Davenport, H. W. and Chavré, V. J. (1951). Relation between substrate disappearance and acid secretion in mouse stomach *in vitro*. *Amer. J. Physiol.*, **166**, 456
101. Kidder, G. W. III (1971). Effects of exogenous ATP on acid secretion in frog gastric mucosa, *Amer. J. Physiol.*, **221**, 421
102. Kidder, G. W. III, Curran, P. F. and Rehm, W. S. (1966). Interactions between cytochrome system and H ion secretion in bullfrog gastric mucosa, *Amer. J. Physiol.*, **211**, 513
103. Kidder, G. W. III (1970). Cytochrome c as site of action of thiocyanate in frog gastric mucosa, *Amer. J. Physiol.*, **219**, 641
104. LeFevre, M. E., Gohman, E. J. Jr. and Rehm, W. S. (1964). A hypothesis for discovery of inhibitors of gastric acid secretion, *Amer. J. Physiol.*, **207**, 613
105. Mitchell, P. (1966). Chemiosmotic coupling in oxidative and photosynthetic phosphorylaton, *Biol. Rev.*, **41**, 445
106. Sernka, T. J. (1972). *Gastric Secretions*, 293 (G. Sachs, E. Heinz and K. J. Ullrich, editors) (New York: Academic Press)
107. Onsager, L. (1969). The motion of ions: principles and concepts. *Science*, **166**, 1359
108. Hersey, S. J., High, W. L. and Jobsis, F. F. (1972). *Gastric Secretion*, 239 (G. Sachs, E. Heinz and K. J. Ullrich, editors) (New York: Academic Press)
109. Kidder, G. W. III (1971). *Gastric Secretion*, 273 (G, Sachs, E. Heinz and K. J. Ullrich, editors) (New York: Academic Press)
110. Durbin, R. P. and Michelangeli, F. (1972). *Gastric Secretion*, 307 (G. Sachs, E. Heinz and K. J. Ullrich, editors) (New York: Academic Press)

3
Principles of Electrophysiology and their Application to Epithelial Tissues

STANLEY G. SCHULTZ
University of Pittsburgh, Pennsylvania

3.1   INTRODUCTION

The secretion and absorption of salts and water by the gastrointestinal tract and the presence of spontaneous electrical potentials across several gastrointestinal tissues have been recognised for more than a century. Only within the past 25 years, however, has it become clear that these processes are

69

inextricably interwoven. While numerous techniques are currently available to measure ion transport and bioelectric properties of a wide variety of epithelial tissues, attempts to understand one set of phenomena without the other are futile. The mechanisms responsible for transepithelial ion movements cannot be understood without a knowledge of the associated bioelectric processes and vice versa.

In this chapter, we will first briefly outline the various approaches toward relating ionic diffusion, membrane properties and trans-membrane electrical potential differences (p.d.) across simple, single membranes. Next, we will consider the problem of biological membranes that may be characterised by non-diffusional 'current-generating' transport processes. These considerations will then be applied to the problem of epithelial tissues that are characterised by at least two limiting membranes arranged in series, often possessing significant 'shunt' or extracellular pathways for ion movements. This section of the text will focus largely on the representation and interpretation of the electrophysiology of epithelial tissues in terms of equivalent electrical circuits. Finally, the principles under discussion will be illustrated by an analysis of the relations between ion transport and bioelectric properties of the gastric mucosa and small intestinal epithelium, two tissues that have been studied intensively for more than two decades.

Needless to say, space limitations permit no more than an outline of basic principles and the major current avenues of investigation. Readers interested in more comprehensive information should consult the original literature. For a review of basic principles of electrolyte solutions and electrochemistry, the classic monograph by MacInnes[1] probably remains unsurpassed. In addition, excellent theoretical treatments of ion transport across artificial membranes appear in the monographs by Helfferich[2] and Lakshminarayanaiah[3]. Detailed discussions of microelectrode techniques, their shortcomings and the short-circuit technique may be found elsewhere[4-6].

3.2 ION FLUXES AND THE FLUX-RATIO EQUATION

The three general approaches to the analysis of ionic movements across membranes share a common principal objective. They all relate trans-membrane electrical potential differences and ionic fluxes to the concentrations of ions in the surrounding media and the properties of the intervening membrane. The first is a combined kinetic–thermodynamic approach, commencing with a consideration of the Nernst–Planck equation. The second is based on the principles of irreversible thermodynamics and starts with an analysis of the general differential equation for a liquid junction potential originally derived by Nernst[7, 8]. The third is based on the more recent theory of reaction rate processes[9]. Useful expressions for diffusion potentials and ionic fluxes have been derived using each of these approaches. Often these expressions closely resemble one another. Here, we will limit ourselves to the Nernst–Planck equation, which is the most frequently used starting point for a consideration of ionic movements. Excellent descriptions of the irreversible thermodynamic and the reaction rate approaches may be found in the cited references, as well as in Ref. 3.

The Nernst–Planck equation relates the flux of an ion (J_i) to the product of the concentration of the ion within the membrane at any point ($\bar{c}_i$), the mobility of the ion within the membrane (i.e. the velocity per unit driving force) ($\bar{u}_i$) and the conjugate driving force. The latter is the gradient of the electrochemical potential, $d\bar{\mu}/dx$, and is expressed as:

$$d\tilde{\mu}_i/dx = RT(d \ln \bar{c}_i/dx) + z_i\mathfrak{F}\,(d\bar{\psi}/dx)$$

where $\bar{\psi}$ is the electrical potential at any point within the membrane, x is the thickness of the membrane and z_i, $\mathfrak{F}$, R and T are the ionic valence, Faraday constant, gas constant and absolute temperature, respectively. Thus,

$$-J_i = \bar{c}_i\bar{u}_i\,(d\tilde{\mu}_i/dx) = \bar{c}_i\bar{u}_i\,[RT(d \ln \bar{c}_i/dx) + z_i\mathfrak{F}(d\bar{\psi}/dx)] \qquad (3.1)$$

One should note that this equation uses concentrations rather than thermodynamic activities and thus assumes ideal solution conditions. A more rigorous treatment would include activity coefficients, but the resulting expressions would not differ substantially. Moreover, convective flow due to possible interactions between the ion i, volume flow (i.e., solvent drag) and/or the flow of other solutes are neglected.

By considering equation (3.1) along with Figure 3.1, one gets an idea of the difficulties involved in relating ion fluxes and trans-membrane potentials

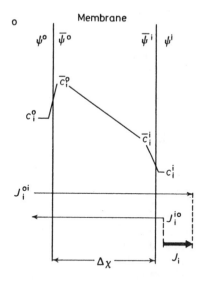

Figure 3.1 Schematic diagram for a single membrane illustrating the symbols to be used throughout this chapter. Overbars designate intramembrane parameters. The superscripts o and i designate the two interfaces of the membrane with the surrounding solutions. Also shown are the bidirectional fluxes of species i across the membrane and the net flux

to external concentrations. First, equation (3.1) applies to diffusional events *within* the membrane (designated by the overbars which will be used to denote parameters within the membrane phase). Thus, to relate these events to external, measurable parameters, one must have some information or make some assumptions regarding the partition coefficient (β_i) which relates c_i to $\bar{c}_i$ at both membrane–solution interfaces. As we shall see, these relations depend upon the nature of the membrane and, particularly, upon whether the membrane is 'neutral' or 'charged' (cf. 3.2.3). Second, the relation between $\bar{u}_i$ and both $\bar{c}_i$ and $\bar{\psi}$ is unknown. Finally, equation (3.1) cannot be integrated without some assumption regarding the electrical potential gradient (or electrical field) $d\bar{\psi}/dx$. Consequently, several approaches to the solution of equation (3.1) have been offered. These will be outlined below.

Despite the fact that the Nernst–Planck equation cannot be solved explicitly for J_i without additional assumptions, the relation between the bidirectional tracer fluxes across the membrane (J_i^{oi} and J_i^{io}) can be derived directly from equation (3.1). This relation has had profound impact on the analysis of ion movements across epithelial tissues. Thus, as demonstrated by Ussing[10] (see also Behn[11] and Teorell[12]):

$$J_i^{oi}/J_i^{io} = (c_i^o/c_i^i) \exp (z_i \mathfrak{F} \, \Delta\psi/RT) \qquad (3.2)$$

where $\Delta\psi = \psi^o - \psi^i$.

Five assumptions underlie the so-called Ussing flux-ratio equation. First, the membrane is considered to separate two well-mixed compartments and the ion, i, is assumed to be in thermodynamic equilibrium across the membrane-solution interfaces; i.e., diffusion through the membrane must be the rate-limiting step in the bidirectional movements. Second, the chemical state of i within the membrane must be the same as that in the surrounding solutions; i.e., there can be no chemical reactions, associations, complex formation, or binding within the membrane. Third, the membrane is in a steady state with respect to i, so that the flux is constant and the same at every point within the membrane in the direction of flow (i.e., $dJ_i/dt = 0$ and $dJ_i/dx = 0$). Fourth, both unidirectional fluxes traverse the membrane through pathways having identical properties. Fifth (and finally), the flow of i does not interact with the flows of other solutes or solvent (including interactions between the flows of tracer and abundant species).

These assumptions have been discussed in detail by Kedem and Essig[13] and Hoshiko and Lindley[14], and both groups have derived equation (3.2) using the phenomenological equations of irreversible thermodynamics.

Thus, if the bidirectional fluxes of an ion across a single membrane or a complex barrier such as an epithelial tissue conform to equation (3.2), one may conclude that the movements of this ion are due to strict, uncomplicated ionic diffusion driven by differences in concentration and electrical potential alone. However, failure to conform to equation (3.2) does not justify the conclusion that the net movement of the ion in question is not attributable to simple diffusion. Processes such as 'exchange diffusion' or 'single-file' diffusion will perturb the flux-ratio despite the fact that J_i may still be given by equation (3.1)[15].

An examination of equation (3.2) provides insight into the so-called 'short-circuit' technique[6] that has contributed immeasurably to the study of ion transport across a wide variety of epithelia. If a membrane or epithelial tissue is clamped between two half-chambers (Figure 3.2) and is bathed on both surfaces with identical solutions, a spontaneous electrical potential difference (p.d.) will be detected across the tissue by the electrodes labelled A and A'. (There are a few exceptions to this, such as rabbit gall bladder.) Sufficient current may be passed across the tissue using an external circuit and the current-passing electrodes (B and B') to 'null' the spontaneous p.d. to zero. According to equation (3.2), since $J_i = J_i^{oi} - J_i^{io}$

$$J_i = J_i^{io}[(c_i^o/c_i^i)\exp(z_i\mathfrak{F}\,\Delta\psi/RT) - 1]$$

The current flow across the tissue attributable to the *net* flow of i is given by

$$I_i = z_i\mathfrak{F}J_i$$

so that

$$I_i = z_i\mathfrak{F}J_i^{io}[(c_i^o/c_i^i)\exp(z_i\mathfrak{F}\,\Delta\psi/RT) - 1]$$

Clearly, if $c_i^o = c_i^i$ and $\Delta\psi = 0$, then I_i will equal zero for any ion whose movement conforms to equation (3.2). Stated another way, under 'short-circuit' conditions, when $c_i^o = c_i^i$ and $\Delta\psi = 0$, $J_i^{io} = J_i^{oi}$ and $J_i = 0$. It follows that under short-circuit conditions, the external current necessary to 'null' the spontaneous $\Delta\psi$ (or, the 'short-circuit current') must be a measure of the sum of the net flows of *all* ions whose movements do not conform

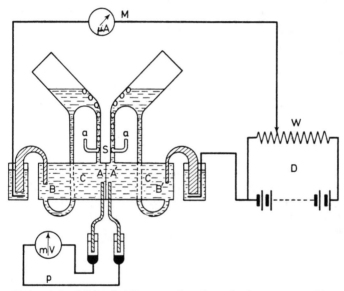

Figure 3.2 Schematic diagram of a short-circuit apparatus. (From Ussing and Zerahn[6] by courtesy of *Acta Physiol. Scand.*)

to equation (3.1) under steady-state conditions. Customarily, such flows are referred to as 'active transport' inasmuch as they cannot be caused by external differences in concentration or p.d. In most cases, this conclusion has proved correct. Strictly speaking, however, the conclusion that ionic flows not conforming to equation (3.1) are the result of active transport processes is contingent upon the exclusion of solute–solvent coupling (solvent drag) and/or solute–solute coupling, as well as the demonstration of a direct dependence upon metabolic energy[15].

We should stress that, apart from the general assumptions given above, the flux-ratio equation and its consequences are independent of the nature of the intervening barrier, the factors governing ion partition into the barrier, or the chemical or electrical potential gradients within the barrier. All of these conclusions are based on thermodynamic considerations. They depend on the initial and final states of the ion (i.e., the properties of the two external solutions) and not on the properties of the intervening barrier.

3.3 SOLUTION OF THE NERNST–PLANCK EQUATION

3.3.1 The Goldman–Hodgkin–Katz (GHK) treatment

Several approaches to the integration of equation (3.1) have been used. Planck[16,17] has provided a solution assuming 'quasi-electroneutrality' (a 'constrained diffusion boundary') throughout the barrier. Somewhat later, Henderson[18] derived an expression for the diffusion potential across a liquid junction assuming constant concentration gradients across the boundary; excellent expositions of these solutions may be found in the MacInnes text[1]. A very general solution for arbitrary electrolyte mixtures, neutral membranes, or charged membranes has been derived by Schlögl[19,20]. No assumptions have been made regarding concentration or electrical potential profiles, but mobilities and fixed charge concentrations are assumed to be constant. However, the applicability of the resulting solution is compromised by its complexity. By far the most popular solution of equation (3.1) was derived by Goldman[21] and later re-derived by Hodgkin and Katz[22], assuming that the electric field across the membrane is constant, or

$$d\bar{\psi}/dx = \Delta\bar{\psi}/\Delta x$$

This approach is popular not only because it permits a rather trivial integration of equation (3.1) and a readily applicable solution, but it has been somewhat successful in describing a number of biological systems. Thus, substituting $\Delta\bar{\psi}/\Delta x$ for $d\bar{\psi}/dx$ in equation (3.1), we obtain

$$-J_i = RT\bar{u}_i \left[(d\bar{c}_i/dx) + z_i\bar{c}_i\mathfrak{F} \, \Delta\bar{\psi}/RT\Delta x \right]$$

Assuming constant $\bar{u}_i$ and J_i (i.e. a steady-state flow), this can be readily integrated to give

$$J_i = \frac{\bar{u}_i z_i \mathfrak{F} \, \Delta\bar{\psi}}{\Delta x} \left[\frac{\bar{c}_i^o \exp\left(-z_i\mathfrak{F} \, \Delta\bar{\psi}/RT\right) - \bar{c}_i^i}{1 - \exp\left(-z_i\mathfrak{F} \, \Delta\bar{\psi}/RT\right)} \right] \tag{3.3}$$

Since the diffusion coefficient of i within the membrane, $\bar{D}_i$, is given by $\bar{D}_i = RT\bar{u}_i$, and since the permeability coefficient within the membrane is simply $\bar{P}_i = \bar{D}_i/\Delta x$,

$$\bar{P}_i = RT\bar{u}_i/\Delta x$$

When substituted into equation (3.3), this gives

$$J_i = \frac{\bar{P}_i z_i \mathfrak{F} \, \Delta\bar{\psi}}{RT} \left[\frac{\bar{c}_i^o \exp\left(-z_i\mathfrak{F} \, \Delta\bar{\psi}/RT\right) - \bar{c}_i^i}{1 - \exp\left(-z_i\mathfrak{F} \, \Delta\bar{\psi}/RT\right)} \right] \tag{3.4}$$

One should note that equation (3.4) describes events *within* the membrane, and additional assumptions are needed to relate intramembrane parameters to measurable external parameters. The simplest approach, used by Hodgkin and Katz[22], is to assume a constant partition coefficient for each ion at both interfaces, so that $\bar{c}_i = \beta_i c_i$ and $\bar{P}_i$ can be replaced with P_i as defined by $P_i = \beta_i RT\bar{u}_i/\Delta x$. In addition, it was assumed that $\Delta\bar{\psi} = \Delta\psi$. Thus, we obtain an equation identical to equation (3.4) except that the overbars designating the membrane phase are omitted.

$$J_i = \frac{P_i z_i \mathfrak{F} \; \Delta\psi}{RT} \left[\frac{c_i^o \exp(-z_i\mathfrak{F}\,\Delta\psi/RT) - c_i^i}{1 - \exp(-z_i\mathfrak{F}\,\Delta\psi/RT)} \right] \tag{3.5}$$

Since in many animal cells the predominant ions involved in determining trans-membrane diffusion potentials are Na, K and Cl, we can readily transcribe equation (3.5) into expressions for the net diffusional fluxes of these ions, J_{Na}, J_K and J_{Cl}. Now, if we assume that all membrane-pump mechanisms are electrically neutral, the maintenance of electroneutrality (or the 'zero-current' condition) restricts the diffusional fluxes of Na, K and Cl so that

$$J_K + J_{Na} = J_{Cl} \tag{3.6}$$

That is, if no net ionic current is attributable to membrane pumps, no net ionic current can result from ionic diffusion. Thus, $I_{Na} + I_K + I_{Cl} = 0$ where $I_i = z_i\mathfrak{F}J_i$. Solving for the conditions described by equations (3.5) and (3.6), we obtain the familiar Goldman–Hodgkin–Katz (GHK) equation:

$$\Delta\psi = \frac{RT}{\mathfrak{F}} \ln \left[\frac{P_{Na}c_{Na}^i + P_K c_K^i + P_{Cl}c_{Cl}^o}{P_{Na}c_{Na}^o + P_K c_K^o + P_{Cl}c_{Cl}^i} \right] \tag{3.7}$$

More generally, when $\Sigma I_+ + \Sigma I_- = 0$, we can write:

$$\Delta\psi = \frac{RT}{\mathfrak{F}} \ln \left[\frac{\sum_+ P_+ c_+^i + \sum_- P_- c_-^o}{\sum_+ P_+ c_+^o + \sum_- P_- c_-^i} \right] \tag{3.8}$$

where the subscripts $+$ and $-$ designate univalent cations and anions, respectively.

If, as in many instances, Cl is distributed at electrochemical equilibrium so that $J_{Cl} = 0$, or if, $P_{Cl} = 0$, equation (3.7) can be reduced to:

$$\Delta\psi = \frac{RT}{\mathfrak{F}} \ln \left[\frac{c_K^i + ac_{Na}^i}{c_K^o + ac_K^o} \right] \tag{3.9}$$

where $a = P_{Na}/P_K$.

The consequences of the 'constant-field treatment' are interesting to examine with respect to the unidirectional fluxes of ions across a membrane. If we view the net flux J_i as the difference between the two unidirectional fluxes so that $J_i = J_i^{oi} - J_i^{io}$, we may sub-divide equation (3.5) into:

$$J_i^{io} = P_i c_i^i \left[\frac{z_i\mathfrak{F}\,\Delta\psi/RT}{\exp(z_i\mathfrak{F}\,\Delta\psi/RT) - 1} \right] \tag{3.10}$$

and

$$J_i^{oi} = P_i c_i^o \left[\frac{(z_i\mathfrak{F}\,\Delta\psi/RT)\exp(z_i\,\mathfrak{F}\,\Delta\psi/RT)}{\exp(z_i\,\mathfrak{F}\,\Delta\psi/RT) - 1} \right]$$

or

$$J_i^{oi} = P_i c_i^o \left[\frac{-z_i\,\mathfrak{F}\,\Delta\psi/RT}{\exp(-z_i\,\mathfrak{F}\,\Delta\psi/RT) - 1} \right] \tag{3.11}$$

The bracketed terms of the right-hand sides of equations (3.10) and (3.11) have the form $x/(e^x - 1)$, which for small values of x can be approximated by $e^{-x/2}$. (When $x \leqslant 2$ or $\Delta\psi \leqslant 52$ mV, the error of this approximation is less than 15%.) Thus,

$$J_i^{io} = P_i c_i^i \exp\left(-z_i \mathfrak{F} \Delta\psi/2RT\right) \qquad (3.12)$$

and

$$J_i^{oi} = P_i c_i^o \exp\left(z_i \mathfrak{F} \Delta\psi/2RT\right) \qquad (3.13)$$

so that

$$J_i = P_i \left[c_i^o \exp\left(z_i \mathfrak{F} \Delta\psi/2RT\right) - c_i^i \exp\left(-z_i \mathfrak{F} \Delta\psi/2RT\right)\right] \qquad (3.14)$$

Equations similar to (3.12), (3.13) and (3.14) have been derived by Kimuzuka and Koketsu[23], starting with Kirkwood's approach based on the theory of irreversible thermodynamics. Similar equations have also been derived by Parlin and Eyring[9] using the theory of rate processes and by Mullins[24] for the condition in which the trans-membrane electrical potential difference, $\Delta\psi$, is the result of two equal boundary potentials. That is, $\Delta\psi = (\psi^o - \bar{\psi}^o) + (\psi^i - \bar{\psi}^i)$ where $(\psi^o - \bar{\psi}^o) = (\psi^i - \bar{\psi}^i)$. Thus an expression of this form would appear to have rather widespread validity, provided that P_i is independent of concentration and $\Delta\psi$ is not much greater than 50 mV. If P_i is concentration-dependent, the concentration terms c_i^o and c_i^i must be multiplied by additional partition factors as described by Jacquez[25].

3.3.2 Analysis of the GHK equations

Because of its simplicity and ease of application, the GHK formulation has gained wide popularity in the analysis of bioelectric phenomena. Consequently in recent years numerous efforts have been made to examine the range of validity of the constant-field assumption[26-28], to extend the validity of equation (3.8) to a family of electrical potential profiles other than the linear profile implied in the constant-field assumption[29, 30], to evaluate the effect of deviations from electroneutrality within the membrane (a space-charge density) on the electrical potential profile[27, 31] and to generalise the solution of the Nernst–Planck equations, thereby removing the need for assumptions regarding intra-membrane concentration or electrical potential profiles[25, 30].

However, perhaps the most relevant question for the electrophysiologist dealing with a membrane whose properties are largely if not entirely unknown is this. Under what conditions can equation (3.8) provide information about relative permeabilities of anions and cations from a knowledge of $\Delta\psi$ and the ion concentrations in the surrounding solutions? This, after all, is the main purpose of equation (3.8). Thus, for Na, K and Cl, we may re-write equation (3.7) in the following form. (This, of course, can be generalised to all univalent anions and cations.)

$$\Delta\psi = \frac{RT}{\mathfrak{F}} \ln\left[\frac{c_K^i + (P_{Na}/P_K)c_{Na}^i + (P_{Cl}/P_K)c_{Cl}^o}{c_K^o + (P_{Na}/P_K)c_{Na}^o + (P_{Cl}/P_K)c_{Cl}^i}\right] \qquad (3.15)$$

The important question is: under what conditions will the permeability ratios (*not* the individual permeability coefficients) be constant and independent of external concentrations and $\Delta\psi$? Sandblom and Eisenman[32], using a thermodynamic approach without assumptions regarding concentration or electrical profiles, demonstrated that equation (3.15) is generally valid *only* when the total concentrations of univalent-univalent salts in the surrounding solutions are equal or when the membrane is permeable to species of only one sign. Thus, if the membrane is permeable only to Na and K, equation (3.9) is *always* valid. Furthermore, it was possible to identify the permeability ratios as the products of the mobility ratios and the ratio of partition coefficients. For example,

$$P_{Na}/P_K = (\bar{u}_{Na}/\bar{u}_K)(\beta_{Na}/\beta_K)$$

so that constancy of the permeability ratio does not imply constancy of individual mobilities or individual partition coefficients. Thus, although the individual permeability coefficients may not be constants, the permeability ratios will be constant under the two conditions defined above, regardless of the nature of the membrane. It follows that conformity with equation (3.8) under these special conditions does not imply the presence of a constant electric field.

3.3.3 The Teorell–Meyer–Sievers (TMS) approach

Two simplifying assumptions lead to the readily applicable and popular GHK equation (3.8). First, the partition coefficients into the membrane are constant and equal at both interfaces. Second, the electric field within the membrane is constant (i.e., $\bar{\psi}$ is a linear function of x). Although the latter assumption has been extended to include a family of non-linear potential profiles that are antisymmetric about the midpoint of the membrane, the GHK assumptions are not generally valid[12, 33] and are particularly inapplicable to membranes that bear a high density of fixed charges (so-called ion-exchange membranes). The classic approach toward the treatment of these membranes was proposed simultaneously by Teorell[34] and Meyer and Sievers[35], and later revised by Teorell[36], and is outlined in Figure 3.3. First, ionic partition from the solution phase into the membrane phase is assumed to be governed by the Donnan equilibrium distribution, so that

$$\beta = -\left(\frac{\omega\bar{X}}{2c}\right) + \left[1 + \frac{\omega\bar{X}^2}{4c^2}\right]^{1/2} \tag{3.16}$$

where c designates the total concentration of univalent-univalent salts in the solution and $\omega\bar{X}$ designates the fixed-charge concentration in equivalents per litre. Thus, β_i will be a function of the fixed-charge concentration and the concentration in the external solution. Obviously, if $c^o \neq c^i$, $\beta^o \neq \beta^i$, so that, in general, the partition coefficients for the same ion may differ at the two interfaces of the membrane. One should note that if the distribution is governed entirely by the Donnan equilibrium, β is the same for all univalent cations and $1/\beta$ is the partition coefficient for all univalent anions. Thus,

$$\beta^o = \bar{c}^o_+/c^o_+ = c^o_-/\bar{c}^o_-$$

and

$$\beta^i = \bar{c}^i_+/c^i_+ = c^i_-/\bar{c}^i_-$$

for all univalent anions and cations. The implicit assumption here, of course, is that factors other than the fixed-charge density do not influence partition into the diffusion pathway (e.g., electrostatic or steric factors). This assumption would not be valid for partition into a charged pore whose radius approaches ionic dimensions, so that larger ions are excluded; these ions

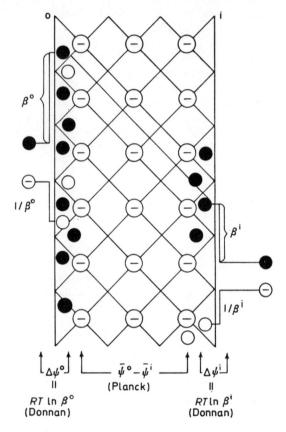

Figure 3.3 Schematic representation of the TMS approach toward the analysis of ion movements across a membrane bearing a fixed negative charge. Solid circles (●) designate cations and open circles (○) designate anions.

would then behave essentially as fixed charges in the external solution, and equation (3.16) would have to be modified. In addition, partition in accordance with a Donnan equilibrium does not discriminate among different cations or different anions. That is, because the same β applies to all univalent cations, the selectivity characteristics of a number of ion-exchange membranes are overlooked in the TMS model. Eisenman and co-workers[37, 38] have derived theoretical expressions for diffusion across ion-exchange membranes following the general approach of TMS but using ion-exchange equilibrium constants to describe partition into the membrane phase. This approach admirably accounts for the ion selectivity characteristics of a variety of membrane models containing fixed or mobile charged groups, as well as neutral ion-carriers or ionophores.

After partition into the membrane, diffusional events within the membrane are described by the Planck solution or variants thereof. Thus, the trans-membrane electrical potential difference is given by the sum of the two boundary potentials and the internal diffusion potential as given by the Planck equation. Since the resulting expressions for diffusion potentials and ion fluxes are rather complex and difficult to apply, the reader is referred to the literature cited above for further detail. The reader should note that, although the approaches employed by TMS, Eisenman and his co-workers, and Barry et al.[31] are more rigorous and generally valid than the GHK approach, all yield expressions of similar form, particularly when the fixed-charge density of the membrane is low. One major disadvantage of the TMS approach is that its application requires more information about membrane properties than is currently available for biological membranes. To date, no compelling evidence exists that this approach (or variants thereof) is distinctly superior to the GHK formulation, which has been moderately successful in interpreting bioelectric phenomena and ionic movements.

3.4 DIFFUSION POTENTIALS ACROSS BIOLOGICAL MEMBRANES AND THE EFFECTS OF RHEOGENIC PUMPS

Although ionic asymmetries between the cell interior and the exterior milieu have long been known to be consequences of active ion-transport mechanisms, until recently most evidence (or lack of opposing evidence) suggested these mechanisms to be electrically neutral, producing a 'forced exchange' of one ion for another with no net displacement of charge. In some systems at least, persuasive evidence to the contrary has been reported. That is, some carrier mechanisms are apparently not electrically neutral[39]. While such mechanisms have been frequently called 'electrogenic', this term is unfortunate and has led to considerable confusion and unnecessary debate. All electrical potentials in living systems that are displaced from equilibrium as the result of exergonic metabolic processes (e.g., all electrical potentials that are not a consequence of a simple Donnan equilibrium) are dependent upon steady-state ionic asymmetries. These, in turn depend upon active ion-transport processes. In this sense all active ion-transport processes are electrogenic despite the fact that they may be mechanistically electroneutral. They are responsible for the 'genesis' of trans-membrane electrical potential differences in biological systems. Without them these p.d.s would be dissipated. For this reason, the term 'rheogenic', proposed recently by Schwartz[30], seems more appropriate to distinguish 'current-generating' carrier mechanisms from electroneutral carrier mechanisms that bring about no net displacement of charge.

In deriving the constant-field equation (3.8), one assumes the sum of the currents due to ionic diffusion to be zero. This implicitly assumes that the sum of ionic currents resulting from carrier-mediated (or, more generally, non-diffusional) processes is zero, or that there are no rheogenic pumps.

Recently, attempts have been made to incorporate the effects of rheogenic pumps into expressions for the trans-membrane electrical potential difference and, thereby, to arrive at relations that may be more generally appropriate for biological systems.

The general approach is to introduce the net pump flows, $_pJ_i$, as ionic currents, $_pI_i = z_i \mathfrak{F} \, _pJ_i$, where the subscript p designates net flows of i due to a carrier (or pump) mechanism. Then one can impose the 'zero-current' or electroneutrality restriction which is generally applicable to epithelial tissues under all experimental conditions.

Let us focus on the movements of Na, K and Cl across the mucosal membrane into the epithelial cell illustrated in Figure 3.4. For simplicity's sake,

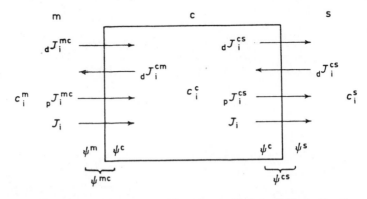

Figure 3.4 Schematic representation of an epithelial cell illustrating the bidirectional fluxes of a species i across the mucosal (m) and serosal (s) membranes. The symbols for the concentrations of i in the mucosal (m), intracellular (c), and serosal (s) compartments are also defined, as well as the electrical potential differences across the two limiting membranes.

we will assume that the unidirectional diffusion fluxes are given by equations (3.12) and (3.13). Later we will see that similar results are obtained using more general, though more complicated, approaches. We may then write a general equation describing the net flux of i resulting from combined diffusional flows (designated by the subscript d) and pump flows (designated by the subscript p).

$$_dJ_i^{mc} + \, _pJ_i^{mc} - \, _dJ_i^{cm} = J_i \tag{3.17}$$

where

$$_dJ_i^{mc} = P_i^m c_i^m \exp(z_i \mathfrak{F} \, \Delta\psi/2RT) \tag{3.18}$$

$$_dJ_i^{cm} = P_i^m c_i^c \exp(-z_i \mathfrak{F} \, \Delta\psi/2RT) \tag{3.19}$$

and $\Delta\psi = \psi_c - \psi_m$. We may now write expressions for J_{Na}, J_K and J_{Cl} in the form of equation (3.17) using equations (3.18) and (3.19). The electroneutrality restriction states that $J_{Na} + J_K - J_{Cl} = 0$. Solving the three equations for this condition, we obtain

$$\Delta\psi = \frac{RT}{\mathfrak{F}} \ln \left[\frac{(P_{Na}^m c_{Na}^c + P_K^m c_K^c + P_{Cl}^m c_{Cl}^m) - \xi^{\frac{1}{2}}(_pJ_{Na}^{mc} + \, _pJ_K^{mc} - \, _pJ_{Cl}^{mc})}{P_{Na}^m c_{Na}^m + P_K^m c_K^m + P_{Cl}^m c_{Cl}^c} \right] \tag{3.20}$$

where $\xi = \exp{(\mathfrak{F}\,\Delta\psi/RT)}$. One should note that the direction of the pump flow can be reversed by the relation ${}_pJ_i^{mc} = -{}_pJ_i^{cm}$.

Clearly, equation (3.20) reduces to the GHK equation (3.7) when the combined net pump flows are electrically neutral, i.e., ${}_pJ_{Na}^{mc} + {}_pJ_K^{mc} = {}_pJ_{Cl}^{mc}$.

More generally, it can be shown that

$$\Delta\psi = \frac{RT}{\mathfrak{F}}\ln\left[\frac{(\Sigma P_+^m c_+^c + \Sigma P_-^m c_-^m) - \xi^{\frac{1}{2}}(\Sigma_p J_+^{mc} - \Sigma_p J_-^{mc})}{\Sigma P_+^m c_+^m + \Sigma P_-^m c_-^c}\right] \quad (3.21)$$

where the subscripts $+$ and $-$ designate all univalent cations and anions, respectively. A similar expression, has been derived by Schwartz[30] which is not restricted to the constant-field condition but is applicable to a family of electrical potential profiles that are antisymmetric about the midpoint of the membrane. In addition, a generalisation of the Goldman equation for steady-state diffusion of univalent ions across a membrane with arbitrary potential profile and in the presence of rheogenic pumps has been derived by Jacquez[25]. These expressions all have one shortcoming, however. They cannot be solved explicitly for $\Delta\psi$ because $\Delta\psi$ appears on both sides of the equation. Still, this presents no serious obstacle to the experimenter, since $\Delta\psi$ is usually one of the measured parameters.

3.5 EQUIVALENT ELECTRICAL CIRCUIT OF EPITHELIAL TISSUES

Up to this point, we have been concerned primarily with ion fluxes and electrical potentials across single membranes or barriers. These considerations apply directly to artificial membranes as well as biological membranes that surround non-polar or symmetrical cells. The extension of these considerations to epithelial tissues is complicated by the polar or asymmetric properties of the cells that comprise these multicellular 'membranes'. Net *trans-cellular* ion movements involve movements across at least two limiting cell membranes arranged in series. Were it not for the differences in ion permeabilities and/or carrier mechanisms of these membranes, net movements in the absence of, or against, trans-epithelial gradients of electrochemical potential would be impossible. Furthermore, convincing evidence now exists that all epithelia possess extracellular routes or 'shunt pathways' for trans-epithelial ion movements. These routes parallel the trans-cellular route, and thereby circumvent the limiting cell membranes. The single common structural feature possessed by all of these epithelia is the series array formed by the junctional complexes, responsible for binding the individual cells together at their apical ends to form a multicellular sheet, and the underlying inter-cellular spaces. Currently, the histological evidence suggesting that the tight junctions and the lateral intercellular spaces are the anatomic counterparts of the trans-epithelial shunt pathway is compelling[40-42] and this author has little doubt that future data will corroborate this conclusion.

The relative roles played by the trans-cellular route and the shunt pathway with regard to ion movements and the accompanying bioelectric phenomena across gastrointestinal epithelia appear to cover a wide spectrum[43]. One extreme is exemplified by tissues such as the salivary gland ducts and frog stomach. These tissues are characterised by relatively large trans-epithelial p.d.s, high trans-epithelial resistances and low hydraulic conductivities; they are capable of sustaining large trans-epithelial ion gradients and the salivary gland ducts are characterised by hypertonic absorbates. These features strongly suggest that the shunt pathways in these tissues offer a high resistance to the trans-epithelial diffusion of ions and osmotic water flow. At the other extreme are tissues such as the gall bladder and small intestine that are characterised by low and often negligible trans-epithelial p.d.s, low trans-epithelial resistances and high hydraulic conductivities. These tissues cannot sustain large trans-epithelial ionic gradients and the absorbate is virtually isotonic with the luminal fluid. It has now been demonstrated conclusively that the shunt pathway across these tissues offers an extremely low resistance to ionic diffusion so that these epithelia are, to a large extent, 'self-short-circuited'.

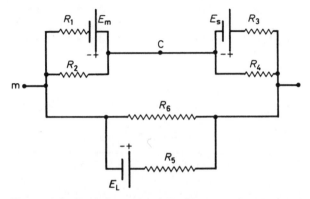

Figure 3.5 Equivalent electrical circuit applicable to all epithelia. Refer to text for details.

Thus, there are, in general, at least three sites at which electrical potential differences can originate in epithelial tissues: (a) the two limiting cell membranes which may display diffusion potentials as well as potentials secondary to rheogenic pumps; and (b) the shunt pathway which may give rise to diffusion potentials in the presence of trans-epithelial ionic assymmetries.

Consequently, the electrophysiology of epithelial tissues can be most easily analysed by examining the equivalent electrical circuit model illustrated in Figure 3.5[44]. In this model, E_m is an electromotive force or a 'battery' operating across the mucosal or apical membrane; R_1 is the internal resistance of this battery and R_2 is the shunt resistance across the membrane. E_s, R_3 and R_4, and E_L, R_5 and R_6 are the parameters for the serosal (basolateral) membranes and shunt pathway, respectively.

Before analysing this circuit, we should consider the relationship between the electrical analogues (i.e., batteries and resistances) and the electrodiffusional parameters (i.e., concentration gradients and permeabilities) with which we have been concerned up to this point. We will follow the general procedure outlined by Finkelstein and Mauro[28], using the constant-field assumption for purposes of simplification. Thus equation (3.1) may be written as

$$-J_i = \bar{c}_i \bar{u}_i z_i \mathfrak{F} \left[(RT/z_i \mathfrak{F})(\mathrm{d} \ln \bar{c}_i/\mathrm{d}x) + \Delta\bar{\psi}/\Delta x) \right]$$

or

$$I_i (\mathrm{d}x/\bar{c}_i \bar{u}_i z_i^2 \mathfrak{F}^2) = -[(RT/z_i \mathfrak{F}) \, \mathrm{d} \ln \bar{c}_i - (\Delta\bar{\psi}/\Delta x)]\mathrm{d}x \qquad (3.22)$$

Under steady-state conditions, I_i is independent of x so that we may integrate equation (3.22) and obtain

$$I_i \int_0^{\cdot i} (\mathrm{d}x/\bar{c}_i \bar{u}_i z_i^2 \mathfrak{F}^2) = -(RT/z_i\mathfrak{F}) \ln (\bar{c}_i^i/\bar{c}_i^o) - \Delta\bar{\psi} \qquad (3.23)$$

Although integration of the expression on the left-hand side of equation (3.23) requires assumptions regarding the concentration profile, it can be shown that this integral has the units of specific resistance (ohm cm^2) so that we may define the 'integral resistance' R_i of the membrane to i as

$$R_i = \int_0^{\cdot i} (\mathrm{d}x/\bar{c}_i \bar{u}_i z_i^2 \mathfrak{F}^2)$$

Furthermore, the first term on the right-hand side of equation (3.23) is simply the Nernst (equilibrium) potential of the ion, i, so that we may write

$$E_i = -(RT/z_i\mathfrak{F}) \ln (\bar{c}_i^i/\bar{c}_i^o)$$

Thus, equation (3.23) is simply a statement of Ohm's law

$$R_i I_i = (E_i - \Delta\bar{\psi})$$

where $(E_i - \Delta\bar{\psi})$, the difference between the equilibrium potential of i and the actual p.d., provides the net driving force for the current flow, I_i. Obviously when $E_i = \Delta\bar{\psi}$, $I_i = 0$. Clearly, the 'integral conductance' of the membrane to i is given by $G_i = 1/R_i$.

Thus, for every ion that is distributed asymmetrically across the membrane, one may insert an electrical analogue consisting of a battery and a resistance in series (Figure 3.6 (a)). Similarly, the effects of a rheogenic pump may be introduced by a current source and a resistance. Finally, the effects of per-meant ions distributed symmetrically across the membrane may be represen-ted by the parallel resistance (R_{sh}), since these ions do not serve as a source of e.m.f. but their flows through the membrane 'shunt' and reduce the effect of other batteries on the trans-membrane p.d. (Figure 3.6 (b)). Clearly, each element in the electrical circuit has an analogue in terms of the equations of electrodiffusion. Thus, we may lump these parallel elements together as shown in Figure 3.6 (c). The p.d. from o to i is simply $E_m R_m$ where $R_m = R_2/(R_1 + R_2)$. The value of $E_m R_m$, is given by the *appropriate* expression for the diffusion potential with or without rheogenic pumps (e.g., equations (3.8) or (3.21)). The paper by Finkelstein and Mauro[28] should be consulted for a detailed and general treatment of the relation between ionic systems and equivalent electrical circuits.

The equivalent circuit illustrated in Figure 3.5 may be readily solved for ψ^{mc} and ψ^{ms} under zero-current conditions (i.e., when there is no net current flow from m to s)[44]. Thus,

$$\psi^{mc} = [E_m R_m (R_3 R_s + R_5 R_L) - (E_s R_s - E_L R_L) R_1 R_m]/R_t \quad (3.24)$$

and

$$\psi^{ms} = [(E_m R_m + E_s R_s) R_5 R_L/R_t] + [E_L R_L (R_1 R_m + R_3 R_s)/R_t] \quad (3.25)$$

where $\psi^{ms} = \psi^s - \psi^m$; $\psi^{mc} = \psi^c - \psi^m$; $R_m = R_2/(R_1 + R_2)$; $R_s = R_4/(R_3 + R_4)$; $R_L = R_6/(R_5 + R_6)$ and $R_t = R_1 R_m + R_3 R_s + R_5 R_L$.

We should stress that this solution takes into account the orientations of the batteries illustrated in Figure 3.5, so that the E's in equations (3.24) and (3.25) represent absolute values. One may reverse the polarity of any battery simply by changing the sign preceding that E in equations (3.24) and (3.25).

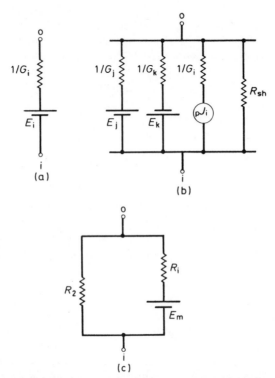

Figure 3.6 Electrical analogues of concentration gradients, ionic permeabilities and rheogenic pumps that permit the analysis of electrophysiological phenomena in terms of equivalent electrical circuits.

The role of the shunt pathway in influencing the electrophysiologic properties of epithelial tissues can be easily appreciated if we consider the two extreme conditions exemplified first, by a very high shunt resistance, so that

$$R_5 R_L >> (R_1 R_m + R_3 R_s) \text{ and } R_5 R_L \cong R_t \quad (3.26)$$

and second, by a very low shunt resistance, so that

$$R_5 R_L << (R_1 R_m + R_3 R_s) \text{ and } (R_5 R_L/R_t) \cong 0 \quad (3.27)$$

For the high-resistance tissues defined by equations (3.26), equation (3.25) reduces to

$$\psi^{ms} \cong E_m R_m + E_s R_s \tag{3.28}$$

and equation (3.24) reduces to

$$\psi^{mc} \cong E_m R_m \tag{3.29}$$

Thus, the trans-epithelial p.d. is simply the algebraic sum of the e.m.f.s across the two limiting membranes. The intracellular p.d. determined with microelectrodes is simply the p.d. resulting from the e.m.f. across the punctured membrane. A change in ψ^{mc} can result only from a change in $E_m R_m$ so that changes in ψ^{mc} in response to changes in the ionic composition of the mucosal solution may provide information regarding the permselective properties of the mucosal membrane[45].

In contrast, for the extremely low resistance tissues defined by equations (3.27)

$$\psi^{mc} \cong [E_m R_m R_3 R_s - (E_s R_s - E_L R_L) R_1 R_m]/R_t \tag{3.30}$$

and

$$\psi^{ms} \cong E_L R_L \tag{3.31}$$

Thus, in the presence of a very high shunt conductance (compared with the conductance of the trans-cellular pathway), ψ^{mc} is a function of all three e.m.f.'s and is not a direct measure of $E_m R_m$. Moreover, the low resistance parallel shunt markedly attenuates (and, in the extreme, abolishes) the contribution of $E_m R_m$ and $E_s R_s$ to the trans-epithelial p.d. (ψ^{ms}) so that the latter simply measures diffusion potentials in the extracellular pathway and provides no information regarding the e.m.f.s across the limiting membranes of the trans-cellular pathway. When such an epithelial tissue is bathed on both surfaces by solutions having identical ionic compositions, $E_L R_L = 0$ and $\psi_{ms} \cong 0$! The latter situation is most closely approached by the gall bladder[43,46], where it is estimated that close to 96% of the total tissue conductance is attributable to the shunt pathway, so that $(R_s R_L/R_t) = 0.04$. Under these conditions $(E_m R_m + E_s R_s)$ may be enormous but simply will not be reflected in ψ^{ms}. The implications of equations (3.24) and (3.25) with respect to the interpretation of electrophysiologic data on tissues with low or intermediate resistance shunt pathways are distressing. The value of the microelectrode, one of the most powerful tools of the electrophysiologist, is severely compromised by the fact that intracellular p.d.s are the *composite results* of the e.m.f.s originating at the two limiting membranes and the shunt pathway. Thus, the effect of a change in the composition of the mucosal solution alone on ψ^{mc} may reflect changes in $E_L R_L$ and $E_s R_s$, as well as $E_m R_m$. If the compositions of the mucosal and serosal solutions are changed simultaneously in an identical fashion, the change in ψ^{mc} may reflect a change in $E_s R_s$ as well as $E_m R_m$. Under these conditions $E_L R_L = 0$. Furthermore, if the change in intracellular p.d. is elicited under conditions in which the compositions of both bathing solutions are constant and identical (e.g., by the addition of actively transported sugars or amino acids to the mucosal solution of short-circuited rabbit ileum[44] or by neural stimulation of salivary acinar cells[47]) the mechanism responsible for the change in trans-membrane p.d. cannot be unequivocally localised to the punctured membrane.

Information that may assist in localising the mechanism responsible for a change in intracellular p.d. in a tissue characterised by low or intermediate resistance shunt pathways can be obtained by simultaneous measurements of the intracellular p.d. (say, ψ^{mc}) and the trans-epithelial p.d. (ψ^{ms}). Then three criteria can be deduced[44].

First, if the change in ψ^{mc} is due to a change in E_mR_m *alone*

$$\Delta\psi^{ms}/\Delta\psi^{mc} = 1/[1 + (R_3R_s/R_5R_L)] \tag{3.32}$$

so that $\Delta\psi^{ms} < \Delta\psi^{mc}$ whenever $R_5R_L < \infty$. Clearly, $\Delta\psi^{ms} \cong \Delta\psi^{mc}$ when $R_5R_L >> R_3R_s$.

Second, if the change in ψ^{mc} is due to a change in E_sR_s *alone* (e.g., activation of a rheogenic pump)

$$\Delta\psi^{ms}/\Delta\psi^{mc} = -(R_5R_L/R_1R_m) \tag{3.33}$$

so that, in response to an increase in E_sR_s (more positive), ψ^{ms} will become more positive, but ψ^{mc} will become more negative, and vice versa.

Third, if the change in ψ^{mc} is due to a change in E_LR_L *alone* (i.e., the establishment of a diffusion potential)

$$\Delta\psi^{ms}/\Delta\psi^{mc} = 1 + (R_3R_s/R_1R_m) \tag{3.34}$$

so that the effect on ψ^{ms} will be greater than the effect on ψ^{mc} and in the same direction.

These criteria permit one to exclude certain possibilities, and in some instances, to infer others. However, if more than one e.m.f. is changed by a given procedure, the interpretation of a change in intracellular p.d. is fraught with uncertainties.

Finally, the presence of high conductance shunt pathways not only confounds the interpretation of changes in trans-epithelial and intracellular p.d.s, but also severely complicates the analysis of the resting or steady-state trans-epithelial electrical potential profile[45]. When one drives a microelectrode from the outer or mucosal solution through the cell into the serosal or inner solution, the resulting electrical potential profile either resembles that illustrated by Figure 3.7(a) or that illustrated by Figure 3.7(b). High-resistance tissues such as isolated frog skin[48], toad urinary bladder[49], toad skin[50] and the frog gastric parietal cell[51] display a profile that conforms to Figure 3.7(a), where the trans-epithelial p.d. is the sum of two or more potential steps in the *same* direction. In all instances, the cell interior is electrically positive with respect to the luminal or outer solution. In contrast, low-resistance tissues, such as the small intestine[45,52] and proximal renal tubule[53], display a profile that conforms to Figure 3.7(b), where the transepithelial p.d. is the difference between two potential steps in *opposite* directions. In all instances, the cell interior is electrically negative with respect to the luminal solution. As shown by equation (3.30), for the case of a low-resistance tissue bathed on both surfaces with identical solutions, the p.d. across the luminal membrane is a function of both E_mR_m and E_sR_s so that neither its magnitude nor its orientation need directly reflect E_mR_m alone. Indeed, it can be shown[45] that even if E_mR_m is orientated with the cell interior positive as shown in Figure 3.5

$$\psi^{mc} > 0 \text{ when } E_s R_s < [(R_3 R_s + R_5 R_L)/R_1 R_m] E_m R_m \qquad (3.35)$$

whereas

$$\psi^{mc} < 0 \text{ when } E_s R_s > [(R_3 R_s + R_5 R_L)/R_1 R_m] E_m R_m \qquad (3.36)$$

Thus, when $R_5 R_L = \infty$, ψ^{mc} will always be positive and will have the same orientation as the $E_m R_m$ shown in Figure 3.5. However, if $R_5 R_L$ is sufficiently low, ψ^{mc} may have a polarity opposite that of $E_m R_m$. Thus, the fact that the cell interior is negative in a variety of low-resistance epithelia does not

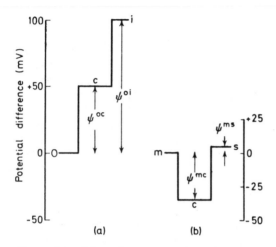

Figure 3.7 Schematic representation of electrical potential profiles across some high-resistance epithelia (a) and low-resistance epithelia (b). (From Schultz[45] by courtesy of the Rockefeller University Press.)

necessarily mean that the e.m.f. across the mucosal membrane is also orientated in the interior-negative direction. Clearly, inferences regarding the relative ionic permeabilities, etc. of the mucosal (and basolateral) membranes of low-resistance epithelia cannot be safely based on measurements of the electrical potential profile.

These considerations point to the necessity of characterising epithelial tissues with respect to the relative conductances of their transcellular and extracellular pathways before the results of electrophysiological studies can be interpreted definitely. Failure to take into account the profound influences of the shunt pathway may result in qualitative as well as quantitative errors.

3.6 THE ELECTROPHYSIOLOGY OF THE GASTRIC MUCOSA[54,55]

Although the existance of an electrical potential difference across the gastric mucosa was first recognised by Donné in 1834, only within the past two decades has the relation between this p.d. and HCl secretion become the subject of intensive investigation. Much of our current information derives from *in vitro* studies on frog gastric mucosa, using the short-circuit apparatus described in Figure 3.2. When isolated frog gastric mucosa is mounted in this 'Ussing chamber', the mucosal (secretory) solution is approximately 30 mV negative with respect to the serosal (nutrient) solution. The external current necessary to reduce this spontaneous p.d. to zero (that is, the short-circuit current) is approximately $80\mu A\ cm^{-2}$, so that the trans-epithelial resistance is approximately 350 ohm cm^2. In 1951, Hogben[56] demonstrated conclusively that under short-circuit conditions both Cl and H are actively transported from the serosal to mucosal solutions and that the short-circuit current (I_{sc}) is equivalent to $J_{Cl} - J_H$. Thus, the trans-mural p.d. is a consequence of the fact that active Cl transport into the mucosal solution exceeds that of active H secretion. The I_{sc} is simply the difference between these two ionic currents. Under short-circuit conditions, net trans-epithelial movements of Na and K across the frog gastric mucosa are negligible. Moreover, the bidirectional fluxes of Na and K across short-circuit frog gastric mucosa are very small, suggesting that extracellular shunt pathways probably do not contribute significantly to trans-epithelial ion movements. Indeed, the studies of Hogben suggest that the entire tissue conductance can be attributed to ion movements (primarily Cl and H) through the trans-cellular route.

Subsequently, two sets of observations have complicated what originally seemed to be a relatively clear picture. The resulting controversies still remain unsettled.

First, it was demonstrated that in the resting stomach, the I_{sc} is completely accounted for by J_{Cl}. However, when acid secretion is then stimulated by histamine, both J_H and J_{Cl} increase in a one-for-one manner, so that the I_{sc} is still entirely due to the basal (resting) active Cl secretion and is unrelated to the rate of acid secretion. Similarly, inhibition of active HCl secretion by thiocyanate does not affect the basal rate of active Cl secretion or I_{sc}[57,58].

Second, Heinz and Durbin[59] demonstrated that active H secretion can proceed in the absence of Cl. When Cl in the bathing solutions is replaced with sulphate, the orientation of the trans-epithelial p.d. is reversed. The mucosal solution becomes approximately 8 mV positive with respect to the serosal solution and the I_{sc} is now completely due to the rate of active H secretion. Thus, the mechanism responsible for active H secretion can function in the absence of a transportable anion and under these conditions appears to be rheogenic.

Therefore, the active Cl secretory process is apparently rheogenic and independent of H secretion, and the active-secretory process is apparently rheogenic and independent of concomitant Cl secretion. Yet, under physiological conditions, the stimulation of H secretion is accompanied by an equivalent increase in Cl secretion, so that active H secretion and active Cl secretion must be somehow coupled.

On the basis of these observations, the total active Cl secretion by the gastric mucosa may be divided into a 'non-acidic' rheogenic component J_{Cl} and a component that accompanies acid secretion J_{HCl} which does not contribute to the I_{sc}. Three questions arise from these observations. First, if the active H secretory process can function independently of Cl, why is H secretion under physiological conditions always accompanied by an equivalent secretion of Cl? Second, is the active Cl secretory mechanism that operates in the absence of H secretion also responsible for the increment in active Cl secretion which accompanies active H secretion after stimulation with agents such as histamine? Third, are there two independent active transport mechanisms, one that accounts for the rheogenic 'non-acidic' J_{Cl} and another that causes a chemically-coupled secretion of HCl via a ternary complex (H and Cl combining with a common carrier) but which can be uncoupled in the absence of Cl and pump H alone? These questions are incompletely resolved to date.

One can better appreciate the alternative proposals to resolve this problem by referring to the mucosal membrane schematised in Figure 3.8. Good evidence exists that the mucosal membrane of amphibian gastric mucosa is

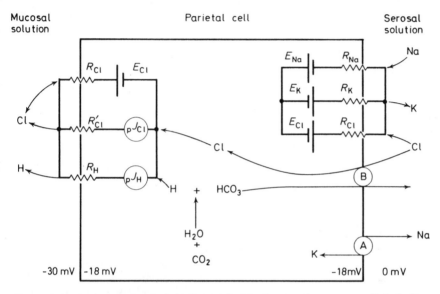

Figure 3.8 Equivalent electrical circuit model of the frog gastric secretory cell, including the apparent electrical potential profile.

virtually impermeable to Na and K inasmuch as varying the concentrations of these ions in the mucosal solution has no effect on the trans-epithelial p.d.[55]. On the other hand, the mucosal membrane does appear to be permeable to Cl[55]. Thus, an *independent* rheogenic H pump at the mucosal membrane, $_pJ_H$, could generate an electromotive force across the membrane that would have to drive Cl across the mucosal membrane through the Cl 'leak' pathway, causing HCl secretion. In other words, this mechanism rests on the need to maintain electroneutrality and the fact that the mucosal membrane is virtually impermeable to all ions except Cl[55]. The main shortcoming of this mechanism is that the onset of acid secretion has frequently been shown to have little or no effect on the trans-epithelial p.d. or resistance[54]. Thus if an independent rheogenic H pump were to draw Cl through a passive leak pathway, the permeability of this pathway to Cl would have to be exceedingly large to permit tight coupling without a change in trans-epithelial p.d.

An alternative proposal, strongly supported by the equivalent electrical circuit analyses of Rehm and his collaborators[61-64], is that the active Cl secretory mechanism that operates rheogenically in the absence of H secretion is accelerated by the activation of the rheogenic H secretory mechanism via a current-loop process. Our principal objection to the Rehm model is that it is based entirely on an analysis of electrical circuits. Although the approach is sound for passive ion movements driven by forces that can be translated into electrical analogues, there is no evidence that a like approach can be applied to carrier processes, which probably involve the binding of a transported ion to a membrane component followed by a translocation process (the mechanism of which is entirely unknown). Thus, although the Rehm position is electrically feasible, its translation into biochemical mechanisms poses difficult problems.

Finally, the possibility that the mucosal membrane possesses a rheogenic Cl secretory process and an independent carrier mechanism capable of transporting HCl or H alone is exceedingly attractive. Certainly it is compatible with all available data on frog gastric mucosa. A carrier model possessing these characteristics has been proposed by Forte[55] (Figure 3.9) The model, involves the formation of a ternary carrier-H—Cl complex, and resembles the model proposed by Curran et al.[65] for the coupling between amino acid and Na transport across the brush border of rabbit ileum. Clearly, in the absence of Cl this mechanism is capable of effecting the rheogenic secretion of H. If the affinity of XH for Cl is high, the presence of Cl could result in a tight coupling between H secretion and Cl secretion in the form of a neutral complex that would affect neither trans-epithelial p.d. nor I_{sc}. In short, this model is capable of accounting for a tight coupling between H and Cl secretion, the fact that exchange diffusion of Cl across the mucosal membrane depends upon H secretion, the possibility of H secretion in the absence of Cl, and the fact that certain inhibitors (e.g. SCN) inhibit HCl secretion without affecting the 'non-acidic' component of Cl secretion[55]. In addition, this model is formulated in biochemical rather than electrical analogues, thereby circumventing some of the problems discussed above.

The foregoing discussion should make it clear that, although many experimental observations on frog gastric mucosa have been repeatedly confirmed, the interpretation of these observations in terms of underlying mechanisms of H and Cl secretion remains in dispute.

The properties of the serosal (nutrient) membrane of frog gastric mucosa are also schematised in Figure 3.8. In brief, this membrane seems to possess an active Na–K exchange mechanism resembling that observed in a wide variety of animal tissues. This causes extrusion of Na from the cell and the active accumulation of K by the cell[55]. In addition, evidence has been presented for the presence of a neutral $Cl-HCO_3$ exchange mechanism (B) that results in the uptake of Cl by the cell and the extrusion of HCO_3 into the plasma[66]. Finally, the serosal membrane appears to be permeable to K, Cl and Na[60, 64].

Studies of diffusion potentials indicate that the permeability to K and Cl is much greater than that to Na. Thus, the electrical potential difference across the serosal membranes would appear to be dominated by the trans-membrane gradients of K and Cl[60]. On the other hand, micropuncture studies of frog gastric mucosa parietal cells by Villiegas[51] indicate that the cell interior is electrically negative with respect to the serosal solution by only 18 mV. A much greater value would be expected if the p.d. were determined primarily by K and Cl. This suggests that the microelectrode studies may be incorrect that the estimated intracellular ion concentrations are wrong, or that the permeability to Na has been significantly underestimated. Recently, Blum et al.[67] have reported that the p.d. across the serosal membrane of *Necturus* gastric mucosa is approximately 45 mV, cell interior negative. These values

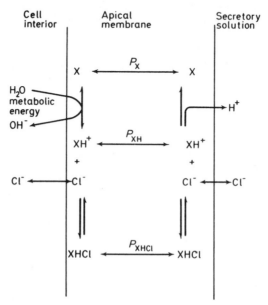

Figure 3.9 Carrier model proposed by Forte[55] to permit tight coupling between H and Cl secretion by the gastric mucosa. (Reproduced by courtesy of Wiley-Interscience)

are closer to those expected for a membrane that behaves as a KCl electrode, but they are still much smaller than expected. Clearly, the problem of the passive ionic permeabilities and electrical potential difference across the serosal membranes is still unresolved, and further study of these properties is needed. The observation by Villiegas[51] that the mucosal solution is electrically negative with respect to the cell interior is obviously consistent with the operation of a rheogenic Cl pump at the mucosal membrane whose activity exceeds that of the rheogenic H pump.

Until now, we have focused attention entirely on the properties of amphibian gastric mucosa. More recent studies on mammalian gastric mucosa indicate many similarities with respect to H and Cl secretion, but there is a distinct difference with respect to Na transport. Thus, for isolated gastric mucosa of rat, cat, dog and monkey, complete removal of Na from the mucosal solution abolishes or markedly reduces the trans-epithelial p.d. In contrast to amphibian stomach, these preparations bring about a significant active Na transport from mucosa to serosa. Two mechanism have been proposed to account for this phenomenon. The first is a forced Na–H exchange at the mucosal membrane followed by active Na extrusion across the serosal membrane: however, evidence against this possibility has been presented. The second is that the mucosal membrane of mammalian stomach has a much greater passive permeability to Na than that of the amphibian stomach. Thus, Na could enter the cell across the mucosal membrane down an electrochemical potential gradient and subsequently be extruded by the active Na–K exchange pump at the serosal membrane. This matter is still controversial, however. The reader is referred to the reviews by Durbin and Forte for a more detailed discussion[54, 55].

Finally, we should point out that almost all attempts at a mechanistic interpretation of ion transport by the gastric mucosa have focused attention on the parietal (oxyntic) cell which is clearly responsible for HCl secretion, but which accounts for less than 10% of the total cell population of the gastric mucosa. Quite possibly, the 'non-acidic' active Cl secretion, as well as the active Na absorption that is a prominant feature of *in vitro* mammalian gastric mucosa, are carried out by other cell types. Thus attempts to generate models linking all of these processes within the parietal cell may be groundless. The difficulties of mechanistic modelling of the transport processes of an epithelial tissue consisting of several cell types most certainly present a formidable challenge to the investigator.

3.7 THE ELECTROPHYSIOLOGY OF SMALL INTESTINAL EPITHELIUM[68, 69]

In the absence of activity transported sugars or amino acids, *in vitro* preparations of mammalian small intestine are characterised by small trans-epithelial p.d.s, ranging between 3–6 mV, with the serosal solution electrically positive with respect to the mucosal solution[68]. Studies on short-circuit preparations, using either the modification of the Ussing chamber described by Schultz and Zalusky[70] or the apparatus described by Clarkson and Toole[71], indicate that the tissues behave like an ohmic resistor. The trans-epithelial resistance ranges between approximately 100 ohm cm^2 for unstripped rabbit and rat ileum and approximately 40 ohm cm^2 for stripped preparations of rabbit ileum[72] and unstripped rat jejunum[43]. It is now abundantly clear that these extremely low trans-epithelial resistances do not result from unusually leaky or expansive cell membranes, but rather, from the presence of high-conductance (low-resistance) extracellular shunt pathways whose anatomic counterparts appear to be the 'tight junctions' and lateral intercellular spaces[43]. The properties of this shunt pathway and its consequences will be outlined below.

Since the relation between the I_{sc} and net trans-epithelial ion movements under short-circuit conditions has been most extensively investigated in rabbit and rat ileum, our discussion will be limited to these preparations. In unstripped preparations of rabbit[70] and rat ileum[71, 73], the I_{sc} appears to be almost entirely attributable to active Na transport from mucosa to serosa. Under these conditions, no significant net transepithelial Cl transport occurs and the bidirection fluxes of Cl appear to conform to the Ussing flux-ratio equation (3.2) for an ion whose movements are entirely attributable to strict ionic diffusion[73, 74]. Similar findings have been reported for human ileum *in vitro*[75]. On the other hand, when the muscle layers of rabbit ileum are removed as described by Field *et al.*[72] and a low concentration of glucose is included in the bathing medium (1–5 mM), although most of the I_{sc} can still be attributed to active Na transport from mucosa to serosa, there is a small but significant component of active Cl absorption and a residual current probably caused by HCO_3 secretion. Stripping the ileum of its underlying serosal tissues and muscle layers has been shown to provide better oxygenation of the epithelial layer. This preparation may more closely mimic the behaviour of mammalian ileum *in vitro*, in which active Cl absorption and HCO_3 secretion are well established[76-79]. Thus, the I_{sc} across an 'optimal' preparation of rabbit ileum would seem to consist of the algebraic sum of ionic currents due to active Na and Cl absorption and active HCO_3 secretion. Trans-epithelial K movements seem entirely due to simple passive ionic diffusion and largely, if not entirely restricted to the high conductance shunt pathway.

The present picture with respect to the cellular mechanisms involved in active Na and Cl absorption and active HCO_3 secretion may be analysed with reference to Figure 3.10. Recent studies on rabbit ileum have shown that at

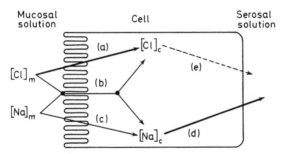

Figure 3.10 Schematic illustration of pathways of Na and Cl movements across the absorptive epithelium of rabbit ileum

least three pathways are responsible for the influx of Na and Cl into the epithelial cells from the mucosal solution in the absence of sugars or amino acids. One pathway (b) is shared by both Na and Cl[80].

Let us first focus attention on pathways (b) and (c). The intracellular concentration of Na in mucosal strips of rabbit ileum is approximately 40–50 mM[81]. Recent studies by Lee and Armstrong[82] indicate that the thermodynamic activity coefficient of intracellular Na in bullfrog small intestine is approximately 0.5. This is consistent with values in studies on other tissues, which indicate that the thermodynamic activity of intracellular Na is significantly lower than its bulk concentration. Measurements of the electrical potential profile across rabbit ileal cells indicate that the cell interior is, on the average, 36 mV negative with respect to the mucosal solution[44]. Thus, Na entry into the cell from the mucosal solution, though to a large degree carrier-mediated[83], is directed down its electrochemical potential gradient and must be considered a passive movement. The finding that Na influx is unaffected by metabolic inhibitors or ouabain corroborates this[84]. Extrusion of Na from the cell into the serosal solution (d) appears to be mediated by the Na–K-activated, ouabain-sensitive ATPase that has been localised largely, if not exclusively, in the basolateral membranes of the absorptive cells[85]. This localisation is entirely consistent with the finding that the presence of ouabain in the serosal solution alone abolishes active Na absorption whereas the presence of ouabain in the mucosal solution alone is ineffective[70]. Thus, as in many other epithelia, Na entry into the cell appears to be a passive process whereas extrusion from the cell into the serosal solution is an active process dependent upon a supply of metabolic energy and mediated by a Na–K-activated ATPase.

In contrast with Na, the intracellular Cl concentration of mucosal strips of rabbit ileum is approximately 55 mM[86]. This, together with the intracellular p.d. of -36 mV, suggests that the electrochemical activity of intracellular Cl exceeds that of the mucosal solution. Thus, entry of Cl into the cell from the lumen is an active transport process. Although the interpretation of intracellular concentrations is clouded with many uncertainties, including the fact that the epithelium consists of at least five cell types, this concept is supported by the finding that Cl influx across the mucosal membrane is a saturable, carrier-mediated process that is competitively inhibited by other halide anions and is markedly inhibited by metabolic inhibitors. The current overall picture is that entry of Cl into the cell from the lumen is an active transport process resulting in an intracellular electrochemical potential for Cl which exceeds that in the mucosal and serosal solutions[86]. Although the mechanism by which Cl leaves the cell across the basolateral membranes is not established simple diffusion down an electrochemical potential gradient might suffice. At present a more complex mechanism probably need not be invoked.

About 25% of the total Na and Cl influxes across the brush border of rabbit ileum are mediated by a neutral coupled NaCl influx process that is not dependent upon metabolic energy but is completely inhibited by theophylline or an elevation of intracellular cyclic-AMP concentration[80]. The significance of the remaining Cl influx via route (a) is as yet unclear. It is a saturable function of the Cl concentration in the mucosal solution, is diminished in the presence of metabolic inhibitors and may be involved in an exchange for intracellular HCO_3. Although the last point has not been established for *in vitro* preparations, *in vivo* studies on rat[76] and human ileum[87] have provided strong evidence for a $Cl–HCO_3$ exchange process. It seems likely that the HCO_3 is formed within the cell as suggested by the findings of Carlinsky and Lew for isolated colonic mucosa of *Bufo arenarum*[88]. The fate of the resulting H^+ ion is not established. It may exit from the cell across the basolateral membranes or engage in an exchange process with Na at the mucosal membrane as postulated by Turnberg *et al.*[87]. Finally, it should be stressed that although route (b) has been directly implicated in trans-epithelial Na and Cl transport, much if not all of the Na influx via route (c) and the Cl influx via route (a) may enter cells or compartments that are not involved in the trans-epithelial movements of these ions. Indeed, the principal influx pathway for Na and Cl absorption may be the coupled pathway (b) which could also bring about a Cl–HCO$_3$ exhange as well as possibly a Na–H exchange. The roles of pathways (a) and (c) in trans-epithelial Na and Cl transport remain to be defined explicitly. (See Note added in proof.)

Active Na absorption by *in vivo* as well as *in vitro* preparations of small intestine from a variety of animal species is markedly enhanced by the presence of actively transported sugars or amino acids in the mucosal solution[89]. Studies on *in vitro* preparations of rabbit ileum, rat jejunum and goldfish small intestine clearly indicate that the presence of actively transported sugars or amino acids in the mucosal solution enhances Na influx into the cell across the brush border. This probably occurs through the formation of a ternary complex involving a membrane component (carrier), Na and the

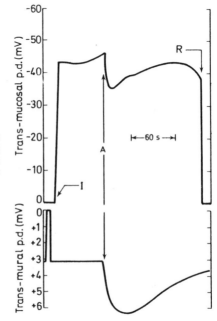

Figure 3.11 Effects of alanine on the trans-mucosal (ψ^{mc}) and transmural (ψ^{ms}) electrical potential differences in rabbit ileum. (From Rose and Schultz[44] by courtesy of the Rockefeller University Press.)

organic solute. The kinetics of these coupled processes have been recently described in detail[89]. Na efflux out of the cell is apparently associated with the same Na–K active transport mechanism that operates in the absence of actively transported sugars or amino acids. The overall process is associated with an increase in the trans-epithelial p.d. and I_{sc} that appears to be due to the increased active flow of Na from mucosal to serosa.

Studies on the effect of actively transported sugars or amino acids on the electrical potential profile across isolated rabbit ileum have helped elucidate the electrophysiology of this low-resistance tissue as well as the mechanism responsible for the extrusion of Na out of the cell into the serosal solution[44]. As shown in Figure 3.11, the cell interior is approximately 35–40 mV negative with respect to the mucosal solution, and the serosal solution is approximately 3 mV positive with respect to the mucosal solution. The addition of alanine (A) to the mucosal solution results in an immediate depolarisation of the mucosal membrane of approximately 10 mV and a simultaneous increase in the trans-epithelial p.d. of only 3 mV. Thus $\Delta\psi^{ms}/\Delta\psi^{mc}$ is less than unity; for rabbit ileum it averages 0.3–0.4. Similar findings have been reported by White and Armstrong[52] for bullfrog small intestine. As discussed above, this can only result from the presence of a shunt pathway across the tissue that attenuates the effect of a change in $E_m R_m$ on ψ^{ms}. In the absence of a shunt, $\Delta\psi^{ms} = E_m R_m + E_s R_s$ and $\psi^{mc} = E_m R_m$, so that, all other factors remaining constant, any change in $\Delta\psi^{mc}$ resulting from a change in $E_m R_m$ *alone* must be reflected in an identical change in ψ^{ms}. That is, in the absence of a shunt, $\Delta\psi^{ms}/\Delta\psi^{mc}$ must be unity. Thus, the observations of Rose and Schultz[44] and White and Armstrong[52] strongly suggest, first, that the coupled influx of Na with sugars or amino acids across the brush border is rheogenic and, second,

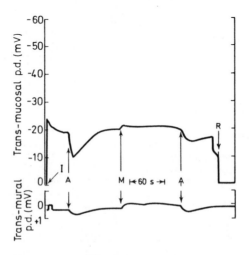

Figure 3.12 Effects of alanine on the trans-mucosal (ψ^{mc}) and transmural (ψ^{ms}) electrical potential differences across rabbit ileum poisoned with metabolic inhibitors and/or ouabain. (From Rose and Schultz[44] by courtesy of the Rockefeller University Press.)

that a low-resistance shunt pathway must be present across the tissue that attenuates the effect of $\Delta\psi^{mc}$ on $\Delta\psi^{ms}$.

These conclusions were further corroborated and extended by studies on the effect of amino acids or sugars on simultaneously recorded $\Delta\psi^{mc}$ and $\Delta\psi^{ms}$ in the presence of ouabain and/or metabolic inhibitors[44]. As shown in Figure 3.12, the addition of alanine (A) to the mucosal solution still results in a sizeable depolarisation of the p.d. across the brush border but only a minimal increase in ψ^{ms}. These results suggest that the coupled entry of Na and sugars or amino acids across the brush border is rheogenic but that the resulting $\Delta\psi^{ms}$ is markedly attenuated by the low-resistance shunt across this tissue. They also suggest that an additional process, dependent upon metabolic energy and inhibited by ouabain, is responsible for the major component of the increase in ψ^{ms} in response to sugars or amino acids. It seems reasonable that the latter represents the active Na extrusion mechanism. This implies that the Na–K exchange process is not electrically neutral. Indeed, the extrusion of three Na ions in exchange for the active uptake of two K ions (a stoichiometry suggested for this coupled Na–K pump in erythrocytes and muscle) would satisfy these findings[93]. However, further study is needed to clarify this issue definitively.

3.7.1 The shunt pathway across rabbit ileum

Trans-epithelial shunt pathways of extremely low resistance are clearly possessed by at least two gastrointestinal organs, the gall bladder and small intestine. Fromter[46] has convincingly shown that at least 96% of the total tissue conductance across *Necturus* gall bladder is attributable to this shunt pathway. The presence of a very high conductance shunt is implied in the findings of Barry et al.[90] on rabbit gall bladder but precise estimates of its total ionic conductance are unavailable. Nonetheless, it seems safe to guess that at least 90% of the total tissue conductance is due to this pathway across rabbit gall bladder.

Recent studies by Frizzell and Schultz[83] indicate that the shunt pathway across rabbit ileum (unstripped) accounts for at least 85–90% of the total tissue conductance, so that the main route for trans-epithelial ionic diffusion is not trans-cellular but extracellular. Clearly, under short-circuit conditions and in the absence of significant solvent drag, ionic movements through the shunt would not result in a net trans-mural flux. Instead, large bidirectional ionic fluxes through the shunt, equal in both directions, would be superimposed upon relatively small ionic movements through the trans-cellular route. This seriously complicates the experimental determination of net ionic movements under short-circuit conditions, inasmuch as these now represent small differnces between large numbers. Moreover, in the presence of a high conductance shunt, relatively large net movements of ions through this pathway can be driven by small and often-overlooked driving forces such as a trans-mural p.d. or solvent drag. Thus, the common practice of ignoring the trans-mural p.d. in studies of ion movements across small intestine because it is generally small (i.e., 3–5 mV) is, at best, hazardous. For example, one can readily show that when the serosal solution is only 5 mV positive with respect to the mucosal solution, the diffusional backflux of Na through the shunt from mucosa to serosa represents approximately 30% of the active transport of Na from serosa to mucosa via the trans-cellular route. Under conditions in which the serosal solution is 12 or more mV positive with respect to the mucosal solution, net Na absorption may be completely masked or even reversed, simply due to Na diffusion through the shunt.

Studies on the absolute ionic permeabilities of Na, K and Cl through the extracellular pathway across isolated rabbit ileum indicate that this shunt is cation-selective and that the value for P_{Cl}/P_{Na} is 2.5 times lower than that which one would expect on the basis of their free-solution mobilities[83]. A similar cation selectivity appears to characterise the shunt pathway across rabbit gall bladder[90] and the proximal renal tubule of rat[91] and dog[92]. Moreover, it is implied by studies of diffusion potentials across normal human ileum[87]. The precise biochemical basis for this selectivity remains to be unequivocally established.

Elucidation of the permeabilities of the shunt pathway across rabbit ileum have clarified three important problems with respect to ion transport and the electrophysiological properties of this preparation.

First, the unidirectional flux of Na from serosa to mucosa (J_{Na}^{sm}) appears to be attributable to diffusion through the extracellular route. No significant trans-cellular route for this back flux is discernible. Since Na is apparently exchanged rapidly across the brush border (i.e. $J_{Na}^{cm} \neq 0$), this can mean only that the basolateral membranes are virtually impermeable to Na and that the active Na extrusion mechanism is rectified.

Second, unpublished data (kindly provided by Dr. Michael Field and Mr. Robert Schooley) suggest that the bidirectional fluxes of K across short-circuited rabbit ileum are probably restricted to the shunt pathway. That is, little or no trans-cellular component of transmural K movements is apparent. This strongly suggests that the mucosal membrane is at most only minimally permeable to K.

Finally, as predicted by equation (3.31), in the presence of a high-conductance shunt, diffusion potentials across the tissue will be determined primarily if not exclusively by the permselective properties of the shunt pathway. (The extreme case is exemplified by rabbit gall bladder.) Thus, little or no information is provided regarding the permeabilities of the limiting cell membranes. This prediction has been experimentally verified by Frizzell and Schultz[83]. Thus, previous efforts at inferring the permselective properties of the mucosal and basolateral membranes of small intestinal epithelia from trans-epithelial diffusion potentials must be considered invalid. Needless to say, this complicating feature of a high-conductance shunt places the analysis of the permselective properties of the limiting cell membranes beyond the realm of the classical electrophysiological approach. For the moment, one is forced to rely upon inferences drawn from studies of ion fluxes.

This discussion will be concluded with a speculative picture of the electrophysiological properties of the limiting membranes of the rabbit ileal absorptive cell, based on inferences drawn from a variety of studies. The purpose here is to present a working hypothesis rather than an 'established' fact in the hope that it will stimulate investigation. Validation or dismissal of this hypothesis will present a formidable experimental challenge. The bases of this 'picture' (Figure 3.13) are the inferences alluded to above. First, Na contributes to the conductance of the mucosal membrane[44]. Second, since replacement of Cl in the musocal solution does not affect ψ^{mc}, it appears that Cl does not contribute to the conductance of the mucosal membrane[44]. The same conclusion appears to apply to HCO_3[44]. Third, since the intracellular K concentration is much greater than that in the mucosal solution, whereas K is not actively secreted, and trans-mural movements of K appear to be restricted to the shunt pathway, the mucosal membrane would appear to be impermeable to K.

These considerations suggest that the e.m.f. across the mucosal membrane is largely due to the Na gradient across the boundary, as is apparently the case for a variety of high-resistance epithelia (e.g., isolated frog skin and toad urinary bladder).

The serosal or basolateral membranes seem to be impermeable to Na[83]. If the mucosal membrane is impermeable to K, the maintenance of a steady-state intracellular K concentration must rely on the pump-leak system at the serosal membranes, so that this boundary is permeable to K and the K gradient must contribute to $E_s R_s$. We have no information regarding the permeability of the serosal membrane to Cl. However, if P_{Cl} is not negligible, it would contribute to $E_s R_s$ in the same direction as the K gradient. A rheogenic Na extrusion mechanism apparently operates at the serosal membranes that would also contribute to the $E_s R_s$ in the same direction as the K gradient[44, 83]. All these points suggest that the cell interior should be electrically negative with respect to the serosal solution, as is found experimentally.

These considerations suggest that the electrical potential profile across rabbit ileum (Figure 3.13) should resemble that illustrated in Figure 3.7(a). That

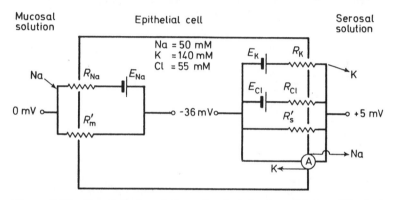

Figure 3.13 Hypothetical equivalent electrical circuit model for rabbit ileal cells in the absence of actively transported sugars or amino acids. Included are the apparent intracellular concentrations of Na, K and Cl in the presence of a modified Ringer's solution, and the observed electrical potential profile. The rheogenic Na–K pump is designated by A. R'_m and R'_s designate unspecified shunt pathways across the mucosal and serosal membranes.

is, the cell interior should be electrically positive with respect to the mucosal solution. However, microelectrode studies indicate that the cell interior is electrically negative with respect to the mucosal solution. To explain this apparent discrepancy we invoke the argument discussed in detail by Schultz[45], that is, in the presence of a high-conductance shunt pathway, transmembrane p.d.s need reflect neither the magnitude nor the direction of the trans-membrane e.m.f.s. Thus, the electrical profile predicted by the equivalent circuit illustrated in Figure 3.13 may be reconciled with experimental observations by recourse to the presence of a high-conductance shunt pathway.

Note added in proof

With reference to Figure 3.10, recent studies by Nellans, Frizzell and Schultz (unpublished observations) suggest that the Na-independent Cl influx process (a) does not participate in Cl absorption and probably represents movement(s) into cells or compartments that are not involved in transepithelial transport. Active Cl absorption as well as the short-circuit current are abolished in the absence of Na, so that the coupled NaCl influx process (b) appears to be exclusively responsible for transepithelial Cl transport under short-circuit conditions. Further, this process appears to be reversible and is capable of mediating a neutral, coupled NaCl and/or $NaHCO_3$ efflux from the cell into the mucosal solution. Active Na absorption is reduced but not abolished by removal of Cl and the short-circuit current and ψ^{ms} parallel this reduction in net Na transport from mucosa-to-serosa. Thus, process (c) appears to contribute to transepithelial Na transport.

References

1. MacInnes, D. A. (1961). *The Principles of Electrochemistry* (New York: Dover Press)
2. Helfferich, F. (1962). *Ion Exchange* (New York: McGraw-Hill Book Co.)
3. Lakshminarayanaiah, N. (1969). *Transport Phenomena in Membranes* (New York: Academic Press)
4. Frank, K. and Becker, M. C. (1964). Microelectrodes for recording and stimulation, in *Physical Techniques in Biological Research*, Vol. 5, 22 (W. L. Nastuk, editor) (New York: Academic Press)
5. Spiegler, K. S. and Wyllie, M. R. J. (1968). Electrical potential differences, in *Physical Techniques in Biological Research*, Vol. 2a, 277 (D. H. Moore, editor) (New York: Academic Press)
6. Ussing, H. H. and Zerahn, K. (1951). Active transport of sodium as the source of electric current in the short-circuited isolated frog skin, *Acta Physiol. Scand.*, **23**, 110
7. Nernst, W. (1889). Die electromotorische wirksamkeit der ionen, *Z. Physik. Chem.*, **4**, 129
8. Katchalsky, A. and Curran, P. F. (1965). *Nonequilibrium Thermodynamics in Biophysics* (Cambridge, Mass.: Harvard University Press)
9. Parlin, R. B. and Eyring, H. (1954). Membrane permeability and electrical potential, in *Ion Transport Across Membranes*, 103 (H. T. Clark, editor) (New York: Academic Press)
10. Ussing, H. H. (1949). The distinction by means of tracers between active transport and diffusion, *Acta Physiol. Scand.*, **19**, 43
11. Behn, U. A. R. (1897). Über wechselseitige Diffusion von Electrolyten in verdünnten wässerigen Lösungen, insbesondere über Diffusion gegen das koncentrationsgefälle, *Ann. Physik.*, **62**, 54
12. Teorell, T. (1953). Transport processes and electrical phenomena in ionic membranes, *Prog. Biophys. Chem.*, **3**, 305
13. Kedem, O. and Essig, A. (1965). Isotope flows and flux ratios in biological membranes, *J. Gen. Physiol.*, **48**, 1047
14. Hoshiko, T. and Lindley, B. D. (1964). The relationship of Ussing's flux-ratio equation to the thermodynamic description of membrane permeability, *Biochim. Biophys. Acta*, **79**, 301
15. Curran, P. F. and Schultz, S. G. (1968). Transport across membranes: general principles, in *Handbook of Physiology*, Sec. 6, Vol. 3, 1217. (C. F. Code, editor) (Washington: Amer. Physiol. Soc.)
16. Planck, M. (1890). Über die erregung von electricität und wärme in electrolyten, *Ann. Physik. u. Chem.*, **39**, 161
17. Planck, M. (1890). Über die potentialdifferenz zwischen zwei verdünnten lösungen binarer electrolyte, *Ann. Physik. u. Chem.*, **40**, 561
18. Henderson, P. (1907). Zur Thermodynamik der Flussigkeitsketten, *Z. Physik. Chem.*, **59**, 118
19. Schlögl, R. (1954). Electrodiffusion in freier lösung und geladenen membranen, *Z. Physik. Chem.*, **1**, 305
20. Schölgl, R. (1964). Stofftransport durch Membranen, in *Fortschritte der Physikalischen Chemie*, Band 9 (Darmstadt: Dr. Dietrich Steinkopff Verlag)

21. Goldman, D. E. (1943). Potential, impedance and rectification in membranes, *J. Gen. Physiol.*, **27**, 37
22. Hodgkin, A. L. and Katz, B. (1949). The effect of sodium ions on the electrical activity of the giant axon of the squid, *J. Physiol. (London)*, **108**, 37
23. Kimizuka, H. and Koketsu, K. (1964). Ion transport through cell membrane, *J. Theoret. Biol.*, **6**, 290
24. Mullins, L. J. (1961). The macromolecular properties of excitable membranes, *Ann. N.Y. Acad. Sci.*, **94**, 390
25. Jacquez, J. A. (1971). A generalization of the Goldman equation including the effect of electrogenic pumps, *Math. Biosci.*, **12**, 185
26. Patlak, C. S. (1960). Derivation of an equation for the diffusion potential, *Nature (London)*, **188**, 944
27. MacGillivary, A. D. and Hare, D. (1969). Applicability of Goldman's constant field assumption to biological systems, *J. Theoret. Biol.*, **25**, 113
28. Finkelstein, A. and Mauro, A. (1963). Equivalent circuits as related to ionic systems, *Biophys. J.*, **3**, 215
29. Barr, L. (1965). Membrane potential profiles and the Goldman equation, *J. Theoret. Biol.*, **9**, 351
30. Schwartz, T. L. (1971). Direct effects on the membrane potential due to 'pumps' that transfer no net charge, *Biophys. J.*, **11**, 944
31. Barry, P. H. and Diamond, J. M. (1971). A theory of ion permeation through membranes with fixed neutral sites, *J. Memb. Biol.*, **4**, 295
32. Sandblom, J. P. and Eisenmann, G. (1967). Membrane potentials at zero current: the significance of a constant ionic permeability ratio, *Biophys. J.*, **7**, 217
33. Teorell, T. (1936). A method of studying conditions within diffusion layers, *J. Biol. Chem.*, **113**, 735
34. Teorell, T. (1935). An attempt to formulate a quantitative theory of membrane permeability, *Proc. Soc. Exp. Biol. Med.*, **33**, 282
35. Meyer, K. H. and Sievers, J. F. (1936). La 'permebilite des membranes. I. Theorie de la permebilite ionique, *Helv. Chim. Acta*, **19**, 649
36. Teorell, T. (1951). Zur quantitativen Behandlung der Membranpermeabilität, *Z. Elektrochem.*, **55**, 460
37. Eisenman, G. (1967). On the origin of the glass electrode potential, in *Glass Electrodes for Hydrogen and Other Cations*, 133 (New York: Marcel Dekker)
38. Eisenman, G., Sandblom, J. P. and Walker, J. L., Jr. (1967). Membrane structure and ion permeation, *Science*, **155**, 965
39. Kernan, R. P. (1970). Electrogenic or linked transport, in *Membranes and Ion Transport*, Vol. 1, Chap. 10 (E. E. Bittar, editor) (London: Wiley-Interscience)
40. Ussing, H. H. (1971). Introductory remarks, *Phil. Trans. Roy. Soc. (London)*, **B262**, 85
41. Whittembury, G. and Rawlins, F. A. (1971). Evidence of a paracellular pathway for ion flow in the kidney proximal tubule: electron microscopic demonstration of lanthanum precipitate in the tight junction, *Pflügers Arch.*, **330**, 302
42. Smulders, A. P., Tormey, J. McD. and Wright, E. M. (1972). The effect of osmotically induced water flows on the permeability and ultrastructure of the rabbit gallbladder, *J. Memb. Biol.*, **7**, 164
43. Frömter, E. and Diamond, J. (1972). Route of passive ion permeation in epithelia, *Nature, New Biol.*, **235**, 9
44. Rose, R. C. and Schultz, S. G. (1971). Studies on the electrical potential profile across rabbit ileum: effects of sugars and amino acids on transmural and transmucosal electrical potential differences, *J. Gen. Physiol.*, **57**, 639
45. Schultz, S. G. (1972). Electrical potential differences and electromotive forces in epithelial tissues, *J. Gen. Physiol.*, **59**, 794
46. Frömter, E. (1972). The route of passive ion movement through the epithelium of *Necturus* gallbladder, *J. Memb. Biol.*, **8**, 259
47. Lundberg, A. (1958). Electrophysiology of salivary glands, *Physiol. Rev.*, **38**, 21
48. Ussing, H. H. and Windhager, E. E. (1964). Nature of shunt path and active sodium transport path through frog skin epithelium, *Acta Physiol. Scand.*, **61**, 484
49. Frazier, H. S. (1962). The electrical potential profile of the isolated toad bladder, *J. Gen. Physiol.*, **45**, 515

50. Whittembury, G. (1964). Electrical potential profile of the toad skin epithelium, *J. Gen. Physiol.*, **47**, 795
51. Villiegas, L. (1962). Cellular location of the electrical potential difference in frog gastric mucosa. *Biochim. Biophys. Acta*, **64**, 359
52. White, J. F. and Armstrong, W. McD. (1971). Effect of transported solutes on membrane potentials in bullfrog small intestine. *Amer. J. Physiol.*, **221**, 194
53. Windhager, E. E. and Giebisch, G. (1965). Electrophysiology of the nephron, *Physiol. Rev.*, **45**, 214
54. Durbin, R. P. (1968). Electrical potential difference of the gastric mucosa, in *The Handbook of Physiology*, Sec. 6, Vol. 2, 879 (C. F. Code, editor) (Washington: Amer. Physiol. Soc.)
55. Forte, J. G. (1970). Hydrochloric acid secretion by gastric mucosa, in *Membranes and Ion Transport*, Vol. 3, 111 (E. E. Bittar, editor) (London: Wiley-Interscience)
56. Hogben, C. A. M. (1955). Active transport of chloride by isolated frog gastric epithelium. Origin of the gastric mucosal potential, *Amer. J. Physiol.*, **180**, 641
57. Durbin, R. P. and Heinz, E. (1958). Electromotive chloride transport and gastric acid secretion in the frog, *J. Gen. Physiol.*, **45**, 1035
58. Forte, J. G. (1968). The effect of inhibitors of HCl secretion on the unidirectional fluxes of chloride across bullfrog gastric mucosa, *Biochim. Biophys. Acta*, **150**, 136
59. Heinz, E. and Durbin, R. (1959). Evidence for an independent hydrogen-ion pump in the stomach, *Biochim. Biophys. Acta*, **31**, 246
60. Harris, J. B. and Edelman, I. S. (1964). Chemical concentration gradients and electrical properties of gastric mucosa, *Amer. J. Physiol.*, **206**, 769
61. Rehm, W. S. (1964). Gastric potential and ion transport, in *Transcellular Membrane Potentials and Ion Fluxes*, 64 (F. M. Snell, editor) (New York: Gordon and Breach)
62. Rehm, W. S. (1964). Hydrochloric acid secretion, ion gradients, and the gastric potential, in *Society of General Physiologists. The Cellular Functions of Membrane Transport*, 231 (J. F. Hoffman, editor) (Englewood Cliffs, New Jersey: Prentice-Hall)
63. Rehm, W. S. (1966). Electrogenic mechanisms of the frog's gastric mucosa, *Ann. N.Y. Acad. Sci.*, **137**, 591
64. Rehm, W. S. (1967). Ion permeability and electrical resistance of the frog's gastric mucosa. *Fed. Proc.*, **26**, 1303
65. Curran, P. F., Schultz, S. G., Chez, R. A. and Fuisz, R. E. (1967). Kinetic relations of the Na–amino acid interaction at the mucosal border of intestine, *J. Gen. Physiol.*, **50**, 1261
66. Sanders, S. S., O'Callagan, J., Butler, C. F. and Rehm, W. S. (1972). Conductance of submucosal-facing membrane of frog gastric mucosa, *Amer. J. Physiol.*, **222**, 1348
67. Blum, A. L., Hirschowitz, B. I., Helander, H. F. and Sachs, G. (1971). Electrical properties of isolated cells of *Necturus* gastric mucosa, *Biochim. Biophys. Acta*, **241**, 261
68. Schultz, S. G. and Curran, P. F. (1968). Intestinal absorption of sodium chloride and water, in *Handbook of Physiology*, Sec. 6, Vol. 3, 1245 (Washington: Amer. Physiol. Soc.)
69. Schultz, S. G. and Frizzell, R. A. (1972). An overview of intestinal absorptive and secretory processes, *Gastroenterology*, **63**, 161
70. Schultz, S. G. and Zalusky, R. (1964). Ion transport in isolated rabbit ileum: I. Short-circuit current and Na fluxes, *J. Gen. Physiol.*, **47**, 567
71. Clarkson, T. W. and Toole, S. R. (1964). Measurement of short-circuit current and ion transport across the ileum, *Amer. J. Physiol.*, **206**, 658
72. Field, M., Fromm, D. and McColl, I. (1971). Ion transport in rabbit ileal mucosa. I. Na and Cl fluxes and short-circuit current, *Amer. J. Physiol.*, **220**, 1388
73. Clarkson, T. W. (1967). The transport of salt and water across isolated rat ileum. Evidence for at least two distinct pathways, *J. Gen. Physiol.*, **50**, 695
74. Schultz, S. G., Zalusky, R. and Gass, A. E., Jr. (1964). Ion transport in isolated rabbit ileum. III. Chloride fluxes, *J. Gen. Physiol.*, **48**, 375
75. Al-Awqati, Q., Cammeron, J. L., and Greenough, W. B., III (1972). Electrolyte transport in human ileum: effect of purified cholera exotoxin, *Amer. J. Physiol.*, **224**, 818
76. Hubel, K. A. (1967). Bicarbonate secretion in rat ileum and its dependence on intraluminal chloride, *Amer. J. Physiol.*, **213**, 1409
77. Hubel, K. A. (1968). The ins and outs of bicarbonate in the alimentary tract, *Gastroenterology*, **54**, 647
78. Hubel, K. A. (1969). Effect of luminal chloride concentration on bicarbonate secretion in rat ileum, *Amer. J. Physiol.*, **217**, 40

79. Kinney, V. R. and Code, C. F. (1964). Canine ileal chloride absorption: effect of carbonic anhydrase inhibitor on transport, *Amer. J. Physiol.*, **207**, 998
80. Nellans, H. N., Frizzell, R. A. and Schultz, S. G. (1973). Sodium and chloride fluxes across brush border of rabbit ileum: evidence for a coupled NaCl influx process, *Amer. J. Physiol.*, in press
81. Schultz, S. G., Fuisz, R. E. and Curran, P. F. (1966). Amino acid and sugar transport in rabbit ileum, *J. Gen. Physiol.*, **49**, 849
82. Lee, C. O. and Armstrong, W. McD. (1972). Activities of sodium and potassium ions in epithelial cells of small intestine, *Science*, **175**, 1261
83. Frizzell, R. A. and Schultz, S. G. (1972). Ionic conductances of extracellular shunt pathway in rabbit ileum: influence of shunt on transmural sodium transport and electrical potential differences, *J. Gen. Physiol.*, **59**, 318
84. Chez, R. A., Palmer, R. R., Schultz, S. G. and Curran, P. F. (1967). Effect of inhibitors on alanine transport in isolated rabbit ileum, *J. Gen. Physiol.*, **50**, 2357
85. Fujita, M., Ohta, H., Kawai, K., Matsui, H. and Nakao, M. (1972). Differential isolation of microvillous and baso-lateral plasma membranes from intestinal mucosa: mutually exclusive distribution of digestive enzymes and ouabain-sensitive ATPase, *Biochim. Biophys. Acta*, **274**, 336
86. Frizzell, R. A., Nellans, H. N., Rose, R. C., Markscheid-Kapsi, L. and Schultz, S. G. (1973). Intracellular Cl concentrations and influx across the brush border of rabbit ileum, *Amer. J. Physiol.*, **224**, 328
87. Turnberg, L. A., Bieberdorf, F. A., Morawski, S. G. and Fordtran, J. S. (1970). Interrelationships of chloride, bicarbonate, sodium and hydrogen transport in the human ileum, *J. Clin. Invest.*, **49**, 557
88. Carlinsky, N. J. and Lew, V. L. (1970). Bicarbonate secretion and non-Na component of the short-circuit current in the isolated colonic mucosa of *Bufo arenarum*, *J. Physiol. (London)*, **206**, 529
89. Schultz, S. G. and Curran, P. F. (1970). Coupled transport of sodium and organic solutes, *Physiol. Rev.*, **50**, 637
90. Barry, P. H., Diamond, J. M. and Wright, E. M. (1971). The mechanism of cation permeation in rabbit gallbladder, *J. Memb. Biol.*, **4**, 358
91. Frömter, E., Müller, C. W. and Wick, T. (1971). Permeability properties of the proximal tubular epithelium of the rat studied with electrophysiological methods, in *Electrophysiology of Epithelial Cells*, 119 (Stuttgart: F. K. Schattauer Verlag)
92. Boulpaep, E. L. and Seely, J. F. (1971). Electrophysiology of proximal and distal tubules in the autoperfused dog kidney, *Amer. J. Physiol.*, **221**, 1084
93. Garrahan, P. J. and Glynn, I. M. (1967). The stoichiometry of the sodium pump, *J. Physiol. (London)*, **192**, 217

4
The Gastrointestinal Circulation

J. GRAYSON
University of Toronto

4.1 MORPHOLOGY

4.1.1 Vascular organisation

In the mammal, the splanchnic area receives its arterial blood supply from a series of closely interconnected vessels: the coeliac, superior and inferior

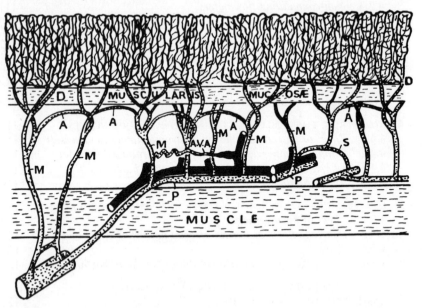

Figure 4.1 The vascular arrangement in the stomach wall of man. M, mucosal arteries arising from the left gastric artery outside the stomach wall. A, anastomosis between two mucosal arteries. D, network in glandular aspect of muscularis mucosae from which capillaries of mucosa arise. A.V.A., arterio-venous anastomosis. P, submucous plexus. S, subsidiary anastomotic channels. (From Barlow *et al.*[1], by courtesy of *Surg. Gynec. Obstet.*)

mesenteric arteries. These vessels form a remarkable system of vascular arcades, communicating freely with each other so that no clearly defined distribution exists for any single vessel and no area of the gastrointestinal tract depends for its nutrition on any one artery[1-3]. Figure 4.1 shows that the vasa recta do not represent the final stage of the arcade system but lead to a continuance of the arrangement within the organ. There are no end-arteries, and an extensive submucous plexus of vessels is derived from the arterial chains on the lesser and greater curvature of the stomach, from which arise the mucosal arteries. Mucosal arteries may also arise directly from the externally situated chains, which anastomose freely as they approach the muscularis muco sa, and

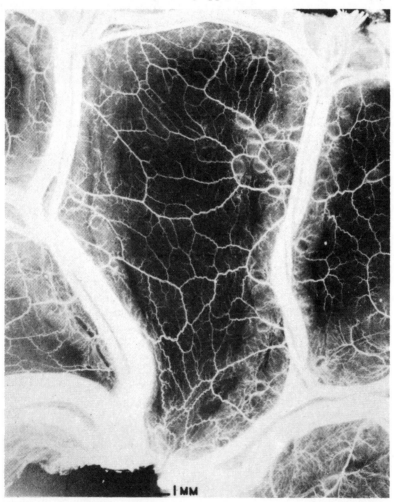

Figure 4.2 Silicone-injected, glycerol-cleared mesentery. Small bowel has been removed along the top edge. The bottom apex is at the posterior line of attachment of the mesentery. A sector is defined as the area between the central two vertical pairs of vessels and the joining primary arcade at the top. (From Frasher and Wayland[4], reproduced by permission of Academic Press.)

again on the glandular aspect of that layer. From this plexus of small arteries, the remarkably rich capillary bed arises. The same kind of arterial distribution is apparently common to the whole gastrointestinal tract. Recently, Frasher and Wayland[4] described a modular arrangement of the microcirculation in the mesentery, which is basically similar (Figure 4.2).

One consequence of the anastomotic network, at least in the stomach, is a substantial functional independence from an exact and intact anatomic supply. Thus, Ivy *et al.*[5] performed experiments in which many of the vessels supplying the stomach were ligated without affecting the ability of the stomach to secrete. One purpose of his experiments was to attempt to reproduce conditions leading to ulceration, but no pathologic changes could be detected. This approach has its limits, however. Heimbecker and Richards[6] observed that a 90% occlusion of the coeliac artery in the conscious dog (using ameroid constrictors) produced marked pathologic changes. These dogs often behaved as though they had gastric pain and showed evidence of bleeding. Their gastric secretion dropped uniformly and dramatically during duodenal infusion. Marked ischaemic changes were apparent in the duodenum, stomach, spleen and liver. Elsewhere in the gastrointestinal tract[7], too, studies have indicated that the integrity of the anastomotic supply is more important than Ivy's experiments imply[5].

4.1.2   Arterio-venous anastomoses in the stomach

The existence of direct communications between arteries and veins has long been known. However, their discovery in skin[8-10] really gave impetus to further study. There were two types: long, direct channels connecting artery and vein (expanded capillary type), and the glomus type (long, tortuous channels). These shunts were thought to serve a homeostatic function, enabling the tissue to carry large volumes of blood without swamping the nutritional vessels of the tissue itself. Since the gastrointestinal tract was thought to have a homeostatic function relative to blood pressure regulation, it seemed reasonable to seek shunts in this region. Clara[11] made passing reference to possible arterio-venous anastomoses in the stomach. DeBusscher[12] described glomus forms in all stomach layers except the mucosa. Although observations failed to confirm his work in detail, the evidence seemed clear that arterio-venous anastomoses of the expanded capillary type (Figure 4.3) do exist in the submucous layers of the stomach. Originally, they were shown in the human stomach by morphologic studies[2, 3], injection of opaque media, microradiography, section and dissection. Injection of glass microspheres, 40–200 μm in diameter, gave a 'substantial' yield in the venous outflow of freshly removed, perfused human stomachs. Since these spheres were too large to pass through capillaries, their appearance in the venous outflow further supported the existence of gastric arterio-venous anastomoses. Sherman and Newman[13] confirmed this in canine experiments by perfusion with glass beads ranging from 100 to 180 μm in diameter. These observations were in no way quantitative, but 'a quantity' of spheres, 180 μm in diameter, was recovered. Because they accepted the view of Krogh[14] that capillaries cannot be dilated to more than 30 μm under the most extreme conditions, Sherman

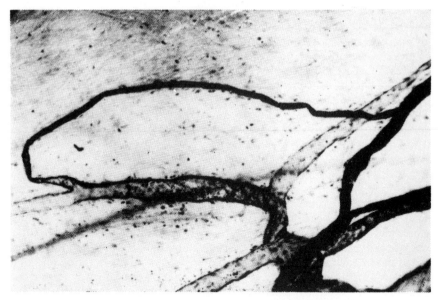

Figure 4.3 Arterio-venous anastomosis in submucosa of human stomach ($\times$ 15). The arteries are dark and the veins light. (Kind permission of Dr. Barlow).

and Newman[13] stated that 'It is our opinion that the presence of arterio-venous anastomoses of far greater than capillary size has been adequately demonstrated histologically and amply confirmed by perfusion of glass spheres'.

Unfortunately, recent work is less emphatic. Using injection methods in the human bowel, Boutler and Parks[15] confirmed the existence of 'profuse' arterio-venous anastomoses 30–35 µm in diameter in all parts of the enteric tract but failed to find any larger communicating vessels. Although Zweifach and Metz[16] found arterio-venous anastomoses in the dog, they were only 20–30 µm in diameter. The retreat from the earlier view gathered more impetus with the introduction of radioactive labelled microspheres. Shoemaker and Powers[17] produced evidence that arterio-venous anastomoses were totally lacking in the stomach of the anaesthetised dog. Their views were confirmed by Buchin and Edlich[18].

The question of arterio-venous anastomoses remains unresolved. The original work of Bentley's group[1,3] in 1951 was convincing. Their histologic studies suggested the existence of arterio-venous anastomoses, probably not more than 50 µm in diameter (though presumably the vessels could be dilated to accept larger glass microspheres). The later negative work could be due to species variation, but large arterio-venous anastomoses have been reported in the dog. Even if one questions the use of glass microspheres for estimating size, smaller channels have also been reported by Zweifach and Metz[16] and by Boulter and Parks[15], using direct methods.

The question arises, then, why were the findings negative from studies involving the labelled microsphere technique? One cannot accept these negative data as final. Too much positive evidence suggests the reality of arterio-venous anastomoses in the stomach. Although the use of labelled microspheres has many advantages, too little is known about the rheology of microsphere suspensions. Even the material from which the microspheres is made is usually undisclosed. Possibly the failure to pass through arterio-venous channels is due to some undisclosed physical interaction with the microcirculation. Much remains to be done before we can finally decide upon the existence or absence of arterio-venous shunts in the gastric circulation. However, the real question may prove to be quantitative. Not, are they absent, but are they present in functional quantity?

4.1.3 Arterio-venous anastomoses in the intestinal tract

The existence of shunts is even more doubtful in the rest of the gastrointestinal tract. It has been stated[19] that arterio-venous anastomoses exist in the small intestinal villi of man, and also in the large intestine[20], although little corroborative evidence has been reported. India ink and latex injections failed to demonstrate arterio-venous anastomoses in the dog or the opposum[21]. Brokis and Moffat[22] considered their presence in the colon as unproved, although a few arterio-venous anastomoses have been reported in the colonic submucosa. These structures were 30–35 μm in diameter and were described as the expanded capillary type[15]. Grim and Lindseth[23] injected labelled microspheres 40 μm in diameter into the superior mesenteric artery and recovered none from the portal vein. Only 3% of similarly injected 20 μm microspheres could be recovered and 17% of 12 μm microspheres[23]. Their findings were substantiated by Delaney[24].

The morphologic evidence in the gut for arterio-venous anastomoses is far less satisfactory than in the stomach and does not really conflict with the microsphere evidence. The best conclusion is that arterio-venous anastomoses may exist, but they are few and probably functionally unimportant. On the other hand, the evidence for functional shunts is convincing. Thus, in the intestine the mucosal and submucosal vasculatures apparently do not always respond the same to a given stimulus. Folkow[25], for example, found that sympathetic stimulation produced a sizeable reduction in mucosal flow with no change in total gut flow. He suggested that this was functional evidence of arterio-venous shunts. Delaney[24] however, noted that Folkow's findings could also be explained by compensatory vasodilation in submucous vessels when the mucosal vessels were constricted.

4.2 METHODS USED TO STUDY GASTROINTESTINAL CIRCULATION

4.2.1 Morphologic studies

Much morphologic information has been obtained from injection procedures (India ink, graphite, gelatin, radio-opaque materials, latex preparations, various plastic agents) combined with light microscopy and microradiography. Such methods have been used to establish the anatomic picture of the gastrointestinal circulation described above. A recent development in injection technique is the use of a silicone-rubber preparation (Microfil*), which can show microcirculatory detail not possible with other methods[26].

4.2.2 Methods of measurement in cannulated vessels

A long succession of flowmeters has followed Ludwig's mechanical strohmuhr[27]. This, like many later methods of flow measurement, necessitated the cannulation of the vessel under examination. Nevertheless, the instrument played a large part in early work on portal and mesenteric artery blood flow estimations[28, 29].

Using portocaval shunts of various kinds, workers have measured portal venous outflow directly[30-33]. However, the main technical effort has been directed toward developing a suitable flowmeter that could be applied directly to a vessel, preferably an intact one in the conscious animal.

Bubble flowmeters[34-36] also have the disadvantage of requiring cannulation and possessing high intrinsic resistance to flow. Rotameters[37] have little resistance but still require vessel cannulation.

4.2.3 Non-cannulating flowmeters

The first of the flowmeters which could be applied to the intact vessel and used in the conscious animal was the thermostrohmur of Rein[38]. It was used extensively by its inventor, as well as by Grindlay et al.[39] and others. In the hands of such workers as these, the thermostrohmuhr was used with success (when one considers that most of their results were later confirmed by other methods). However, it has been severely criticised[40, 41] and seems to be subject to artefact arising from local temperature changes, turbulence, backflow, shifting of the probe, etc.

The electromagnetic flowmeter, introduced first by Kolin[42], is probably the most widely used flowmeter today. It has been applied extensively in many areas[43] and has been used for some time in studies of the gastrointestinal circulation[44]. The method depends upon the induction of voltage in a conductor moving through a magnetic field at right angles to the lines of force. Blood serves as the conductor, the magnetic field is produced by a small electromagnet, and the induced voltage (about one-millionth of a volt) is amplified and recorded. This method records both mean and phasic flow, calibration is linear, and there is a high-frequency response. No cannulation is required, and the technique can be used over long periods in the conscious animal[45]. There are disadvantages, too. Notably, some vessel constriction is needed for accurate recording. Problems arise with zero checks, which, in most commercial probes, still require transient occlusion of the vessel. This type of flowmeter is difficult to use in low-pressure systems, making the measurement of blood flow in the portal vein particularly difficult. The ultrasonic flowmeter introduced recently[46] requires no high intravascular pressure, nor partial occlusion of the vessel. In dimension and shape, the probe is not

* Microfils Canton Biomedical Products, Boulder, Colorado

unlike the electromagnetic flow probe. It uses a high-frequency sound source with a small pickup situated on the opposite side of the vessel. The Doppler effect is used to measure the velocity of moving blood rather than blood flow. Its major disadvantage is that although the vessel need not be occluded, absolutely accurate apposition of the probe and the filling of all gaps is mandatory. It is, in consequence, liable to artefact from shifting of the probe.

Obviously, then, while flow technology has advanced greatly, it is far from perfect.

4.2.4 Volume measurements in the gastrointestinal tract

One of the earliest approaches to the study of gastrointestinal circulation was the use of the plethysmograph to measure gut volume[47]. It was used by many workers[48, 51]. Such methods have their limitations, since volume changes fail to distinguish between flow changes and changes in the amount of blood stored in the organ.

4.2.5 Colour changes in stomach or gut mucosa

The same objections (Section 4.2.4) probably apply to the use of colour change. The first recorded use of colour change as an index of blood flow was probably the classic case of traumatic gastrostomy (Alexis St. Martin) reported by Beaumont in 1833[52]. The same index of flow was used in 1943 by Wolf and Wolff[53] who observed colour changes in the exposed musoca at gastrostomy sites, mainly in children[54]. In the colon and rectum, colour change has been observed[55] by means of a sigmoidoscope; the responses of the colons of normal subjects to vasoactive drugs were investigated.

4.2.6 Temperature methods in bowel blood flow measurements

Shoskes[56] attempted to measure surface temperature of colostomy tissue but failed to secure satisfactory apposition with thermopiles. Grayson[51] used fine gauge needle thermocouples inserted into the mucosa of the exposed colostomy site in human subjects. From isolated gut perfusion experiments, he demonstrated a logarithmic relation between temperature and flow. Grayson argued that the colostomy mucosal temperature, like skin temperature, represented an equilibrium between body core and room temperatures and that mucosal temperature was determined by the volume flow of blood.

4.2.7 Isotope fractionation

This method depends on the assumption that if a substance is injected intravenously in one dose it will be distributed to the organs of the body in proportion to their blood flow. It will then be carried away by their venous drainage. However, for a while the venous drainage will be negligible compared with the arterial delivery, and during this time the fractional distribution of the substance among the organs will correspond to the fractional distribution of cardiac output. Sapirstein[58] found that rubidium (^{86}Rb) transfers completely to the tissues. The method is simple: after injection of ^{86}Rb, cardiac output is quickly measured, the animal is killed and the radioactivity of the various tissues is determined. A major difficulty, of course, is that only one set of observations can be made on any one animal. Sapirstein[59] has also pointed out that the presence of arterio-venous shunts may constitute a potential source of error.

4.2.8 Clearance methods

The criteria for the use of clearance techniques in blood flow measurement were clearly delineated by Homer Smith in 1951[60]. One criterion is that the substance concerned must be cleared from the blood by the organ in one passage and that it must be capable of simple measurement. Clearance methods have been widely used in the liver: bromsulphalein typifies the many clearance indicators used from time to time. Probably none of these substances really meets all of Smith's criteria, and even stronger objections arise from sampling errors. Sapirstein[58] states, 'we were forced to the conclusion that dye methods as generally used are, at best, semi-quantitative. There is a potential positive error (extrasplanchnic extraction) . . . and a potential negative error which is, in all probability, so dependent on the minute details of technique in cannula placement that its magnitude cannot be properly evaluated'. Probably these remarks also apply to other clearance methods used in the splanchnic area.

Blood flow in the stomach has been measured by analogous methods. Thus, fractionation of the cardiac output, using labelled potassium (^{32}K), has been used for mucosal and total measurement. Again, one doubts whether Homer Smith's criteria are really met. Delaney and Grim[61] list a formidable series of objections to the use of ^{32}K. Another method in vogue is the use of labelled microspheres. These are small plastic spheres (16–20 µm) labelled with radioactive sodium. After arterial injection, most of the microspheres lodge in the small vessels of the microcirculation, and the accumulated radioactivity is used as a measure of blood flow. Most workers using labelled microspheres failed to obtain a significant yield of microspheres in the venous effluent, although evidence exists that some of the radioactive sodium may elute and appear in the venous effluent[18], constituting a potential source of error. The importance of this evidence in interpreting the presence or absence of arterio-venous shunts has already been discussed. Labelled microspheres apparently pass in no significant quantities through any existing shunts. This probably favours the validity of the method in measuring tissue flow. Nevertheless, any technique depending for its effectiveness on the blockage of small blood vessels cannot be regarded as ideal.

Probably no single 'ideal' method exists for measuring flow in the stomach. To the author, by far the most satisfactory technique is the aminopyrine clearance method, introduced by Jacobson in 1966[45, 62]. The method evolved from the earlier observations of Carryer and Ivy[63] and of Davenport[64] relating to the secretion of sulphonamide drugs into the stomach; the method is based upon the pH partition hypothesis of Shore et al.[65] Its use depends on the ability of the un-ionised form of a weak base, like aminopyrine, which is its usual state in the plasma, to traverse the gastric mucosa readily. However, at the pH of gastric juice, aminopyrine ionises and cannot be reabsorbed in this form. The result is an effective gastric 'clearance' of aminopyrine. The only samples required are plasma and gastric contents, and the gastric volume secretion must be measured. Jacobson and his colleagues have done much to validate the method[66]. Other groups have also used aminopyrine, and Harper and his co-workers[67] have independently confirmed its validity. The method can be used repeatedly in the conscious animal.

4.3 AUTOREGULATION OF BLOOD FLOW IN THE GUT

Autoregulation of blood flow was first described by Shipley and Study[68], who recognised that renal blood flow was constant over a wide range of systemic arterial blood pressures (140–60 mmHg). The essence of the response was vasodilatation, a decrease in vascular resistance when the blood pressure fell, or conversely, an increase in vessel tone when the transmural pressure was raised. The phenomenon could be demonstrated in the isolated perfused organ and was shown to be independent of extrinsic factors such as nerves or hormones. Grayson and others recognised a similar phenomenon in the hepatic arterial bed[69, 74, 76, 77] and in the grey matter of the brain[70]. Later it was described in skeletal muscle[71] and in small intestine[72]. The concept of autoregulation generated a view of circulatory control quite different from orthodox concepts, which stressed central regulation through nerves or hormones.

Autoregulation may partly be related to the basic property of all muscle to develop a greater contractile force with an increase in stretch[73]. Folkow and Öberg[71] provided a substantial basis for this myogenic view, making the added point that autoregulation depends on the pre-existence of relatively normal myogenic tone in the vascular bed. After all, vessels which are already fully dilated cannot be expected to dilate further. This may explain the frequent failure to demonstrate the phenomenon. Factors such as depth of anaesthesia, operative trauma and haemorrhage have also been shown to be important to its successful demonstration[72, 75]. Nonetheless, the evidence for the reality of autoregulation in many intact tissues is now unequivocal. That there is a myogenic factor, i.e. a reaction to transmural pressure initiated in the smooth muscle of the blood vessels is also probable. It is equally probable that metabolic factors arising in the tissue itself play the largest role in the autoregulatory response to altered perfusion pressure.

In the splanchnic area, most evidence supports autoregulation in the hepatic artery[69, 72, 75, 78], a reduction in hepatic arterial resistance when systemic arterial blood pressure falls. Beyond this, matters are unclear. Most authors agree that autoregulation cannot be demonstrated in the portal vein or its branches. Portal vein flow declines when the systemic arterial pressure falls[75, 78, 79]. Early papers based on the use of electromagnetic flowmeters for measuring blood flow in the superior mesenteric artery of the dog[80, 81] described pressure–flow relationships that were non-linear (convex to the pressure axis), that is to say, pressure–flow relationships similar to those reported for the portal vein. However, Johnson[82] and Texter et al.[83] produced evidence indicating the presence of autoregulation in the superior mesenteric artery of the dog.

Folkow et al.[84] supported the concept of intestinal autoregulation. Most of his arguments were based on 'autoregulatory escape', in which continued stimulation of sympathetic nerve caused transient reduction in bowel blood flow after which flow returned toward normal despite maintenance of the stimulation. The return was thought to be due to autoregulation over-riding the vasoconstrictor drive. Apparently autoregulatory escape is an independent event[85], in no way indicating the presence of autoregulation.

A body of evidence also suggests that no autoregulation exists in the gastrointestinal tract. Thus Jacobson et al.[86] found no evidence of autoregulation in the dog stomach. Nor was there evidence for autoregulation in the dog colon[87]. Hinshaw[88], using perfused intestinal loops of the dog, failed to find evidence of autogulation in the small intestines; he noted that 'the findings of the present investigation appear to be at variance with those of others (Folkow, Johnson and Texter). However, the present experiments were carried out in the identical manner of those on kidney (which did show autoregulation)'.

Whether the data published by Johnson[82] and by Texter et al.[83] support their interpretations may be questioned. Both groups studied small numbers of dogs and the results were variable. It is true that flow–pressure curves were obtained for individual dogs which could justifiably be interpreted as autoregulatory, but whether this represents the mean for the group is somewhat doubtful. Boley and Gliedman[7] presented further evidence supporting autoregulation in the gut by partially occluding the superior mesenteric artery to reduce blood flow by 50%; in some experiments, the drop in pressure distal to the occlusion cuff was even greater. However, the mean pressure decline for the series was 48%. Autoregulation being an adjustment of vessel resistance to altered perfusion pressure[68], Boley's findings cannot be interpreted to favour the existence of autoregulation, at least as a regular phenomenon, in the gut.

In any case, most investigators in the field agree that portal outflow (and, therefore presumably portal inflow) shows no autoregulation relative to arterial pressure change. Since (apart from the splenic contribution) portal inflow is the same as gastrointestinal outflow, it is doubtful that the gastrointestinal tract as a whole exhibits autoregulation. One might agree with Johnson that the tendency to autoregulate is a ubiquitous property of vascular smooth muscle, but it seems to play a minor role in the gut and is easily overshadowed by other factors.

4.4 ADRENERGIC CONTROL OF GASTROINTESTINAL BLOOD VESSELS

4.4.1 Effect of catecholamines on gastrointestinal blood vessels

In 1895, Oliver and Schafer[89] stated that 'It may be fairly assumed that, although we are unable to record any plethysmographic observations upon the intestine, the great rise in blood pressure which invariably follows the injection of the extract (suprarenal gland) is in all cases due very largely to contraction of the arterioles in the splanchnic area'. From this statement arose two concepts which have long influenced physiological thought. One is that the gastrointestinal tract participates with other regions of the body, such as skin or kidneys, in controlling peripheral resistance and blood pressure. The second concept, which received early support from Brodie and Dixon[90] (and which to this day dies hard), is that epinephrine is a powerful splanchnic vasoconstrictor. Both ideas have contributed heavily to many theories concerning shock and haemorrhage; both were integral to Cannon's views on the redistribution of blood in emotional disturbance.

In truth, the literature concerning the action of the catecholamines on gastrointestinal blood flow has shown considerable divergence of opinion for 50 years. The acceptance of epinephrine as a powerful intestinal vasoconstrictor was challenged as early as 1917, when Hoskins and Cunning[91] used gut volume and outflow measurements in the dog to show that the action of epinephrine was inconstant and could cause either vasoconstriction or vasodilatation. Clarke[50], using volume measurements on cat and rabbit gut, showed initial vasoconstriction followed by dilation with epinephrine. The vasodilatation persisted after denervation and was considered at least partly a direct effect of epinephrine on the vessels. However, in later experiments, using drop recorders instead of volume measurements, Clarke[92] found constant vasoconstrictor effects with epinephrine which were reversed by ergotoxin. He deduced the presence of both vasodilator and vasoconstrictor nerve endings. These findings were confirmed first by Bülbring and Burn[93] and later by Green et al.[94], using electromagnetic flowmeters on the canine superior mesenteric artery. Both epinephrine and norepinephrine were vasoconstrictors. The effect of epinephrine but not norepinephrine could be reversed by adrenergic blockade with azaptine phosphate (Ilidar). Isopropylnorepinephrine was a vasodilator.

In terms of Ahlquist's receptor theory[95] both a and β receptors are present in the gastrointestinal tract, since both ergotoxine and azaptine phosphate block a receptors, unmasking the vasodilator effects of β stimulation.

Epinephrine has both vasoconstrictor and vasodilator effects in the gastrointestinal circulation. Although much of the early work indicated primarily a vasoconstrictor effect with epinephrine, most of the recent work supports Clarke's[50] original view that epinephrine increases total blood flow to the gut. Mills and Moyer[96] (measuring superior mesenteric artery blood flow in the dog) and Greenway and Lawson[97] (measuring portal venous flow in the cat) found predominantly vasodilator responses to systemic epinephrine. Ross[98], using both systemic and closed arterial administration, found a transient vasoconstriction superseded by vasodilatation (autoregulatory escape); β blockade increased the vasoconstrictor effect but did not totally abolish the dilator effect. Norepinephrine was an unequivocal vasoconstrictor.

For intestinal mucosa, epinephrine is clearly vasoconstrictor[100]. Ross[98] found total intestinal blood flow increased, but the mucosa remained ischaemic throughout epinephrine administration. In man, colour changes in the human bowel[99, 101] indicate that epinephrine caused constriction of colonic vessels. Using temperature measurements on exposed human colostomy and

ileostomy sites, Grayson and Swan[102] showed that both epinephrine and norepinephrine produced vasoconstriction. Moreover, during infusion, stable
plateaus were obtained.

There is less agreement concerning the effect of epinephrine on the gastric
mucosa. Delaney and Grim[103] used labelled microspheres and found a vasodilator action both in the gastric mucosa and in the stomach as a whole.
Jacobson et al.[62] and Rudick et al.[104] reported that epinephrine was a vasoconstrictor in the stomach. Apparently the circumstances of measurement
greatly affect the findings, and epinephrine must be regarded as capable of
either dilating or constricting stomach blood vessels.

Which vessels are responsible for the overall vasodilator action of epinephrine on gastrointestinal total outflow remains unclear. Direct evidence in
the stomach[62, 103] indicates that mucosal blood flow accounts for 60–70%
of total gastric flow. No comparable direct measurement is available for the
bowel, but the assumption seems reasonable that the mucosa accounts for a
considerable proportion of the total flow. Since intestinal mucosal vessels
appear to constrict with epinephrine (and norepinephrine), it is also unclear
which vessels could account for the overall increase in intestinal blood flow
accompanying epinephrine administration. The possibility that functional
shunts may be involved was suggested by Folkow[25], since the extent of dilation is difficult to explain except in terms of redistribution of blood flow.

4.4.2 Sympathetic nerves supplying the gastrointestinal tract

The gastrointestinal region down to the descending colon is supplied by the
thoracic sympathetic outflow (T5 to T12). The rest of the colon and rectum
are supplied by the lumbar outflow (L1 to L3). The thoracic sympathetic
nerves comprise three principal paired nerves: the greater, the lesser and the
lowest splanchnic nerves. These consist of preganglionic myelinated fibres that
have emerged from the lateral column of grey matter in the spinal cord and
pass without a relay through the relevant sympathetic ganglion in the corresponding intra-abdominal plexus. Of these plexuses, the coeliac is the most
important. Postganglionic fibres supply nerve plexuses in the gastrointestinal
wall, the submucous plexus (Meissner's), and one lying between the muscle
layers (Auerbach's). Fibres from these plexuses supply the muscle and mucosal
region of the gastrointestinal tract and probably account for the major innervation of the blood vessels.

4.4.3 Sympathetic control of gastrointestinal blood vessels

Agreement is general that splanchnic nerve stimulation initially increases
gastrointestinal vascular resistance. In early studies, Bayliss and Starling[49]
observed pallor, Bunch[105] recorded a volume decrease, and Burton-Opitz[29]
showed a large reduction in portal flow. However, there was also some
evidence of vasodilator fibres in the splanchnic nerves. Thus, weak stimulation
could increase blood volume[105, 106] although there was disagreement on this
finding[49]. However, Bülbring and Burn[93] showed that splanchnic stimulation
alone reduced gut volume, but after ergotoxine administration it increased

gut volume. This could not have been a cholinergic response since the increased volume was unaffected. These authors related the response to the action of adrenaline (which was then thought to be the sympathetic transmitter) on blood vessels. After adrenalectomy or adrenergic blockade, splanchnic stimulation slightly enhanced portal flow or mesenteric artery flow[107].

No cholinergic fibres seem to supply the blood vessels of the bowel. Since the experiments of Bülbring and Burn[93] were performed after adrenalectomy, the adrenaline reversal they found after ergotoxine administration could not be attributed to epinephrine released from the adrenal gland. However, Folkow et al.[107] suggested that the rise in blood flow found by them and others might well be due to reduction of intestinal muscular extravascular compression, since sympathetic stimulation relaxes the gut wall. In summary, the major effect of sympathetic nerve activation in the gastrointestinal tract is vasoconstriction.

One wonders, then, are such nerves tonically active and under what circumstances can they be activated? Considerable evidence points to tonic activity of gastrointestinal sympathetic nerves. Thus, in the dog and cat vasodilation occurs in the bowel after splanchnic section[48, 108, 109]. Most of these observations, however, were based on changes in volume or colour that might not truly reflect flow. Richens[110] produced direct evidence of vasodilation on splanchnic sections on the rat. In conscious human colostomy subjects, Grayson[102] found various degrees of resting vasomotor tone. Like Wolf and Wolff[101] and Almy and Tulin[55] he concluded that autonomic control of mucosal blood flow in the human bowel is unstable and highly responsive to emotional stimuli.

4.4.4 Autoregulatory escape

This term was introduced by Folkow et al.[113] to describe the effects of continued stimulation of the sympathetic supply to the gut or continued infusion of noradrenaline. With both, initial vasoconstriction was marked, followed by a return of blood flow toward or beyond initial levels. Folkow thought that escape from the vasoconstrictor effect was due to autoregulation, which, in this context, would seem to be a powerful factor in local resistance control. Folkow suggested that the anatomical locus of the escape phenomenon was in submucosal vessels; in this parallel circuit explanation the mucosal vessels remain constricted but the submucosal arterioles dilate[113]. A second view holds that precapillary structures in series with the constrictor elements of the vascular bed are the site of both autoregulation and autoregulatory escape[85]. A third view is that the same elements which initially constrict later dilate; the dilatation is envisaged as due to accumulation of metabolites[114, 115].

Richardson and Johnson[85] have provided compelling arguments that escape from adrenergic vasoconstrictor drive and autoregulation are unrelated. Escape can occur in situations where no autoregulation exists. Moreover, autoregulation depends upon the initial state of the vascular bed, whereas escape does not. The same workers also argue forcibly against the concept of a 'series vascular element'. The view that the same elements constrict and then relax is also unlikely since much evidence suggests that no escape occurs in the mucosa. Continuous noradrenaline or adrenaline infusion in man produced marked intestinal mucosal vasoconstriction that was dose-dependent and was maintained at a steady plateau throughout the infusion[116]. Similarly, in canine experiments, mucosal vasoconstriction produced either by catecholamine infusion or by splanchnic nerve stimulation did not 'escape'[117].

In summary, the gastrointestinal mucosa appears not to escape from the constrictor effect of sympathetic stimulation. Total blood flow to the gut does escape, either by the opening of submucosal shunts[121] or by a compensatory dilatation in submucosal microcirculatory beds[115]. Thus, escape is limited to the submucosa. It is associated with infusion of epinephrine, norepinephrine, angiotensin, or sympathetic stimulation[115]. It does not occur in relation to haemorrhage. Escape does not depend on pH levels[122]. During the escape phase, intestinal oxygen consumption in the cat rises.

The mechanisms and functional importance of the phenomenon remain obscure, but two consequences are apparent. First, escape is hard to reconcile with effective, central control of gastrointestinal blood vessels integrated with regulation of total body peripheral resistance. The net outcome of autoregulatory escape is that sympathetic stimulation has little effect on total gastrointestinal vascular resistance.

The second, more positive, consequence is that autoregulatory escape restores an initially depleted portal inflow to its initial prestimulation levels. The value of this during a period of sympathetic activity is obvious. The close link is often overlooked between circulatory function and other homeostatic mechanisms, such as glucose homeostasis. An interesting speculation is raised: although autoregulatory escape in the gut may run counter to the role of the intestinal circulation in peripheral vascular homeostasis, escape may facilitate regulation of blood glucose. Catecholamines and sympathetic activity influence glucose release from the liver and utilisation of sugar.

Another mechanism besides autoregulatory escape offsets the homeostatic usefulness of the gastrointestinal circulation in the control of blood pressure: the reciprocity between arterial and portal venous blood flows, in which decreasing portal blood flow is accompanied by increasing hepatic arterial flow, and vice versa[118]. This reciprocity, together with escape and the probable operation of submucosal shunts, means that the gastrointestinal tract does not show central sympathetic control of peripheral vascular resistance and blood pressure[123].

4.5 LOW-PRESSURE STATES AND THE GASTROINTESTINAL CIRCULATION

4.5.1 Effect of haemorrhage

A fall in blood pressure leads to reduced intestinal blood flow in all species studied to date. Some disagreement exists, however, concerning the relative importance of active vasoconstriction and the passive effects of reduced perfusion pressure.

The bowel vessels themselves do not respond directly to altered perfusion pressure, as shown by the experiments of Boley and his co-workers[7]. They used partial occlusion of the superior mesenteric artery to produce a 50% drop in flow and a proportional change in pressure distal to the occlusion. The systemic pressure did not change, but the perfusion pressure supplying much of the gut was lowered substantially. Their evidence indicated no significant change in mesenteric vascular resistance.

The data conflict, however, about the mesenteric response to the fall in perfusion pressure in haemorrhage. Selkurt et al.[122] showed an overall increase in splanchnic resistance with haemorrhage but could find no evidence of this in the mesenteric circulation, a finding confirmed with electromagnetic flowmeters by Brobmann et al.[123] However, their experiments involved extensive surgery in the anaesthetised dog, procedures which may interfere with the response to blood loss. In contrast, Gregg and Fisher[43] used electromagnetic flowmeters in the conscious dog and showed a threefold increase in mesenteric vascular resistance. Grayson and Swan[124] produced evidence of mucosal vasoconstriction in man during fainting. Greenway et al.[125] reported that a decline in systemic blood pressure produced a fall in portal flow, the result of vasoconstriction in the mesenteric bed, although the effect was partially countered by vasodilatation in the hepatic arterial bed (a confirmation of the portal-hepatic reciprocity shown previously[126, 127]). McNeill et al.[127] showed that sympathetic nerves were uninvolved in the mesenteric response to haemorrhage, but that circulating angiotensin and vasopressin effected intestinal vasoconstriction in the anaesthetised cat. Their concept resembles that described by Gregg and Fisher[43], although the mechanisms involve no sympathetic nerves. Not all workers would agree even on the basic vascular events. Reynell et al.[128] found no change in splanchnic vascular resistance with haemorrhage in anaesthetised dogs, despite a 50% reduction in the volume of blood contained in the splanchnic area. They stated that the splanchnic vasculature does not participate in the generalised vasoconstriction which follows haemorrhage but that it contributes to circulatory homeostasis by a reduction in capacitance. Price et al.[129] using dye dilution techniques in human subjects, measured both splanchnic blood flow and splanchnic blood volume. They removed 15% to 20% of the blood volume in 35 min (and, of course, returned it later). The only effect they could identify with certainty was a reduction in splanchnic blood volume from 1.4–0.85 l, with only a small change in hepatic venous flow. They concluded that 'there is reason to question whether an increase in sympathetic nervous activity did occur. The splanchnic circulation functions as an important blood reservoir in man. It can be preferentially depleted of blood by a mechanism which does not automatically increase vascular resistance'.

The evidence is mounting that in any species, including man, the gastrointestinal tract is not uniform in its response to haemorrhage. Colonic mucosal vasoconstriction has been clearly demonstrated, but it is becoming increasingly clear, too, that shunt mechanisms balance this response within the splanchnic area. The net effect is little change in splanchnic vascular resistance in response to haemorrhage. Increasingly, workers are wondering whether the more important role of the splanchnic area in circulatory homeostasis lies in its ability to alter its venous capacitance. One should recall that 70% of the total blood volume of the body is venous and, of this, 25% is found in the splanchnic area.

4.5.2 Delayed effects of partial arterial occclusion in the bowel

An interesting finding arose from Boley's experiments[5] in which the superior mesenteric artery was partially occluded. At first, mean vascular resistance distal to occlusion did not rise (in some cases it even fell). Eventually, however, intense vasoconstriction supervened, frequently persisting even after removal of the occlusion. The local pathologic consequence included oedema, haemorrhage, ulceration, stenosis, and even bowel necrosis. As yet, this secondary vasoconstriction cannot be explained, but the ability of ganglion blockers to relieve the vasoconstriction indicates a reflex origin.

Gammon and Bronk[130] first proposed the existence of baroreceptors within the mesenteric circulation. Sarnoff and Yamada[131] claimed that coeliac occlusion caused hypertension, a response that could be abolished by ganglion blockade. Selkurt and Roth[132] confirmed this in the cat but not in the dog. However, a number of opposing views have been advanced. Nissen[133] found no evidence of vasoconstriction, but rather a widespread vasodilation after occlusion. Probably baroreceptors as such do not exist in the mesenteric circulation. Local bowel ischaemia can affect the rest of the cardiovascular system another way, probably by producing circulating vasoactive mediators which act elsewhere in the body (including the heart).

4.5.3 Shock

Shock remains a mystery and a constant source of controversy. Unfortunately, space permits only a few brief comments here. The splanchnic circulation is involved in shock, first relative to storage functions or pooling, and, second, as a generator of possible humoral factors acting on organs outside the gastrointestinal tract. Evidence for maintained vasoconstriction in haemorrhagic shock is equivocal. Reynell et al.[128] maintained that the splanchnic area did not participate in the generalised vasoconstriction occurring elsewhere, but participated in homeostasis by a marked reduction in capacitance. Other workers have obtained different results. Greenway et al.[125] showed marked vasoconstriction in the area drained by the portal vein of cats. Abel et al.[134] also found evidence of vasoconstriction in the gastrointestinal tract of monkeys.

Cannon[135] asked the question 'Where is the blood which is out of currency?' For a long time, the splanchnic area seemed to provide the answer. Much of the early work and more recent studies have been done on the dog. In this species, large volumes of blood are sequestered in the splanchnic area (called 'pooling') during development of shock, but probably not as much as is often thought[136]. Nevertheless, while splanchnic pooling as a discrete phenomenon is no longer believed to occur in most mammalian species, splanchnic veins may still represent a major part of the total systemic venous capacity.

Although control of splanchnic venomotor tone has become accepted as important in the regulation of blood volume, workers disagree about its role in the functional disturbances of shock.

Endotoxin shock has also been studied extensively, particularly in the dog, in which gut circulation has been implicated and the evidence for pooling is convincing[137]. In the monkey, no splanchnic pooling occurs; the main features are slow, progressive decline in arterial pressure with a decrease in mesenteric vascular resistance[138].

4.5.4 Generation of vasoactive substances in ischaemic bowel

Ischaemic states of the gastrointestinal tract are important in another way. The liver is no longer thought to produce vasodepressor material, a chemical substance that reduces peripheral vascular resistance in shock. However, interest has continued in the production of agents in the ischaemic bowel which have their effect elsewhere in the cardiovascular system. Lillehei[139] was among the first to suggest an intestinal factor in irreversible shock. Selkurt[140] isolated vasodilators from the portal vein in shock, but the agents failed to enter the systemic blood. More recently Selkurt and Rothe[141] concluded that such substances were not the lethal agent, prompting the comment from Alexander[74] that 'It would seem high time to call off the search for something which has never been shown to exist and which has been proven not to be there'. Despite this injunction, the search continues. Thus, Fine[142] has advanced much evidence that endotoxin is absorbed from the lumen of the gut across a mucosal barrier damaged by ischaemia. He has also emphasised the importance of the hepatic reticulo-endothelial system in dealing with the supposedly absorbed endotoxin. Again, species differences may exist (the primate gut is not ischaemic[138]), and the dog may experience a unique pathophysiological response in endotoxin shock. Vyden and Corday showed that superior mesenteric vascular occlusion in the dog markedly affects circulation of brain, myocardium and kidney, and depresses both arterial blood pressure and cardiac output[144]. Lefer et al.[145] showed that a myocardial depressor factor (MDF) was generated in the wall of the ischaemic pancreas and gut. They contend that MDF is a peptide with a molecular weight of 800–1000. Similar findings were reported by Williams and Grindlinger[146]. Neither these workers nor Lefer et al.[145] found any evidence of endotoxin involvement in the dog. Thus, the data suggest that ischaemic bowel and pancreas produce blood-borne agents which act on the heart and on peripheral blood vessels. Nevertheless, how important these substances are in the wider picture of shock remains unclear, and what their relation is to Selkurt and Rothe's non-lethal vasodilators is uncertain.

4.6 EFFECT OF ACETYLCHOLINE AND THE VAGUS NERVE ON GASTROINTESTINAL BLOOD FLOW

4.6.1 Effect of acetylcholine

The effect of acetylcholine on the gastrointestinal circulation is controversial. Dale,[147] using plethysmography, was probably the first to show increased gut volume in response to acetylcholine. Nechelles et al.[148] reported that acetylcholine reduced gastric blood flow in the rat, without affecting motility. In dogs, small doses of acetylcholine decreased and large doses increased blood flow. In the canine gut, the results reported by Bülbring and Burn[51] varied, the more common response being a reduction in volume on administration of acetylcholine. According to Gotsev[149], close intra-arterial injections in the dog caused local vasodilatation, but systemic infusions reduced blood flow, partly through mechanical causes and partly via a reflex. In the isolated perfused human stomach, Walder[150] confirmed the variability: in a total of fifteen stomachs, vasoconstriction occurred in seven and vasodilation in eight.

The problem is complex. Many factors can affect blood flow: the direct action of acetylcholine on vascular smooth muscle, the metabolic response to acetylcholine, and the effect of altered gut motility. These have still not been satisfactorily balanced, and it is illogical to postulate a uniform action throughout the whole gastrointestinal tract. However, much evidence has been reported for a predominantly vasodilator action for acetylcholine. Using isolated intestinal segments of the dog, Sidky and Bean[33] showed vasodilatation and a rise in blood flow preceding alterations in motility, which persisted after cessation of movement. Atropine eliminated the motor effects but was not a strong drive nor a primary mechanism. Price et al.[151] had similar results in intact anaesthetised dogs. They demonstrated that the effects of acetylcholine on the bowel wall and on the arterioles were separate: norepinephrine decreased both flow and motility, further confirming the independence of vessel control from bowel movements. Recently, Brobmann et al.[152], using isolated canine gut segments, showed that acetylcholine has a direct vasodilator action on the blood vessels of the gut. In vivo, this action is opposed in various degrees by mechanical factors such as passive or active changes in intraluminal pressure.

4.6.2 Effect of the vagus nerves

In the stomach, the vagus nerve seems to have a direct vasodilator action on mucosal blood vessels[153], whereas it acts on intestinal blood flow predominantly by increasing vascular resistance[153, 154].

Opinions, of course, are not unanimous. Ballinger et al.[155] proposed an action of cholinergic parasympathetic nerves in opposing the sympathetics. In their experiments, vagal section reduced flow through the common mesenteric vein by 42%, much of this being intestinal, although the fall in flow could also have been merely due to abolition of extravascular muscle squeeze.

Vatner et al.[156] studied responses to physiologic activities such as feeding or exercise in conscious dogs. They showed that vasodilator responses in the gastrointestinal tract occurring within 15 min of presenting food were blocked by cholinergic blocking agents but not by thoracic vagotomy, nor by α- and β-adrenergic blocking agents. This still does not specifically demonstrate a vasodilator action of acetylcholine directly on the vessels.

Much of the difficulty would seem to lie in the separation of purely vascular from extravascular responses. In the stomach, the added possibility exists that the vasodilatation associated with vagal stimulation[104] results from secretory activity involving a metabolic intermediary. (The plasma kinins histamine and prostaglandins have naturally been suggested.)

In summary, evidence suggests that acetylcholine is mainly an intestinal and possibly also a gastric dilator, but the evidence for direct participation of the vagus nerve in gastrointestinal vasodilator responses is slight.

4.7 PANCREATIC BLOOD FLOW

4.7.1 Methods and resting values

The pancreatic circulation has been difficult to study, partly because we lack a really satisfactory technique. Until recently, no one seemed to agree on pancreatic blood vessel control. Most early reports were based on plethysmographic studies of pancreatic volume. Unfortunately, while volume may be related to flow, it may not. Direct measurements (often venous outflow) were also made in the early days of pancreatic blood flow research. Later, the thermostrohmuhr applied to the arterial supply enjoyed extended popularity. Recently, electromagnetic flowmeters have come into fashion. However, all these methods involve extensive surgery. With a few exceptions, such as the studies of Delaney and Grim[61] observations have been made on the anaesthetised, freshly operated upon, and partially shocked animal. Clearance techniques have proved elusive. ^{42}K and ^{86}Rb have been used in the Sapirstein fashion[157], but an enormous disadvantage attends the use of these isotopes. Only one observation can be made per animal, imposing obvious limitations on experimental design. A more recent method, which seems to have had some success, is local hydrogen clearance[158]. Heat conductivity has also been used but the results are not truly quantitative.

Most estimations of pancreatic blood flow in the resting animal have ranged between 61 and 129 ml min^{-1} (100 g)$^{-1}$ of tissue. Aune and Semb[158] obtained mean values in the conscious dog of 76 ml min^{-1} (100 g)$^{-1}$, whereas in anaesthetised preparations this fell to 42.8 ml min^{-1} (100 g)$^{-1}$ tissue. Rappaport et al.[159] reported similar values for pancreatic blood flow in the anaesthetised dog. These estimations may be misleading, since the pancreas and the duodenum effectively share the same blood supply and probably the reported values are high. By means of a complex surgical procedure, Rappaport et al.[159] attempted to separate the pancreas from the duodenum. With intact pancreaticoduodenal communications they obtained values close to those of Aune and Semb[158] (using widely different methods). When the duodenal fraction was obliterated, the residual pancreatic flow was greatly reduced to values ranging from 0.08 to 0.16 ml min^{-1}(100 g)$^{-1}$.

4.7.2 Pancreatic blood flow and external secretion

Claude Bernard[160] was perhaps the first to examine pancreatic circulation in relation to its exocrine function. He observed flushing and congestion of the pancreas during digestion. The participation of blood flow in secretory events gained confirmation as the years progressed. Bernstein[161] showed that stimulation of the central end of the cut vagus appeared to inhibit secretion; he thought the mechanism involved reflex vasoconstriction. Heidenhain[162] showed that when the blood pressure in the dog rose, pancreatic secretion fell; when the blood pressure fell, secretion resumed. He interpreted these findings as effects of vasoconstriction or vasodilatation on pancreatic secretion. Gottlieb[163] added further evidence in 1894 (of no more certain calibre than the rest), concluding that the flow of pancreatic juice 'unquestionably is dependent on the supply of blood'. Maltesos and Watson[164] added to the chorus of affirmation with thermostrohmuhr measurements of pancreatic blood flow changes in response to hydrochloric acid administered intraduodenally or secretin given intravenously. They concluded that an initial abrupt rise in flow preceded the secretion and thereafter flow and secretion followed a parallel course.

A complication appeared when Bennett and Still[165] showed that increased pressure in the pancreatic duct itself had a marked dilator effect on pancreatic vessels, probably through reflex pathways. They measured venous outflow directly and concluded that when secretion was unaccompanied by some impairment of pancreatic duct outflow, blood flow did not change during secretion.

Gayet and Guillaume[166] used both a plethysmograph and a thermostrohmuhr to measure volume and flow increases during secretin administration. While these were initially coincident, the increase in volume outlasted the increase in flow, suggesting duct retention. If one accepts the interpretation of Bennet and Still[165], the initial flow increment may have nothing to do with the actual process of secretion. Not surprisingly, Tankel and Hollander[167] remarked, 'There is no conclusive evidence that an increase in glandular activity is invariably accompanied by an increase in blood flow'.

More recent work using more refined methods has helped clarify the situation, though it is still far from satisfactory. Holton and Jones[168] used a light transmission technique to measure pancreatic blood flow. Although this method depends more on blood volume than on flow, they argued that their data could be better interpreted in vascular than secretory terms. They showed that pancreozymin and secretin produced prompt increases in tissue volume, which disappeared within a few minutes and were not abolished by atropine. Delaney and Grim[61], in studies on the conscious dog, reported essentially the same results with secretin, but they found no marked effect for pancreozymin. However, Aune and Semb[158], using hydrogen gas clearance, reported immediate vasodilatation with both secretin and pancreozymin. The effects were transient and flow returned to normal within 20 min, although secretion continued unchanged. These changes are strikingly similar to those of Gayet and Guillaume[166] 36 years earlier. One gets the overall impression that both secretagogues, secretin and pancreozymin, produced marked, brief vasodilator effects in the pancreas.

4.7.3 Pancreatic blood flow and extrinsic nerve control, catechol amines and other vasoactive agents

This aspect of pancreatic circulatory function, too, is clouded by the lack of precise data. For example, no information is available to indicate whether pancreatic blood vessels possess resting vasomotor tone. Workers even disagree on the action of the catecholamines. Barlow et al.[169] produced evidence that, with both epinephrine and norepinephrine administration, pancreatic blood flow first fell and exocrine secretion was inhibited, and then it rose above resting levels while secretion returned to resting levels. During the initial phase of the response, the action of epinephrine on blood flow could be blocked by phenoxybenzamine with no alteration in the inhibition of secretion. Thus, secretion could be inhibited by a direct action of the catecholamines on the secreting cells of the pancreas, or it could result from the opening of unidentified shunts.

These results do not agree entirely with those of Delaney and Grim[61], who found that pancreatic blood flow was increased by norepinephrine and decreased by epinephrine. However, Rappaport et al.[159] recently produced evidence resembling that of Barlow et al.[61], showing that both norepinephrine and epinephrine had marked initial vasoconstrictor effects.

Apparently pancreatic blood flow and secretory activity are not necessarily linked directly. An intact nutrient flow may not be needed for secretion to begin, since the excised rabbit pancreas secretes in vitro at respectable rates. Whether a change in blood flow is a prerequisite for a change in secretory level is uncertain. Beyond this, no secure evidence exists for linearity between flow and secretion. Reports of work involving other pancreatic stimuli clarify matters little. Gayet and Guillaume[166], using a plethysmographic method, reported an increased pancreatic volume with vagal stimulation. Anrep[170] found that vagal stimulation produced no change in flow in his decerebrate animals. On the other hand, Kuznetsova[171] reported increased secretory and blood flow activity during sham feeding in conscious dogs; the blood flow changes were prolonged. Feeding, of course, is a non-specific vasodilator, and these observations may reflect no more than generalised vasodilatation. Histamine reportedly had little effect on pancreatic blood flow, although its effect on pancreatic secretion is known to be marked. Tankel and Hollander[172] claim that it acts directly on the secretory cells. The possible involvement of the plasma kinins, especially kallikrein has, of course, been invoked[168], but any functional importance of these products remains unsubstantiated.

4.7.4 Pancreatic blood flow and endocrine secretion in the pancreas

Rappaport et al.[159] used a preparation in which the pancreas was entirely isolated from the duodenum and gastrointestinal tract. They altered pancreatic flow by norepinephrine administration and established a nearly linear relation between pancreatic blood flow and insulin production. When blood flow was altered by mechanical means, the results were not so clear-cut and there was some suggestion of intrapancreatic shunts. Present evidence indicates that the perfusion of the islets of Langerhans may be important to their secretory activity.

4.8 GASTRIC BLOOD FLOW AND SECRETION

Since the classical observations of Beaumont[52], it has been widely recognised that blood flow in the gastric mucosa increases when secretion is induced.

For years, little more could be said. With time, it became apparent that the stomach (like the rest of the gastrointestinal tract) was not a homogeneous organ and the location of blood flow changes in response to secretion became important. Although technical difficulties hampered experimental work for a long time, recent improvements in flow technology have permitted real advances.

Menguy[173] showed that the distribution of blood to the stomach wall was greatest in the antrum but shifted to the fundus with hypersecretion. Later, electromagnetic flowmeters were placed on individual arteries supplying the stomach and vagal stimulation was shown to cause a 60% increase in blood flow in the corpus but not in the antrum. Histamine, on the other hand, had a widespread effect on both regions. However, measurements of blood flow involving all the tissue layers of the stomach wall could be misleading, since mucosa and muscle need not necessarily react in the same way to a given stimulus, least of all one so specific as secretory stimulus.

A better approach to this problem was found only recently. Delaney and Grim[174] reported the first substantial evidence that secretory flow changes were confined to the mucosa. Using the newly developed aminopyrine clearance technique, Jacobson et al.[175] evaluated the problem quantitatively. They measured mucosal flow and total flow with an electromagnetic blood flowmeter in the conscious dog[45]. Using graded doses of histamine, they showed that secretory rates and blood flow were related. Histamine had little predictable effect on total flow except in large doses, when it produced an increase in blood flow (not temporally linked with the secretory effects). The conclusion was drawn that flow to non-mucosal tissues might even be reduced to compensate for the increase in mucosal flow.

Numerous questions arise. For example, does secretion depend on blood flow at all? Could it occur in the living animal in the absence of blood flow? Evidence indicates that secretion can occur without an effective circulation. Ivy et al.[5] ligated most of the vascular supply to the stomach and only temporarily decreased gastric secretion; mucosal blood flow was not measured. The isolated gastric mucosa has been shown to be capable of secretory activity, but secretory rates are miniscule compared with those of the stomach in situ.

Past pharmacological evidence gave conflicting answers to the question of whether the secretory or the circulatory change is primary, mainly it seems because of a failure to distinguish mucosal from total flow to the stomach. Recently, secretagogues (histamine, gastrin, and bethanecol) have been shown to increase mucosal blood flow and secretion in a dose–response relationship; this is as true for blood flow as for secretory rates[175]. Results with the gastric secretory inhibitors vasopressin, catecholamines, secretin, atropine, prostaglandin E[1] and isoproterenol (all of which depress both flow and secretion) support a positive correlation between flow and secretion[62, 66, 175, 176]. Nevertheless, Jacobson and his colleagues[175] presented reasons why the blood flow changes might not be primary and are not in themselves the cause of the increased secretory rates. Rather, it seems the other way round. The ultimate link between secretion and blood flow is still unknown, but it may be increased H^+ secretion as suggested by Harper et al.[67].

The effect of epinephrine in the active compared with the inactive stomach has generated some interest. Jacobson *et al.*[62] showed that epinephrine inhibited both gastric secretion and gastric blood flow. Delaney and Grim[174,177] using [42]K, showed that epinephrine enhanced mucosal flow and secretion. Cowley and Code[178] attempted to resolve the difficulty using a modification of the aminopyrine clearance method for the non-secreting stomach (the canine Heidenhain pouch). Like previous workers, they found that pitressin, norepinephrine, and a single rapid injection of gastrin all reduced mucosal flow. However, epinephrine increased mucosal flow. They suggested that possibly the difference could be explained by the fact that, in Jacobson's experiments, secretion had already been stimulated by histamine and that the mucosal circulation was already fully vasodilated. The only action remaining to epinephrine would be vasoconstrictive, with epinephrine presumably acting on α receptors.

4.9 INTESTINAL BLOOD FLOW

4.9.1 Intestinal function and blood flow

Until recently, little information was available concerning the relation between blood flow, secretion, digestion, or other metabolic activity in the bowel mucosa. Even today, the field has been inadequately explored.

Reactions to the anticipation and ingestion of food have been clearly described by Vatner *et al.*[156]. Mesenteric flow increases within 5–15 min of presentation of food, reaching a maximum of 115% to 300% of control values within 30–90 min and returning to control levels in 3–7 h. These effects are far too large to be part of the general, non-specific responses to eating. The vasodilator effects are prevented by cholinergic blockade, but not by α- or β-adrenergic blockade, nor by thoracic vagotomy. In dogs that could smell and see, but not eat, the responses were attenuated. The implication is that sympathetic cholinergic transmission might be involved. The critical experiments remain to be done.

These findings are not entirely consistent with those of Grim and Lindseth[23], using labelled microspheres. They reported an increase in total flow of 31%, no increase in mucosal capillary flow, a large increase in arteriovenous anastomotic flow and increased muscularis flow. However, their data should be viewed cautiously, since control experiments could not be performed in the same animals.

Evidence abounds (summarised recently by Bynum and Jacobson) that instillation of hypertonic glucose or foodstuffs into the gut causes an increase in splanchnic blood flow[179]. In our laboratory, we recently found that intravenously injected glucose has powerful gastrointestinal dilator effects[180], probably maximal in the duodenum or upper small intestine. Ample evidence exists that blood flow and oxygen consumption show parallel changes during intestinal absorption of nutrients[181].

The nature of the circulatory–absorptive relationship is unclear. One is tempted to assume that oxygen consumption under these conditions is related to absorption. However, it may be equally involved with the metabolic changes attending absorption, for it is becoming increasingly apparent that the duodenum and upper part of the small intestine, at least, possess endocrine and metabolic functions quite distinct from the processes of secretion, digestion, or absorption.

Glucagon is a potent gastrointestinal vasodilator, producing a 100% rise in hepatic blood flow[181] with a fourfold increase in hepatic glucose output. Portal flow[181] increases dramatically, and marked vasodilation of the superior mesenteric arterial bed occurs[182]. Interestingly despite this increase in mesenteric and hepatic outflows, hepatic arterial resistance rises with glucagon administration. Ross[182] has localised the vascular effects of glucagon specifically to the splanchnic area. In contrast, glucose has widespread effects throughout the body. The action of glucagon is independent of activation of β receptors.

4.9.2 Intensity of intestinal flow responses and capillary filtration in the functioning gut

In the acutely denervated intestine of the cat, Folkow et al.[183] showed the resting blood flow to be between 40 and 60 ml min^{-1}(100 g)$^{-1}$ of tissue. The capillary filtration coefficient was 0.17 ml min^{-1} (100 g)$^{-1}$ tissue. With maximal dilation produced by isoproterenol, flow increments reached levels of 270 ml min^{-1}(100 g)$^{-1}$, at which level the capillary filtration coefficient was about 0.4 ml min^{-1}(100 g)$^{-1}$ [183]. These values are 10 times those reported for skeletal muscle and are for flow in the full thickness of the bowel. Folkow et al.[183] postulated that maximal flow in the mucosa was more likely to be about 500 ml min^{-1} (100 g)$^{-1}$, and that filtration resembles that in the renal glomeruli.

These blood flow variations shed some light on the possible functional importance of shunting mechanisms. It has been said that 'arterio-venous anastomoses are an anatomical expression of functional lability'[184]. Applying this to the bowel, the existence of arterio-venous anastomoses would enable wide variation in mucosal flow in response to local demand, while permitting the continuance of a fairly steady portal blood flow. The contradictory demands of mucosal function and homeostasis could thus be met.

4.9.3 Vascular responses to intraenteric pressure

Mall[185] suggested that raised tension in the bowel wall would decrease blood flow. This conjecture was strengthened by the findings of Anrep et al.[186]. However, Lawson and Chumley[187], using isolated loops of dog ileum, were the first to obtain quantitative evidence. Moderate increments of pressure in the lumen up to 30 mmHg had little effect on blood flow. Further elevation of pressure in the lumen up to mean mesenteric artery pressure had transient effects. Actually, stretching a segment of gut wall directly, although it has a greater effect, still permitted some recovery, and they postulated local vasodilator reflexes.

These results have not been confirmed in vivo, and workers generally agree that raised intraluminal pressure in rats[188], rabbits[189] and dogs[190] reduces bowel wall blood flow. Bean and Sidky[190] pointed out that when bowel tonus was high, blood flow was reduced. Decreased tonus would allow high flow even without contractions, but the presence of rhythmic contractions had a pumping action on bowel wall vessels. Peristalsis was concluded to be an important factor in the propulsion of blood through the intestine[151, 152, 190].

4.9.4 Effect of blood pO_2 and pCO_2 levels on gastrointestinal blood flow

Reactive hyperaemia after release of a vascular occlusion is a dramatic challenge to the vasculature of any organ. In the bowel, it is sluggish and un-remarkable, beginning slowly and lasting much longer than in most other tissues[191]. Repayment of the metabolic debt is slow. During the period of occlusion, then, no spectacular dilation of vessels occurs. The effects that take place are thought to be metabolic and probably not specifically linked to oxygen deficiency.

Many reports of the effects of controlled hypoxia are vague and contradictory. In their isolated perfused preparation, however, Bean and Sidky[190] found marked vasodilation in the bowel when it was perfused with blood containing 7% oxygen. However, when the whole animal was rendered anoxic, blood flow was reduced. This probably represents a reflex through the chemoreceptors[192]. With asphyxia, if the blood pressure rose, the constrictor effect was over-riden and vasodilation occurred. The possible relation of hypercapnia and anoxia to functional activity in the intestine was also investigated by Svanik et al.[193], who found both interventions to be vasodilator, probably having their maximum effect on precapillary sphincters. However, neither was thought to be of major importance for the mediation of functional hyperaemia during digestion.

Seemingly, then, the local effect of hypoxia is vasodilation, but this can be reversed by chemoreceptor-initiated activity or enhanced by receptor stimulation.

Bowel blood vessel responses to hypercapnia have not been extensively studied. Still, good evidence exists[194, 195] that with raised blood CO_2 levels, intestinal vasodilatation occurs independently of tonus or motility. Infusing CO_2 into the lumen of intestinal loops also has marked vasodilator effects.

4.9.5 Effect of other vasodilator agents

Recently, prostaglandins have been shown to exert a marked effect in depressing gastric secretion. Jacobson[176] reported experiments relating secretion to blood flow in the stomach with prostaglandin E_1. After stimulating secretion, either with pentagastrin or with histamine, he observed that both norepinephrine and prostaglandin E_1 inhibited secretion. However, the prostaglandin is a vasodilator, unlike norepinephrine which constricts gastric vessels. He concluded that prostaglandin E_1 inhibited secretion by a direct action on the secretory cells. In the rat, too, locally administered prostaglandin E_2 was shown to be a powerful vasodilator[196], successfully antagonising the constrictor actions of norepinephrine and vasopressin. Prostaglandin E_1 also dilates the mesenteric artery[197].

Other interesting vasodilators in the gut are the plasma kinins: bradykinin kallidin II, and eledoisin[198]. Eledoisin is six times more powerful than bradykinin, but the kinins as a group are among the most effective intestinal vasodilators.

The functional importance of these powerful dilators is hard to assess at this stage. One is tempted to assume that they are tissue hormones operating in circulatory and secretory regulation, but concrete evidence is still lacking.

4.9.6 Effects of exercise and environmental temperature

Exercise seems to cause an initial decrease in bowel blood flow[198], followed by slow compensation, so that blood flow and splanchnic resistance have returned to normal after 30 min. Exercise performed in a warm environment produces long-lasting depression of splanchnic resistance and reduction in blood flow. In bowel mucosa elevation of ambient temperature has been shown to produce a primary elevation of skin blood flow with a reduction in bowel blood flow (presumed to be compensatory)[199]. However, with elevated core temperature, sympathetic action on bowel is lost, and with sufficient temperature elevation, dilation occurs also in the mucosa. These findings might fit the observations of the effect of exercise in gastrointestinal blood flow in a warm environment. However, the reservation mentioned earlier still applies, namely, that mucosal flow may not reflect total flow.

References

1. Barlow, T. E., Bentley, F. H. and Walder, D. N. (1951). Arteries, veins and arteriovenous anastomoses in the human stomach. *Surg. Gynec. Obstet.*, **93**, 657
2. Barclay, A. E. and Bentley, F. H. (1949). The vascularization of the human stomach. *Brit. J. Radiol.*, **22**, 62
3. Barlow, T. E. (1951). Arterio-venous anastomoses in the human stomach. *J. Anat.*, **85**, 1
4. Frasher, W. G. and Wayland, H. (1972). A repeating Modular organisation of the microcirculation of cat mesentery. *Microvascular Research*, **4**, 62
5. Ivy, A. C., Grossman, M. I. and Bachrach, W. H. (1950). *Peptic Ulcer*, 69 (The Blakiston Co.)
6. Heimbecker, R. O. and Richards, K. U. (1972). Clinical and experimental studies of the coeliac compression syndrome. *A. C. Surgeon's Forum*, **213**, 390
7. Boley, S. J. and Gliedman, M. (1971). Circulatory responses to mesenteric ischemia. *Vascular Disorders of the Intestine*, 309 (Appleton-Century-Crofts)
8. Grant, R. T. and Bland, E. F. (1931). Observations on arterio-venous anastomoses in human skin and in the bird's foot with special reference to the reaction to cold. *Heart*, **15**, 385
9. Clark, R. E. and Clark, E. L. (1934). Observations on living arteriovenous communications as seen in transparent chambers introduced into the rabbit's ear. *Amer. J. Anat.*, **54**, 229
10. Schumacher, S. S. (1938). Ueber die Bedeutung der arterio-venosen Anastomosen und der epithelioiden Muskelzellen (Quellzellen). *Z. Mikr. Anat. Forsch.*, **43**, 197
11. Clara, M. (1937). *Die arterio-venosen Anastomosen*, (Leipzig: Barth)
12. De Bussacher, G. (1948). Les anastomoses arterio-veineuses de l'estomac. *Acta Ned. Morph.*, **6**, Nos. 1–2, 87

13. Sherman, J. L. and Newman, S. (1954). Functioning arterio-venous anastomoses in the stomach and duodenum. *Amer. J. Physiol.*, **179**, 279
14. Krogh, A. (1929). *Anatomy and Physiology of the Capillaries*, 2nd ed., (New Haven: Yale)
15. Boulter, P. and Parks, A. (1960). Submucosal patterns of the alimentary tract and their significance. *Brit. J. Surg.*, **47**, 546
16. Zweifach, B. and Metz, D. B. (1955). Selective distribution of blood through the terminal vascular bed of mesenteric structures and skeletal muscle. *Angiology*, **6**, 282
17. Shoemaker, C. P. and Powers, S. R. (1966). The absence of large functional arterio-venous shunts in the stomach of the anesthetised dog. *Surgery*, **60**, 118
18. Buchin, R. F. and Edlich, R. F. (1969). Quantitation of gastric arteriovenous blood flow by the microsphere clearance technique. *Arch. Surg. Chicago*, **99**, 579
19. Spanner, R. (1932). Neue Befunden über die Blutwege der Darmwand und ihre funktionelle Bedeutung. *Morph. Jahrb.*, **69**, 394
20. Thamm, M. (1940). Die portcavalen Venenverbindungen des Menschen. *Zbl. Chir.*, **67**, 1828
21. Jacobson, L. F. and Noer, R. (1952). The vascular pattern of the intestinal villi in various laboratory animals and in man. *Anat. Record*, **114**, 85
22. Brokis, J. G. and Moffat, D. B. (1958). The intrinsic blood vessels of the pelvic colon. *J. Anat.*, **92**, 52
23. Grim, E. and Lindseth, E. O. (1958). Distribution of blood flow to the tissues of the small intestine of the dog. *Minn. Med.*, **30**, 138
24. Delaney, J. P. (1969). Arteriovenous anastomotic blood flow in the mesenteric organs. *Amer. J. Physiol.*, **216**, 1556
25. Folkow, B. (1967). Regional adjustments to intestinal blood flow. *Gastroenterology*, **52**, 423
26. Davidson, J. W., Fletch, A. L., Hobbs, D. B., McIlmoyle, G. and Roech, W. (1973). The technique and applications of lymphography. *Can. J. Comp. Med.*, (in press)
27. Ludwig, C. (1863). Quoted from *Howell's Textbook of Physiology*, (1946), 660 (London Saunders)
28. Schmid, J. (1908). Die grosse des Blutstroms in der Pfortader *Arch. fur gescmbe Physiol.*, **122**, 527
29. Burton-Opitz, R. (1911). The vascularity of the liver. Parts I, II, III and IV. *Quart. J. Exp, Physiol.*, **4**, 93
30. Barcroft, J. and Shore, L. E. (1912). The gaseous metabolism of the liver. *J. Physiol.*, **64**, 1
31. MacLeod, J. J. R. and Pearce, R. G. (1914). The outflow of blood from the liver as affected by variations in the condition of the portal vein and the hepatic artery. *Amer. J. Physiol.*, **35**, 87
32. Blalock, A. and Mason, M. F. (1936). Observations on the blood flow and gaseous metabolism of the liver of the unanesthetised dog. *Amer. J. Physiol.*, **117**, 328
33. Sidky, M. and Bean, J. W. (1958). Influence of rhythmic and tonic contraction of intestinal muscle on blood flow and blood reservoir capacity in dog intestine. *Amer. J. Physiol.*, **193**, 386
34. Bruner, H. D. (1948). Bubble flow meter. *Methods Med. Res.*, **1**, 80
35. Selkurt, E. E. (1948). Measurement of renal blood flow. *Methods Med. Res.*, **1**, 191
36. Cull, T. E., Scibetta, M. P. and Selkurt, E. E. (1956). Arterial inflow into the mesenteric and hepatic vascular circuits during hemorrhagic shock. *Amer. J. Physiol.*, **185**, 365
37. Shipley, R. E. and Wilson, C. (1951). An improved recording rotameter. *Proc. Soc. Exp. Biol. N.Y.*, **78**, 724
38. Rein, H. (1928). Die Thermo-strohmuhr. Ein Verfahren zur fortlaufenden Messung der mittleren Absoluten durch Flussmengen in uneroffneten Gefassen in situ. *Z. Biol.*, **87**, 384
39. Grindlay, J. H., Herrick, J. F. and Mann, F. C. (1941). Measurement of blood flow of the liver. *Amer. J. Physiol.*, **132**, 489
40. Barcroft, H. and Loughridge, W. M. (1938). On the accuracy of the thermostromuhr method for measuring blood flow. *J. Physiol.*, **93**, 382
41. Shipley, R. E., Gregg, D. E. and Wearn, J. T. (1942). Operative mechanism of some errors in the application of the thermostromuhr method to the measurement of blood flow. *Amer. J. Physiol.*, **136**, 263

42. Kolin, A. (1936). An electromagnetic flowmeter. Principle of the method and its application to blood flow measurements. *Proc. Soc. Exp. Biol. N.Y.*, **35**, 53
43. Gregg, D. E. and Fisher, L. C. (1963). *Handbook of Physiology*, Vol. II, 1533, (Amer. Phys. Soc. Washington)
44. Ottis, K., Davis, J. E. and Green, H. C. (1957). Effects of adrenergic and cholinergic drugs on splenic inflow and outflow before and after adrenergic blockade. *Amer. J. Physiol.*, **189**, 599
45. Jacobson, E. D., Eisenberg, M. M. and Swan, K. G. (1966). Effects of histamine on gastric blood flow in conscious dogs. *Gastroenterology*, **51**, 466
46. Franklin, D. L., Schlegel, W. and Rushmer, R. F. (1961). Blood flow measured by Doppler frequency shift of back scattered ultra sound. *Science*, **134**, 564
47. Bayliss, W. M. (1893). On the physiology of the depressor nerve. *J. Physiol. London*, **14**, 303
48. Hallion, L. and Francois-Franck, C. A. (1896). Recherches experimentales executees a l'aide d'un nouvel appareil volumetrique sur l'innervation vaso-motrice de l'intestin. *Arch. dePhysiol.*, **8**, 478
49. Bayliss, W. M. and Starling, E. H. (1899). The movement and innervation of the small intestine. *J. Physiol.*, **24**, 99
50. Clarke, G. A. (1930). The selective vasoconstrictor action of adrenaline. *J. Physiol.*, **69**, 171
51. Bülbring, E. and Burn, J. H. (1936). Sympathetic vasodilation in skin and intestine of the dog. *J. Physiol.*, **87**, 254
52. Beaumont, W. (1833). *Experiments and observations on the gastric juice and the physiology of digestion*, (Plattsburge: Allen)
53. Wolf, S. and Wolff, A. G. (1943). *Human Gastric Function*, (New York: Oxford Univ. Press)
54. White, B., Cobb, S. and Jones, L. (1939). Mucous colitis. *Psychosomatic Medicine*, **1**, 18, (New York: Nat. Res. Council Monograph)
55. Almy, T. P. and Tulin, M. (1947). Alterations in colonic function in man under stress. Experimental production of changes simulating irritable colon. *Gastroenterology*, **8**, 616
56. Shoskes, M. (1948). Responses of colonic muscle to local application of drugs. *Gastroenterology*, **10**, 305
57. Grayson, J. (1949). Vascular reactions in the human intestine. *J. Physiol.*, **109**, 439
58. Sapirstein, L. A. (1956). Fractionation of the cardiac output of rats with isotopic potassium. *Circulation Res.*, **4**, 689
59. Sapirstein, L. A. (1958). Indicator distribution methods in the measurement of splanchnic blood flow of the normal dog. *Liver Function*, **4**, 93 (R. W. Brauer, editor) (Amer. Inst. Biol. Sci. Monograph)
60. Smith, H. W. (1951). *The Kidney: Structure and function in health and disease*, (New York: Oxford Univ. Press)
61. Delaney, J. P. and Grim, E. (1966). Influence of hormones and drugs on canine pancreatic blood flow. *Amer. J. Physiol.*, **211**, 1398
62. Jacobson, E. D., Linford, R. H., Grossman, M. I. (1966). Gastric secretion in relation to mucosal blood flow studied by a clearance technique. *J. Clin. Invest.*, **45**, 1
63. Carryer, H. M. and Ivy, A. C. (1939). Studies on the secretion of sulfanilamide by the digestive glands. *J. Pharmacol. Exp. Ther.*, **66**, 302
64. Davenport, H. S. (1942). The mechanism of the secretion of sulfanilamide drugs in gastric juice. *Yale J. Biol. Med.*, **14**, 589
65. Shore, P. A., Brodie, B. B. and Hogben, C. A. M. (1957). The gastric secretion of drugs: a pH partition hypothesis. *J. Pharmacol. Exp. Ther.*, **119**, 361
66. Jacobson, E. D. (1968). Clearances of the gastric mucosa. *Gastroenterology*, **54**, 434
67. Harper, A. A., Reed, J. D. and Smy, J. R. (1968). Gastric blood flow in anesthetised cats. *J. Physiol.*, **194**, 795
68. Shipley, R. E. and Study, R. S. (1951). Changes in renal blood flow, extraction of inulin, glomerular filtration rate, tissue pressure and urine flow with acute alterations of renal artery blood pressure. *Amer. J. Physiol.*, **167**, 676
69. Ginsburg, M. and Grayson, J. (1964). Factors controlling liver blood flow in the rat. *J. Physiol.*, **123**, 574
70. Carlyle, A. and Grayson, J. (1956). Factors involved in the control of cerebral blood flow. *J. Physiol.*, **133**, 10

71. Folkow, B. and Oberg, B. (1961). Autoregulation and basal tone in consecutive vascular sections of skeletal muscles in reserpine treated cats. *Acta Physiol. Scand.*, **53**, 105

72. Johnson, P. C. (1969). Myogenic nature of increase in intestinal vascular resistance with venous pressure elevation. *Circulation Res.*, **7**, 992

73. Bayliss, W. M. (1902). On the local reaction of the arterial wall to changes in internal pressure. *J. Physiol.*, **28**, 220

74. Alexander, R. S. (1963). The systemic circulation. *Annu. Rev. Physiol.*, **25**, 213 (Annu. Rev. Inc. California)

75. Schmid, H. E. and Spencer, M. P. (1962). Characteristics of pressure flow regulation by the kidney. *J. Appl. Physiol.*, **17**, 201

76. Torrance, H. B. (1961). The control of the hepatic arterial circulation. *J. Physiol.*, **158**, 39

77. Hanson, J. M. and Johnson, P. C. (1966). Local control of hepatic arterial and portal venous flow in the dog. *Amer. J. Physiol.*, **211**, 712

78. Greenway, C. V., Lawson, A. E. and Start, R. D. (1967). The effect of hemorrhage on hepatic artery and portal vein flows in the anesthetised cat. *J. Physiol. (London)*, **193**, 375

79. Grayson, J. (1954). The role of the portal vein in the integration of splanchnic blood flow. *L'Hypertension portale. Le 'Dumping syndrome'. IVe Congres de Gastro-enterologi* 1 (Paris: Masson)

80. Selkurt, E. E., Scibetta, M. P. and Cull, T. E. (1958). Hemodynamics of intestinal circulation. *Circulation Res.*, **6**, 92

81. Trapold, J. H. (1956). Effect of ganglionic blocking agents upon blood flow and resistance in the superior mesenteric artery of the dog. *Circulation Res.*, **4**, 718

82. Johnson, P. O. (1960). Autoregulation of intestinal biood flow. *Amer. J. Physiol.*, **199**, 311

83. Texter, E. C., Jr. Merril, S., Schwartz, M., Van Derstapen, G. and Haddy, P. T. (1961). Autoregulation of intestinal blood flow. *J. Clin. Invest.*, **40**, 1084

84. Folkow, B., Lewis, D. H., Lundgren, O., Mellander, S. and Wallentin, W., (1964). The effect of graded vasoconstrictor fibre stimulation on the intestinal resistance and capacitance vessels. *Acta Physiol. Scand.*, **61**, 445

85. Richardson, D. R. and Johnson, P. C. (1969). Comparison of autoregulatory escape and autoregulation in the intestinal vascular bed. *Amer. J. Physiol.*, **217**, 586

86. Jacobson, E. D., Scott, J. B. and Frohlich, E. D. (1962). Hemodynamics of the stomach. I. Resistance–flow relationships in the gastric vascular bed. *Amer. J. Digest. Disease*, **7**, 779

87. Hanson, K. M. and Johnson, P. C. (1967). Pressure–flow relationships in isolated dog colon. *Amer. J. Physiol.*, 574

88. Hinshaw, L. B. (1962). Arterial and venous pressure–resistance relationships in perfused leg and intestine. *Amer. J. Physiol.*, **203**, 271

89. Oliver, G. and Schafer, E. A. (1865). The physiological effects of the suprarenal capsules. *J. Physiol.*, **18**, 230

90. Brodie, T. G. and Dixon, W. E. (1904). Contributions to the physiology of the lungs, Part II. On the innervation in the pulmonary blood vessels and some observations on the action of suprarenal extract. *J. Physiol.*, **87**, 254

91. Hoskins, R. G. and Cunning, R. E. L. (1917). Effects of adrenaline on the distribution of the blood. V. Volume changes and venous discharge in the intestine. *Amer. J. Physiol.*, **43**, 399

92. Clarke, G. A. (1934). The vasodilator action of adrenaline. *J. Physiol.*, **80**, 429

93. Bülbring, E. and Burn, J. H. (1936). Sympathetic vasodilation in skin and intestine of the dog. *J. Physiol.*, **87**, 254

94. Green, H. D., Deal, C. P., Bardhanabaedya, S. and Denison, A. B. (1955). The effect of adrenergic substances and ischemia on the blood flow and peripheral resistance of the canine mesenteric vascular bed before and during adrenergic blockade. *J. Pharmacol. Exp. Ther.*, **113**, 115

95. Ahlquist, R. P. (1948). A study of adrenotropic receptors. *Amer. J. Physiol.*, **153**, 586

96. Mills, L. C. and Moyer, J. H. (1965). Comparative effects of various sympathomimetic amines and angiotensin on cardiac output and renal blood flow. *Shock and Hypertension*. (New York and London: Grimes and Stratton)

97. Greenway, C. V. and Lawson, A. E. (1968). Effect of adrenaline and propranalol on the superior mesenteric artery blood flow. *Can. J. Physiol. Pharmacol.*, **46**, 906

98. Ross, G. (1967). Effects of epinephrine and norepinephrine on the mesenteric circulation of the cat. *Amer. J. Physiol.*, **212**, 1037

99. Friedman, M. H. F. and Snape, W. J. (1946). Colour changes in the mucosa of the colon of children as affected by food and psychic stimuli. *Fed. Proc.*, **5**, 30

100. Drury, A. N., Florey, H. and Florey, M. E. (1920). The vascular reactions of the colonic mucosa of the dog to fright. *J. Physiol.*, **68**, 173

101. Shoskes, M. (1948). Responses of colonic muscle to local application of drugs. *Gastroenterology*, **10**, 305

102. Grayson, J. and Swan, H. J. C. (1950). Action of adrenaline, noradrenaline and dihydroergocornine in the colonic circulation. *Lancet*, **252**, 488

103. Delaney, J. P. and Grim, E. (1964). Canine gastric blood flow and its distribution. *Amer. J. Physiol.*, **207**, 1195

104. Rudick, J., Semb, L. S., Gunteroth, W. G., Mullins, G. L., Harkins, H. N. and Nyhus, L. M. (1965). Gastric blood flow and acid secretion in the conscious dog under various physiological and pharmacological stimuli. *Surgery*, **58**, 47

105. Bunch, J. L. (1899). On the vasomotor nerves of the small intestine. *J. Physiol.*, **24**, 72

106. Bradford, J. R. (1899). The innervation of the renal blood vessels. *J. Physiol.*, **10**, 358

107. Folkow, B., Frost, J. and Uvnas, B. (1948). Action of adrenaline, noradrenaline and some other sympathomimetic drugs on the muscular, cutaneous and splanchnic vessels of the cat. *Acta Physiol. Scand.*, **15**, 412

108. Kremer, M. and Wright, S. (1932). The effects on blood pressure of section of the splanchnic nerves. *Quart. J. Exp. Physiol.*, **21**, 319

109. Izquierdo, J. J. and Koch, E. (1930). Ueber den Einfluss der Nerven splanchnici auf den arteriellen Blutdruck des Kaninchens. *Z. Kreisl. Forsch.*, **22**, 735

110. Richens, C. A. (1948). Use of freeze drying technique for study of vascular activity. *Science*, **107**, 25

111. Wolf, S. and Wolff, A. G. (1943). *Human Gastric Function*, (New York: Oxford University Press)

113. Folkow, B., Lewis, D. H., Lundgren, O., Mellander, S. and Wallentin, I. (1964). The effect of graded vasoconstrictor fibre stimulation on the intestinal resistance and capacitance vessels. *Acta Physiol. Scand.*, **61**, 445

114. Baker, R. and Mendel, D. (1967). Some observations on 'autoregulatory escape' in cat intestine. *J. Physiol. (London)*, **190**, 229

115. Shanbour, L. L. and Jacobson, E. D. (1971). Autoregulatory escape in the gut. *Gastroenterology*, **60**, 145

116. Grayson, J. and Swann, H. J. C. (1960). Action of adrenaline, noradrenaline and dihydroergocornine on the colonic circulation. *Lancet*, **252**, 488

117. Hulten, L. (1969). Extrinsic nervous control of colonic motility and blood flow. *Acta Physiol. Scand.*, Suppl. 335

118. Grayson, J. and Mendel, D. (1965). *Physiology of Splanchnic Circulation* (London: Arnolds)

119. Selkurt, E. E. and Johnson, P. C. (1958). Effect of acute elevation of portal venous pressure on mesenteric blood volume, interstitial fluid volume and haemodynamics. *Circulation Res.*, **6**, 592

120. Johnson, P. C. (1959). Myogenic nature of increase in intestinal vascular resistance with venous pressure elevation. *Circulation Res.*, **7**, 992

121. Folkow, B. (1967). Regional adjustments to intestinal blood flow. *Gastroenterology*, **52**, 423

122. Selkurt, E. E., Alexander, R. S. and Patterson, M. B. (1947). The role of the mesenteric circulation in the irreversibility in hemorrhagic shock. *Amer. J. Physiol.*, **149**, 732

123. Brobmann, G. F., Underwood, L. D., McCoy, J., Price, W. E. and Jacobson, E. D. (1970). Early regional vascular responses to hemorrhage and reinfusion in dogs. *Surg. Gyn. Obst.*, **131**, 409

124. Grayson, J. and Swan, H. J. C. (1950). Intestinal blood flow change in man during fainting. *J. Physiol.*, **112**, 44P

125. Greenway, C. V., Lawson, A. E. and Stark, R. D. (1967). The effect of hemorrhage on hepatic artery and portal vein flows in the anesthetised cat. *J. Physiol. (London)*, **193**, 375

126. Ginsburg, M. and Grayson, J. (1954). Factors controlling liver blood flow in the rat. *J. Physiol. (London)*, **123**, 574

127. McNeil, J. R., Stark, R. D., Greenway, C. V. (1970). Intestinal vasoconstriction after hemorrhage: roles of vasopressin and angiotensin. *Amer. J. Physiol.*, **219**, 1342

128. Reynell, P. C., Marks, P. A., Chidsey, C. C. and Bradley, S. E. (1955). Changes in splanchnic blood volume and splanchnic blood flow in dogs after hemorrhage. *Clin. Sci.*, **14**, 407

129. Price, H. L., Deutsch, S., Marshall, B. E., Stephen, G. W., Behar, M. G. and Neufeld, G. R. (1966). Hemodynamic and metabolic effects of hemorrhage in man with particular reference to the splanchnic circulation. *Circ. Res.*, **18**, 469

130. Gammon, G. D. and Bronk, D. W. (1935). The discharge of impulses from Paccinian corpuscles in the mesentery and its related vascular changes. *Amer. J. Physiol.*, **198**, 985

131. Sarnoff, J. S. and Yamada, I. S. (1959). Evidence for reflex control of arterial pressures from abdominal receptors with special reference to the pancreas. *Circulation Res.*, **7**, 353

132. Selkurt, E. E. and Rothe, C. F., (1960). Splanchnic baroreceptors in the dog. *Amer. J. Physiol.*, **199**, 335

133. Nissen, O. I. (1965). Peripheral resistance response to occlusion of visceral arteries. *Acta Physiol. Scand.*, **63**, 58

134. Abel, F. L., Waldhausen, J. A. and Selkurt, E. E. (1965). Splanchnic blood flow in the monkey during hemorrhagic shock. *Amer. J. Physiol.*, **208**, 265

135. Cannon, W. B. (1923). *Traumatic Shock* (New York: D. Appleton and Company)

136. Bounois, G. (1971). *Vascular Disorders of the Intestine*, 376 (S. J. Boley, editor) (Appleton-Century-Crofts)

137. Bashour, F. A. and McLelland, R. (1967). Splanchnic circulation in shock. *Gastroenterology*, **52**, No. 2, 461

138. Brobmann, G. F., Ulano, H. B., Hinshaw, L. B. and Jacobson, E. D. (1970). Mesenteric vascular responses to endotoxin in monkey and dog. *Amer. J. Physiol.*, **219**, 1464

139. Lillehei, R. C. (1957). The intestinal factor in irreversible hemorrhagic shock. *Surgery*, **43**, 1043

140. Selkurt, E. E. (1959). Intestinal ischemic shock and the protective role of the liver. *Amer. J. Physiol.*, **197**, 281

141. Selkurt, E. E. and Rothe, C. F. (1962). Critical analysis of experimental hemorrhagic shock in animals. *Fed. Proc. 20 Conference on Shock*, 30

142. Fine, J. (1967). *The Intestinal Circulation in Shock*, **52**, 454

143. Vyden, J. K. (1971). The systemic effects of acute superior mesenteric vascular insufficiency. *Vascular Disorders of the Intestine*, 279 (S. J. Boley, editor) (Appleton-Century-Crofts)

144. Vyden, J. K. and Corday, E. (1968). Hemodynamic consequences of acute occlusion of the mesenteric artery. *Circulation*, **37 & 38**, Suppl. 6, 199

145. Lefer, A. M., Cowgill, R., Marshall, F. F., Hall, L. M. and Brand, E. D. (1967). Characterisation of a myocardial depressant factor present in hemorrhagic shock. *Amer. J. Physiol.*, **213**, 492

146. Williams, L. F. Jr. and Grindlinger, G. (1971). Hemodynamic effects of mesenteric ischemia. *Vascular Disorders of the Intestine*, 297 (S. J. Boley, editor) (Appleton-Century-Crofts)

147. Dale, H. H. (1914). The action of certain esters and ethers of choline and their relation to muscarine. *J. Pharmacol.*, **6**, 147

148. Nechelles, H., Frank, R., Kaye, W. and Rosenman, E. (1936). Effect of acetylcholine blood flow through the stomach and legs of the rat. *Amer. J. Physiol.*, **114**, 695

149. Gotsev, T. (1940). Die Bedcutung der Blutgefässe und des Herzens fur die Regulierung des Blutdruckes. *Arch. Exp. Physiol.*, **195**, 26

150. Walder, D. N. (1952). Arteriovenous anastomoses of the human stomach. *Clin. Sci.*, **11**, 59

151. Price, W. E., Shehadeh, Z., Thompson, G. H., Underwood, L. D. and Jacobson, E. D. (1969). Effects of acetylcholine on intestinal blood flow and motility. *Amer. J. Physiol.*, **216**, 343

152. Brobmann, G. F., Jacobson, E. D. and Brecher, G. A. (1970). Effects of distention and acetylcholine on intestinal blood flow *in vivo*. *Angiologica*, **7**, 140

153. Samoilenko, A. V. (1968). Vascular reactions in the systemic circulation during ileal chemoreflexes and the pressor sino-carotid reflex. *Fiziol. Zh. Sechenov*, **54/3**, 329

154. Kewenter, J. (1965). The vagal control of the jejunal and ileal motility and blood flow. *Acta Physiol. Scand.*, **65, Suppl.** 251

155. Ballinger, W. F., Padula, R. T. and Camishton, R. C. (1965). Mesenteric blood flow following total and selection vagotomy. *Surgery*, **57,** 409

156. Vatner, S. F., Franklin, D. and Va Citters, R. L. (1970). Mesenteric vasoactivity associated with eating and digestion in the conscious dog. *Amer. J. Physiol.*, **219,** 170

157. Sapirstein, L. A. (1958). Regional blood flow by fractional distribution of indicators. *Amer. J. Physiol.*, **193,** 161

158. Aune, S. and Semb, L. S. (1969). The effect of secretin and pancreozymin on pancreatic blood flow in the conscious and anesthestised dog. *Acta Physiol. Scand.*, **76,** 406

159. Rappaport, A. M., Kawamura, T., Davidson, J. K., Lin, B. J., Ohira, S., Zeigler, M., Coddling, J. A., Henderson, M. J. and Haist, R. E. (1971). Effects of hormones and blood flow on insulin output of isolated pancreas in situ. *Amer. J. Physiol.*, **221,** 343

160. Bernard, C. (1856). Memoirs sur le pancreas. *C.R. Acad. Sci.* (Paris), Suppl. **1,** 379

161. Bernstein, N. O. (1878). Zur Physiologie der Bauchspeichelabsonderung. *Arch. a. d. Physiol. Anst. Leipzig*

162. Heidenhain, R. (1875). Beiträge zur Kenntnis des Pancreas. *Arch. Ges. Physiol.*, **10,** 557

163. Gottlieb, R. (1894). Beiträge zur Physiologie und Pharmakologie der Pancreassecretion *Arch. Exp. Path. u. Pharmakol.*, **33,** 261

164. Maltesos, C. and Watson, R. H. (1928). Durchblutung und Sekretion des Pancreas bei humoraler Anregung. *Arch. Ges. Physiol.*, **85,** 410

165. Bennett, A. L. and Still, E. U. (1933). A study of the relation of pancreatic duct pressure to the rate of flow through the pancreas. *Amer. J. Physiol.*, **106,** 454

166. Gayet, R. and Guillaume, M. (1933). Effects des stimulations vagales et secretiniques sur les variations de volume du pancreas. *C.R. Soc. Biol. Paris.*, **112,** 1064

167. Tankel, H. and Hollander, F. (1957). The relation between pancreatic secretion and local blood flow. A Review. *Gastroenterology*, **32,** 633

168. Holton, P. and Jones, M. (1960). Some observations on changes in the blood content of cat pancreas during activity. *J. Physiology.*, **150,** 479

169. Barlow, T. E., Greenwell, J. R., Harper, A. A. and Scratcherd, T. (1965). The effects of adrenaline and noradrenaline on the blood flow, electrical conductance and external secretion of the pancreas. *J. Physiol. (London)*, **178,** 9

170. Anrep, G. V. (1961). The influence of the vagus on pancreatic secretion. *J. Physiol.*, **50,** 421

171. Kuznetsova, E. K. (1963). Characteristics of blood supply of the pancreas during different phases of its activity. *Fed. Proc. Transl.*, Suppl. **22,** 99

172. Tankel, H. and Hollander, F. (1957). A study of the pancreatic response to histamine in dogs with total gastrectomies. *Gastroenterology*, **32,** 642

173. Menguy, R. (1962). Effects of histamine on gastric blood flow. *Amer. J. Digest. Dis.*, **7,** 383

174. Delaney, J. P. and Grim, E. (1965). Experimentally induced variations in canine gastric blood flow and its distribution. *Amer. J. Physiol.*, **208,** 353

175. Jacobson, E. D., Swan, K. G. and Grossman, M. I. (1967). Blood flow and secretion in the stomach. *Gastroenterology*, **52,** (part 2), 414

176. Jacobson, E. D. (1970). Comparison of prostaglandin E_1 and norepinephrine in the gastric mucosal circulation (34509) *Proc. Soc. Exp. Biol. Med.*, **133,** 516

177. Delaney, J. P. and Grim, E. (1964). Canine gastric blood flow and its distribution. *Amer. J. Physiol.*, **207,** 1195

178. Cowley, D. J. and Code, C. F. (1970). Effects of secretory inhibitors on mucosal blood flow in nonsecreting stomach of conscious dogs. *Amer. J. Physiol.*, **218,** 270

179. Bynum, T. E. and Jacobson, E. D. (1971). Blood flow and gastrointestinal secretion. *Gastroenterology*, **60,** 325

180. Durotoye, O. A. and Grayson, J. (1972). (unpublished)

181. Shoemaker, W. G., Van Itallie, T. B. and Walker, W. F. (1959). Measurement of hepatic glucose output and hepatic blood flow in response to glucagon. *Amer. J. Physiol.*, **196,** 315

182. Ross, G. (1970). Regional circulatory effects of pancreatic glucagon. *Brit. J. Pharmacol.* **38,** 735

183. Folkow, B., Lundgren, O. and Wallentin, I. (1963). Studies on the relationship between flow resistance, capillary filtration coefficient and regional blood volume in the intestine of the cat. *Acta Physiol. Scand.*, **57**, 270
184. Grayson, J. (1952). Role of the intestinal circulation in the vascular economy of the body. *A CIBA Foundation Symposium. Visceral Circulation*, 236 (Wolstenholme, editor)
185. Mall, F. P. (1896). A study of intestinal contraction. *Johns Hopk. Hosp. Rep.*, **1**, 37
186. Anrep, G., Cerque, S. and Samaan, A. (1934). The effect of muscular contraction upon blood flow in skeletal muscle, the diaphragm and small intestine. *Proc. Roy. Soc. B.*, **114**, 245
187. Lawson, H. and Chumley, J. (1940). The effect of distension on blood flow through the intestine. *Amer. J. Physiol.*, **131**, 368
188. Oppenheimer, M. J. and Mann, F. C. (1943). Intestinal capillary circulation during distension. *Surgery*, **13**, 548
189. Noer, R. J., Robb, J. H. and Jacobson, L. F. (1951). Circulatory disturbances produced by acute intestinal obstruction in the living animal. *A.M.A. Arch. Surg.*, **63**, 520
190. Bean, J. W. and Sidky, M. M. (1950). Intestinal blood flow. *Fed. Proc.*, **9**, 9
191. Selkurt, E. E., Rothe, C. F. and Richardson, D. (1964). Characteristics of reactive hyperemia in the canine intestine. *Circ. Res.*, **15**, 532
192. Bernthal, T. and Schwind, F. J. (1945). Chemoreflex vascular reactions in leg and intestine. *Amer. J. Physiol.*, **143**, 361
193. Svanik, J., Tyllstrom, J. and Wallentine, I. (1968). Effects of hypercapnia and hypoxia on the distribution of capillary blood in the denervated intestinal vascular bed. *Acta Physiol. Scand.*, **74/4**, 543
194. Sidky, M. M. and Bean, J. W. (1951). Local and general alterations of blood CO_2 and influence of intestinal motility in regulation of intestinal blood flow. *Amer. J. Physiol.*, **167**, 413
195. Pals, D. T. and Steggerda, F. R. (1966). Relation of intra-intestinal carbon dioxide to intestinal blood flow. *Amer. J. Physiol.*, **210**, 893
196. Weiner, R and Kaly, G. (1969). Influence of prostaglandin E_2 on the terminal vascular bed. *Amer. J. Physiol.*, **217**, 563
197. Shehadeh, Z., Price, W. E. and Jacobson, E. D. (1969). Effects of vasoactive agents on intestinal blood flow and motility. *Amer. J. Physiol.*, **216**, 386
198. Chou, C. C., Texter, E. C. Jr. and Frohlich, E. D. (1965). A comparative study of the effects of bradykinin, kallidin II and eledoisin on segmental superior mesenteric resistance. *J. Physiol.*, **176**, 1
199. Grayson, J. (1951). Observations on the temperature of the human rectum. *Brit. Med. J.*, **2**, 1379

5
Gastrointestinal Motility

N. W. WEISBRODT
University of Texas Medical School at Houston

5.1 INTRODUCTION

Motility is often used as an inclusive term with many definitions. To the internist, motility may mean the presence of bowel sounds; to the endoscopist, the visualisation of contraction rings; and to the radiologist, the movement of barium. The physiologist frequently defines motility in terms of the temporal and spatial patterns of muscle contractions and electrical activities. This chapter will describe the primary patterns of contraction in each organ of the gastrointestinal tract, discuss what is known about their effects on movement of the luminal contents, and analyse the factors controlling contractions. Most of the discussion will concern the factors controlling contractile activity, including myogenic factors, nervous elements and the effects of hormones and autocoids on muscle and nerve. Each organ of the gastrointestinal tract will be considered separately, since the contractile events differ sufficiently to make generalisations misleading.

For more detail, the reader may consult one of several recent reviews dealing with the entire gastrointestinal tract[1-6] or with particular organs[7,8].

5.2 OESOPHAGEAL MOTILITY

The oesophagus moves material from the pharynx to the stomach. Much of the oesophagus is located in the thorax, where the pressure is lower than that in the pharynx and stomach. Thus, besides transporting material, the oesophagus must withstand entry of air from the pharynx and gastric contents from the stomach[7].

The oesophagus can be divided into three functional parts: the upper oesophageal sphincter (pharyngeoesophageal sphincter), the body of the oesophagus, and the lower oesophageal sphincter (gastro-oesophageal sphincter). All three have characteristic contractile activities at rest and during a swallow.

5.2.1 Patterns of contraction

At rest (between swallows), the upper oesophageal sphincter is closed[7]. If a pressure-sensing device is placed in the sphincteric area, a zone of 1–5 cm is detected where the pressure exceeds that on either side of the zone by several mmHg[9,10]. This pressure varies, but it may reach 60 mmHg. The body of the oesophagus is flaccid at rest. The measured pressure is the same as that of the body cavity in which the oesophagus lies. In the thorax the pressure varies with respiration, dropping with inspiration and rising with expiration. Code et al.[11] found that the pressure changes reverse with respiration as the stomach is neared. From this point, the intraluminal oesophageal pressure equals intra-abdominal pressure. Because the intra-abdominal segment of the oesophagus is short in most species, it is difficult to study. However, in the opossum this segment is several cm in length; thus, in this animal, one can easily study this area as well as the lower oesophageal sphincter[12]. The lower oesophageal sphincter is also closed between swallows. If one measures pressures here, one finds a zone where the pressure may be 40 mmHg higher than that on either side of the sphincter. The length of the zone may vary from several mm to a few cm[9,13].

During a swallow, the three areas of the oesophagus act in concert. Shortly before the distal pharyngeal muscles contract, the upper oesophageal sphincter relaxes. After sphincteric relaxation, it contracts, often to a higher tone than before relaxation. The body of the oesophagus undergoes peristaltic contraction. The oesophageal muscle just below the sphincter contracts shortly after contraction of the sphincteric muscle. The rest of the oesophageal muscle then contracts sequentially, giving the appearance of a contractile wave moving toward the stomach. After the contraction sequence passes along the oesophagus, the body of the organ becomes flaccid again. Shortly

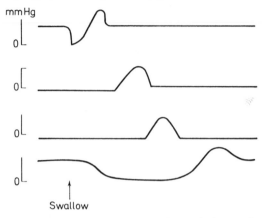

mmHg

Swallow

Figure 5.1 Events in the oesophagus during swallowing. From top to bottom, the tracings represent the upper oesophageal sphincter, the upper thoracic region of the oesophagus, the lower thoracic region, and the lower oesophageal sphincter

before the peristaltic contraction reaches the lower oesophageal sphincter, the sphincter relaxes until the wave of contraction reaches it. It then contracts again, often to a higher level of pressure than before relaxation[9]. This sequence of events is shown in Figure 5.1. Although the time course of these events varies among species, the sequence occurs in all species investigated, despite large differences in the anatomic structure of their oesophagi.

5.2.2 Propulsion of intraluminal material

How a bolus of ingested material traverses the oesophagus depends upon the physical properties of the bolus as well as the contractile activity of the oesophagus. Independent of the properties of the swallowed bolus, both sphincters must relax as the bolus approaches, but peristaltic contraction of the body of the oesophagus is not always necessary for propulsion[7].

Gravity influences movement of fluids down the oesophagus. If a man in an upright position swallows water or other liquids, the bolus actually reaches the stomach several seconds before the peristaltic contraction. For most swallowed material, however, peristaltic contraction is essential for the material to progress normally to the stomach. Often repetitive peristaltic contractions (secondary peristaltic contractions) are required to sweep the bolus fully into the stomach[7].

5.2.3 Control of contractile activity

The upper oesophageal sphincter consists primarily of the cricopharyngeal muscle. This striated muscle is distinct from the rest of the oesophageal muscle and can be identified anatomically as well as physiologically. The mechanisms regulating opening and closure of this sphincter have not been fully defined. Two primary explanations are:

(a) that the sphincter closes passively due to the arrangement of the muscle and is opened by other muscles in the larynx, and

(b) that the cricopharyngeal muscle contracts tonically and relaxes to open the sphincter due to inhibition of muscle activity[14].

The muscle fibres comprising the cricopharyngeus muscle arise from the sides of the cricoid cartilage and pass from one side to the other. Thus, the sphincter consists of the cricoid cartilage anteriorly, and the cricopharyngeus posteriorly. The laryngeal structures to which the sphincter is attached are not stationary but move during deglutition. Upon swallowing, the larynx rises and then descends. In the descended position, the normal elasticity of the sphincteric structures may be responsible for closure; during deglutition, elevation of the sphincter may cause it to open[14].

Electromyographic studies of the cricopharyngeus muscle indicate that, between swallows, the muscle contracts during inspiration but relaxes during expiration[15]. Apparently, then, as long as the pressure differential across the sphincter is small, the muscle does not contract and sphincteric integrity is maintained by structural arrangements of the sphincter. However, alterations of the pressure differential during inspiration can elicit contraction of the cricopharyngeus to facilitate sphincteric closure[10].

During swallowing, the sphincter opens. Although the data are incomplete, the sphincter seems to open by suppression of any cricopharyngeal activity and by displacement of the whole sphincteric area. After relaxation, contraction of the sphincter above resting levels is due to phasic activity of the cricopharyngeus muscle[10,14,15].

Activity of the cricopharyngeus is controlled by motor nerves whose cell bodies lie in the nucleus ambiguus of the medulla. The activity of these neurones co-ordinates with that of the trigeminal, facial, and hypoglossal nuclei. This co-ordinated activity establishes sequential contractions of striated muscle through the pharynx and upper oesophageal sphincter. The nerve cell bodies responsible for this co-ordinated activity have been termed the 'swallowing centre'[14].

The muscle of the body of the oesophagus is arranged in two layers, an outer longitudinal layer and an inner circular layer. The circular muscle probably does most to maintain sphincteric tone and effect peristaltic contraction. The longitudinal muscle contracts and the oesophagus shortens during swallowing. How this contributes to oesophageal function remains uncertain, however[7].

The muscle wall of the oesophagus consists of both smooth and striated fibres. In some species, one type or the other predominates. For example, in dogs almost the whole oesophagus comprises striated muscle. In man, the upper oesophagus consists of striated muscle and the lower of smooth muscle. Despite these remarkable anatomical differences, the contractile activity of the oesophagus is well co-ordinated and is qualitatively similar in all species[7].

The factors controlling peristalsis in the body of the oesophagus could be located at three levels, namely, the central nervous system, the peripheral nerves, and the oesophageal muscle itself. The body of the oesophagus receives extrinsic innervation primarily via the vagus nerves. These nerves are partly of the somatic motor type, arising from the nucleus ambiguus, and are cholinergic. They presumably synapse directly with striated muscle fibres of the oesophagus[14,16]. The visceral motor nerves arise mainly from the dorsal motor nucleus of the vagus and supposedly synapse with the cells of the myenteric plexus[7]. In addition to these cholinergic nerves, the vagus contains adrenergic nerve fibres which arise from the superior cervical ganglion and synapse primarily on the cells of the myenteric plexus[17]. Recently, a third type of nerve, the non-adrenergic inhibitory nerve, has been described in other areas of the gastrointestinal tract[18]. One would not be surprised to find these in the oesophagus, as well.

One of the first theories proposed for the control of oesophageal peristalsis was that a 'centre' in the brain stem sent a series of sequential impulses to progressively distal segments of the oesophagus. This sequential activation resulted in a peristaltic contraction. Evidence favouring this theory was gathered by Kronecker and Meltzer and by Mosso (cited by Ingelfinger[7] and Doty[14]). They found that transection of the canine oesophagus would not interrupt the peristaltic sequence, whereas bilateral vagotomy would. Additional evidence was presented that cooling of carotid blood caused the peristaltic contraction to slow by 20% or more[14]. Perhaps the most convincing experiments supporting central control were performed by Roman[19] in sheep. He demonstrated sequential firing of vagal neurones in the central nervous system (CNS) coincident with oesophageal peristalsis.

These experiments demonstrating CNS control were performed on animals with oesophagi composed exclusively of striated muscle. However, even for striated muscle oesophagi some data indicate that the CNS does not totally control peristalsis. Thus, the explanation that the CNS controls motility predicts that once a contraction has started, it should proceed to completion whether a bolus is swallowed or not. However, Longhi and Jordan[20] reported that in the oesophagus of the conscious dog, peristaltic sequences after swallowing occurred in this striated muscle oesophagus only when a bolus was swallowed. Evidence for the central control of peristalsis in smooth muscle oesophagi is lacking. In fact, some evidence tends to negate a role for the CNS in these oesophagi; e.g. peristaltic contractions still occur in the smooth muscle portions of the feline oesophagus after bilateral cervical vagotomy[7]. Furthermore, Christensen and Lund[12] were able to elicit peristaltic contractions in the smooth-muscle portions of the excised opossum oesophagus which had been placed in an organ bath.

A highly-developed system of nerve cell bodies and endings lies between the longitudinal and circular muscle layers. This is the myenteric plexus. This system resembles that in much of the rest of the gastrointestinal tract. The plexus is especially well represented in the areas of the oesophagus composed of smooth muscle, but it also exists in areas of striated muscle. The cell bodies of the plexus receive input from the extrinsic nerves and from sensory nerves arising in the oesophagus itself. In addition to these nerves, many afferent nerves arise in the oesophagus and flow to the CNS[7]. The nerves of the myenteric plexus could act as modulators of the swallowing centre in the CNS, and/or as a distinct entity capable of initiating and sustaining a peristaltic sequence in the oesophagus. Afferent nerve activity is important in determining the course and character of peristaltic contractions. A ligature tied around the oesophagus will inhibit the passage of a peristaltic contraction[21]. Also, the intensity of contraction of the oesophageal muscle varies with the size of the bolus swallowed[22]. Indeed, afferent stimulation is so important that a peristaltic sequence may not even occur unless a bolus is swallowed to elicit afferent stimulation. Afferent stimulation affects contraction in smooth-muscle oesophagi as well as in striated-muscle organs. Nevertheless, CNS connections are not needed to elicit peristalsis in the isolated oesophagus of the opossum, so afferent stimulation must do something other than simply modulate the swallowing centre.

Experiments have demonstrated that local intrinsic nerves (myenteric plexus) may be able to control peristaltic contractions. In the cat and monkey, the smooth-muscle portions of the oesophagus renew their peristaltic activity 3–7 days after bilateral cervical vagotomy[7]. Furthermore, the smooth muscle portions of the opossum oesophagus undergo peristaltic contraction *in vitro*[12]. An intact myenteric plexus may not be the sole regulator but apparently it is essential for normal peristaltic contractions. In certain diseases, the oesophageal myenteric plexus is destroyed, accompanied by disruption of peristaltic contractions[7].

The third factor controlling peristalsis could lie in the oesophageal muscle itself. Experiments on smooth muscle from the longitudinal and circular muscle layers of the opossum oesophagus have demonstrated gradients of contractile activity along the oesophagus[23]. Strips of longitudinal muscle placed in a bathing medium containing 18 mM KCl contract rhythmically, although the frequency of contraction is not the same for all strips. The frequency decreases progressively for strips taken 6 cm from the lower oesophageal sphincter to strips taken 1 cm from the sphincter. Thus, the longitudinal muscle of the oesophagus has an inherent frequency of contraction. This gradient resembles the frequency gradient in the small bowel (see later). In the small intestine, a characteristic electrical activity accounts for the frequency gradient—termed the basic electrical rhythm (BER) or slow wave. Such an electrical event has not been recorded from oesophageal muscle. Strips of circular smooth muscle do not contract spontaneously. They do contract in response to electrical stimulation. In these unique responses, the contraction does not commence until the stimulus is stopped[12]. This 'off-response' apparently results from stimulation of intrinsic nerves, since it is inhibited by tetrodotoxin (an agent that blocks the activity of many nerves)[24]. The time between the end of the electrical stimulus and the beginning of the contraction is longer for strips taken near the lower oesophageal sphincter than for strips taken more orad. Thus, a gradient also exists in the response of the circular muscle layer (Figure 5.2)[23].

All our information about the control of peristaltic contraction in the body of the oesophagus is difficult to unify. A description that appears reasonable follows: probably the CNS, peripheral nerves, and the muscle itself act in concert to co-ordinate contraction The relative importance of each factor may vary, depending upon the area of oesophagus considered and the type of muscle present. Activity of the upper oesophageal sphincter is co-ordinated with that of the pharyngeal musculature by nerves in the 'swallowing centre' The striated muscle segment of the oesophageal body may also be controlled primarily by the 'centre'. However, afferent and intrinsic nerve activity modulates and may even co-ordinate activity. The smooth muscle portions of the oesophagus may depend upon CNS activity

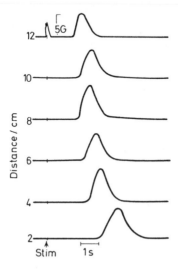

Figure 5.2 Contractile response of isolated strips of circular muscle from different levels of the oesophagus. Arrows and vertical line indicate time of stimulation. Distances are in cm from the gastro-oesophageal junction. (From Weisbrodt and Christensen[23] by courtesy of Williams and Wilkins)

only to initiate a contractile sequence. Once the sequence begins, however, it is co-ordinated by differences in activity of the local nerves and muscles themselves.

The lower oesophageal sphincter comprises the last few cm of muscle of the distal oesophagus. Anatomically, this area is indistinguishable from the rest of the distal oesophagus, and is often described as a 'physiological sphincter'[7]. Much recent work has attempted to answer two questions: what is responsible for sphincteric closure? and, what is the mechanism of sphincteric relaxation?

Normally, the junction between the oesophagus and stomach is closed. If a pressure-sensing device is placed in the area, a pressure of several millimetres of mercury is recorded[7]. There are three likely mechanisms for control of sphincteric closure:

(a) tonic activity of nerves innervating sphincteric muscle,

(b) blood-borne substances acting on sphincteric muscle, and

(c) activity inherent in the muscle cells themselves.

The lower oesophageal sphincter is innervated by fibres of the vagosympathetic trunk. Preganglionic cholinergic fibres arise mainly from the dorsal motor nucleus of the vagus and terminate mainly on cell bodies of the myenteric plexus (see later). Postganglionic adrenergic fibres arise mainly from the superior cervical and celiac ganglion and synapse with cells of the myenteric plexus, as well as with muscle cells. In addition to these classical nerve fibres, a third, non-adrenergic inhibitory fibre may also innervate the lower oesophageal sphincter. The origin and distribution of these fibres is unknown. A dense intrinsic nerve net also exists between the circular and longitudinal muscle fibres. These nerve cell bodies and endings constitute the myenteric plexus. Axons from cell bodies in this plexus innervate the smooth-muscle cells. Nervous activity may help maintain sphincteric closure, but it is not the sole determinant. Bilateral vagal section does not completely cause sphincteric relaxation, and destruction of the myenteric plexus by disease actually heightens sphincteric tone[7].

Recent experiments[25-27] indicate that gastrin is responsible for maintaining sphincteric contraction. Infusion of this hormone or stimulation of its release from the gastric antrum increases sphincteric tone, and removal of the hormone relaxes the sphincter. The hormone may not exert a direct effect upon the muscle cells, however. Instead, acetylcholine may be released from intrinsic nerves in the sphincter[28].

The smooth muscle of the sphincteric region itself possesses properties contributing to its sphincteric action. Although the muscle appears to resemble the rest of the oesophageal smooth muscle anatomically, it responds differently to various stimuli. Christensen[29] and Lipshutz and Cohen[30] found that muscle from the sphincteric region is much more responsive to acetylcholine, norepinephrine and gastrin than is the rest of the oesophageal smooth muscle. The difference in threshold doses needed to produce contraction may approach 100-fold. Sphincteric muscle may also have characteristic electrical activity. Arimori et al.[31] reported the presence of slow, phasic changes of potential of 1.4–2.1 Hz in the dog. These potentials occurred between swallows when the sphincter contracted and disappeared during swallowing when the sphincter relaxed[31]. Thus, the electrical activity of the cells themselves may cause tonic contraction of the lower oesophageal sphincter.

During swallowing, the lower oesophageal sphincter relaxes. The mechanism remains unclear, but probably it is mediated via the nervous system. Stimulation of the vagus nerves or distension of the lower oesophagus causes the sphincter to relax[7]. In addition, isolated sphincteric muscle with the intrinsic nerves intact relaxes with electrical stimulation[32]. This response is blocked by agents that block nervous activity (e.g. tetrodotoxin and local anaesthetics). The sphincter can also be relaxed by means other than swallowing and nervous activity. Recently, secretin has been shown to produce relaxation of the lower oesophageal sphincter, although the mechanism is obscure. However, the hormone does competitively inhibit the contraction produced by gastrin[26,33]. Interactions of gastrin and secretin may determine sphincteric tone between swallows.

Lately, a unifying hypothesis has been proposed for the contractile sequence in the distal oesophagus composed of smooth muscle. According to this hypothesis, after a swallow the responsible nerves to the entire smooth-muscle segment are excited simultaneously. This inhibits the circular muscle. Since all of the muscle, except the distal oesophageal sphincter, is already relaxed, relaxation is noted only at the lower oesophageal sphincter. Upon recovery from this inhibition, the muscle at all levels demonstrates a rebound contraction, and, because of the gradient in latency of the contraction (see above), the contraction appears as a peristaltic sweep down the oesophagus.

5.3 GASTRIC MOTILITY

The musculature of the stomach must contract to perform three main functions. First, the stomach serves as a reservoir to accept large volumes of material during eating. Secondly, it mixes the ingested food with gastric

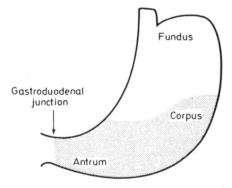

Figure 5.3 Regions of the stomach.
Stippled area indicates caudad region

juice so that digestion can occur. And third, it propels material into the small bowel.

In terms of these motor functions, the stomach can be divided into two parts (Figure 5.3):

(a) the orad portion, consisting of the fundus and part of the corpus, and
(b) the caudad portion, consisting of the distal corpus and antrum[34].

These two areas differ in their contractile activities.

5.3.1 Patterns of contraction

On visual inspection, the orad stomach exhibits little contractile activity, an impression confirmed by measurement of intraluminal pressure and muscle activity. A pressure-sensing device in the orad stomach detects a resting pressure identical to intra-abdominal pressure. Superimposed on the resting pressure are various types of phasic pressure changes. The predominant pressure changes are of low amplitude and long duration (1 min or more)[35]. Some of the pressure changes may reflect activity in the antrum. This activity could be transmitted through the gastric contents to the fundus. However, isolated pouches of the orad stomach are also active[36]. The resting pressure in the orad stomach varies little with the volume of the gastric contents (within limits). The human stomach can accommodate 1600 ml of air with a rise in pressure of less than 10 mmHg[37]. Part of the accommodation may be due to the sliding of cells or layers of cells over one another[3]. However, the increase is at least partly due to relaxation of the muscle cells themselves. Experiments by Cannon and Lieb[33] and later by Lind et al.[36] demonstrated that the orad stomach relaxes upon deglutition. With repetitive swallowing, the orad stomach stays relaxed until the last swallow, after which it recontracts. (A phenomenon called 'receptive relaxation'.) This may play a role in the ability of the stomach to accommodate. As the stomach empties, the orad region contracts, but intragastric pressure stays nearly equal to intraabdominal pressure, presumably due to tonic contraction of the gastric musculature. Whether the muscle merely contracts to accommodate the remaining gastric contents or whether the muscle contracts to propel material into the caudad stomach remains unknown.

The caudad portion of the stomach (distal corpus and antrum) exhibits marked contractile activity. The proportion of time that this area actively contracts varies with the presence and nature of the gastric contents. Contractions can be seen beginning in the midstomach and moving toward the gastroduodenal junction. These contractions usually increase in depth and velocity as they approach the junction. Occasionally, the contractions fail to penetrate the distal antrum, but usually they do, and the terminal antral segment (including the pylorus) contracts almost simultaneously. Thus, the primary contractile event in the stomach, as in the oesophagus, is a peristaltic contraction[35,37]. A pressure-sensing device in the non-contracting distal stomach records a pressure which is near intra-abdominal pressure. With contractile activity, various pressure changes are recorded. These changes have been divided into types I, II and III[35,37]. Types I and II are very similar, differing only in amplitude. They are rhythmic increases in pressure. Their duration and frequency depends upon the species investigated. In man, the durations range between 2 and 20 s and occur at a maximum frequency of 2–4 contractions per minute. Multiple pressure sensors indicate that the pressures occur throughout the caudad stomach with a proximal-to-distal phase lag (Figure 5.4). Thus, types I and II waves probably represent pressures generated by visible peristaltic contractions. Type III waves are described as tonal pressure changes lasting ca. 1 min. They usually occur with superimposed type I or II waves. Since the pressures produced by contractions at any point in the stomach can be transmitted to other areas of the stomach via the gastric contents, some of the tonal waves may represent the summated activities of multiple areas of the stomach. Tonal pressures have been recorded from isolated pouches, but the muscle contractions responsible for these pressures remain unidentified. Bass and his co-workers[39] measured gastric muscle contractions directly, using straingauge transducers. These transducers are sutured to the serosal surface of the stomach and measure activity of the muscle beneath the sensor.

Recordings with these units reaffirm the presence of contractions in the caudad stomach. During the interdigestive and fasting states, the frequency and amplitude of the contractions are sometimes unrelated between the

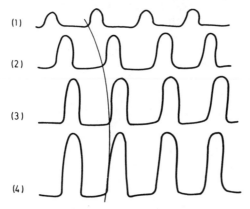

Figure 5.4 Intragastric pressures recorded at multiple sites in the caudad stomach. Traces 1–4 represent progressively distal portions of the stomach. The solid line connecting the beginning of the contractions at multiple sites indicates decrease in phase lag at regions nearer the gastroduodenal junction

distal body and the antrum. Thus, not all contractions sweep over the entire caudad stomach. To date, these units have detected only phasic activity. However, the ability of these transducers to record slow tonal changes is limited.

5.3.2 Propulsion of intraluminal material

As one might expect from the different mechanical behaviours of the orad and caudad regions of the stomach, the movements of the gastric contents also differ in the two areas. Ingested solids tend to accumulate in the orad portion of the stomach. Little mixing occurs here, and the food remains in layers[37]. Liquid tends to flow past the solid material and move toward the caudad stomach. The suggestion has been made that swallowed material follows a definite path along the lesser curvature, but this has not been confirmed. Material in the caudad stomach is actively mixed. Gastric contents in front of a peristaltic contraction are propelled toward the gastroduodenal junction. This includes both liquids and solids. As the contraction approaches the junction, some of the contents are evacuated into the duodenum. However, the contraction does not occlude the lumen, and most of the liquid and practically all of the solid material are propelled back into the proximal portion of the stomach (termed 'retropulsion' by Carlson et al.[40]). These movements thoroughly mix the antral contents. Thus, contractions of the caudad stomach have two purposes: they propel material into the duodenum, and they mix the gastric contents.

5.3.3 Control of contractile activity

Gastric contractions result from the activity of smooth-muscle cells, arranged in three layers: an outer longitudinal layer, a middle circular layer and an inner oblique layer. None of these layers completely envelops the entire stomach. The longitudinal layer is absent on the anterior and posterior surfaces. The circular layer is absent in the paraoesophageal region. The oblique layer is the least complete, being formed from two bands of muscle lying on the anterior and posterior surfaces. These two muscle bands meet orally at the gastro-oesophageal sphincter and fan out to fuse with the circular muscle layer in the caudad part of the stomach. The circular and longitudinal muscle layers thicken as they approach the duodenum. In some animals, thickening is prominent at the junction of the stomach and small bowel (called the 'pyloric sphincter')[16]. In other species, notably the dog, the muscular thickening is minimal[41,42].

The stomach is richly innervated with both intrinsic and extrinsic nerves. Many intrinsic nerve cell bodies lie in various plexuses. The most prominent, the myenteric plexus, lies in a three-dimensional matrix throughout the circular muscle layer. These nerve cells synapse with nerve endings from other intrinsic neurones in the plexus, as well as with endings of extrinsic nerves. Axons from these neurones synapse with the muscle and glandular cells of the stomach. In addition to the plexuses, numerous receptors are present in the mucosal lining and in the muscle wall of the stomach. Cell bodies of these receptors lie within both the plexuses and the extrinsic ganglia. Extrinsically, the stomach is innervated by branches of the vagus nerves and by fibres originating in the celiac plexus. Most fibres in the vagal nerves are afferents rising from receptors in the stomach and small bowel. The efferent fibres are of two main types: cholinergic stimulatory and non-adrenergic inhibitory. Cell bodies of the cholinergic nerves are located in the dorsal vagal nucleus, and their axons synapse primarily with the cell bodies of the intrinsic plexuses. The origin and distribution of the non-adrenergic inhibitory fibres is unknown. The fibres from the celiac plexus are both afferent and efferent. The afferent fibres arise from receptors in the stomach, but little is known of their pathways. The efferent fibres are mainly postganglionic adrenergic fibres which synapse with the neurones of the intrinsic plexuses and with glandular and muscle tissue directly[16,43].

The contractile activity of the stomach can be controlled through at least four mechanisms:

    (a) activity of the extrinsic nerves,
    (b) activity of the intrinsic nerves,
    (c) activity of the smooth-muscle cells themselves, and
    (d) the action of local and blood-borne chemicals.

Because the existence and importance of each of these mechanisms may differ in the orad and caudad stomach, control of these regions will be discussed separately.

Control of the orad stomach has received little study. Apparently, control occurs mainly through nervous and hormonal mechanisms. Several experiments by Jansson and Martinson[44,45] and others[43] have shown that receptive relaxation is due to a nervous reflex having its afferent and efferent pathways in the vagus nerves. If the vagal nerves are transected, receptive relaxation is impaired. Moreover, the stomach becomes less distensible[46]. The inhibitory neurotransmitter at the nerve-smooth muscle junction is unknown, but it appears not to be an adrenergic amine. The response to vagal stimulation depends on many factors, including the strength and frequency of the stimulus and the contractile state of the muscle during stimulation. Both contraction and relaxation of the orad stomach can be induced by stimulating the vagus nerve[44]. Records from vagally-denervated pouches of the orad stomach show contractile activity[47]. Thus, vagal innervation is not absolutely necessary for contraction. However, the activity of these pouches may differ markedly from that of the intact innervated stomach. Sympathetic denervation of the orad stomach is difficult to perform and its effects are unknown. Sympathetic stimulation can lead to relaxation, probably due to the release and effects of catecholamines[48].

Little is known about the activities of the muscle cells of the orad stomach. The cells have resting potentials about the same as those of other smooth muscles and action (or spike) potentials occur periodically that initiate contractions[49]. No spontaneous fluctuations in membrane potential are recorded from muscle cells of the orad stomach either *in vitro* or *in vivo*[50]. This is one of the most striking differences between the muscles of the orad and caudad stomach. Contractile activity of these cells does not depend on neural activity, but is modulated by activity of the intrinsic nerves.

Contractions of the orad stomach are influenced by the gastrointestinal hormones, although the physiological importance of their effects is uncertain. Gastrin stimulates[51] while secretin[47] and cholecystokinin[52] inhibit contractions. The effects of autocoids, such as serotonin, histamine and prostaglandins, depend on the species and will not be discussed here.

In summary, our scant knowledge of the function and control of the motility of the orad stomach permits few conclusions. The best-known function, receptive relaxation, apparently depends upon a reflex whose pathways are via the vagal nerves.

Control of contractions of the caudad stomach is better understood. Since the primary contractile event in this area is a phasic contraction progressing toward the gastroduodenal junction, our discussion will be limited to the control of this type of contraction. The smooth-muscle cells of the distal stomach have a resting membrane potential resembling that of other smooth-muscle cells. In this region, however, the potential fluctuates rhythmically with a cyclic depolarisation and repolarisation of 5–15 mV. This phenomenon, first reported by Alvarez and Mahoney[53] and by Bozler[54], has several names: basic electric rhythm (BER), pacesetter potential, control activity and slow wave. The last term will be used in this discussion. The slow wave is always present, regardless of the presence or absence of contractions. Its frequency varies among species, but in a given animal the frequency is almost constant. Simultaneous recordings of both electrical and mechanical activities have shown that there is no mechanical correlate to the slow wave. Contractions, when they occur, are preceded by a second electrical event. This event is a more-rapid depolarisation of the membrane, going by any of these names: spike bursts, action potentials, second potentials and response activity[55]. Interestingly, recordings made with extracellular electrodes do not always show fast phasic electrical activity. More often, the investigator detects a slower change in potential. The reasons for this are unclear. Spike potentials, when they occur, are always associated with slow waves. One spike burst usually accompanies each slow wave, and it occurs during a specific period of the slow-wave cycle (Figure 5.5). Thus,

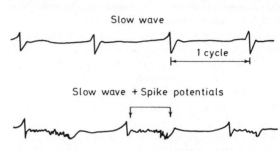

Figure 5.5 Slow waves (top trace) and slow waves accompanied by spike potentials (bottom trace) which are representative of the caudad stomach.

although the slow waves do not directly initiate contractions, this event determines the maximum frequency and timing of the mechanical contraction.

If electrodes are placed along the serosal surface of the stomach, slow waves can be recorded from multiple sites in unanaesthetised animals. The slow waves have the same frequency at all sites, but they do not appear simultaneously at all points along the stomach[50]. Rather, a phase lag occurs so that they seem to pass from an orad point on the greater curvature toward the lesser curvature and toward the gastroduodenal junction[34,56]. The phase lag varies from species to species. In any given animal, the lag between equidistant points becomes less as the gastroduodenal junction is neared

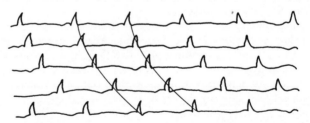

Figure 5.6 Slow waves recorded from multiple sites in the caudad stomach. From top to bottom, tracings are from progressively distal areas of the stomach. Solid lines connecting slow waves indicate the decrease in phase lag in regions nearer the gastroduodenal junction

(Figure 5.6). Thus, slow waves not only determine the timing of a contraction at one locus, they determine the direction and apparent velocity of a 'peristaltic' contraction.

The slow wave appears to be generated by muscle cells in the longitudinal muscle layer and to spread electrotonically into the other layers (mainly circular) to co-ordinate their contractile activities. If the gastric musculature is transected at various levels, slow-wave activity is still recorded at all sites below transections. In these instances, however, the frequencies will not be the same over the entire stomach, nor will the phase lag be constant across a line of transection. The wave frequency in the transected stomach tends to be highest on the greater curvature near the most orad portion of the electrically active stomach. Across lines of transection, the frequency drops progressively as the gastroduodenal junction and lesser curvature are reached[34,56,57]. From these and other experiments, Sarna *et al.*[34] have suggested that slow waves appear as if generated by a matrix of bidirectionally coupled relaxation oscillators. A relaxation oscillator has the capacity to discharge at a constant frequency. Furthermore, it can be influenced within limits by other oscillators, so that its charge–discharge frequency can be altered from its inherent frequency. If relaxation oscillators are placed in a chain and adjusted so their intrinsic frequencies decrease from one end to the other, one has a system resembling the slow-wave pattern seen in the transected stomach. If the oscillators are coupled, however, they oscillate together at the same frequency. In addition, a phase lag would occur in the oscillations from one end of the chain to the other, resembling the orad to caudad slow-wave pattern seen in the intact stomach. Recently, gastric slow waves have been modelled by using a matrix of bidirectionally coupled relaxation oscillators.

Slow waves and spike bursts are generated by the muscle cells themselves. They are influenced by nervous activity and by humoral agents. Vagal nerve transection leads to a decrease in spike-burst activity and fewer contractions. Not only are mechanical contractions less frequent, they are weaker[58]. Vagotomy also affects slow-wave activity. The slow waves become disorganised; i.e. the phase lag varies in both duration and direction. In dogs, Kelly and Code[59] found these alterations to be transient, with the orad-to-caudad phase lag being re-established within a few days. However, the phase lag may be permanently increased. Stimulation of the vagus usually increases the frequency and force of contractions, although the responses are variable. Little is known about the effects of sympathetic nerve section or stimulation on the electrical activity of the caudad stomach. Usually, sympathetic nerve activity depresses contractile activity. The extrinsic nerves provide the pathways for a number of reflexes influencing contractile activity. These reflexes can increase or decrease contractions. Their effects on electrical activity are unknown[48].

The influence of the intrinsic nerves on contractions of the caudad stomach is hard to assess. The stomach does partly recover from vagotomy, perhaps due to the myenteric plexus.

The gastrointestinal hormones, gastrin, secretin and cholecystokinin, influence gastric contractions and electrical activity. Gastrin causes increases in both the frequency and force of contraction[60,61] (although some workers report that force may be decreased)[51,62]. Gastrin also increases the frequency of the slow wave[61,62] (this is one of the few agents or procedures that can alter slow-wave frequency; recently, Kelly and LaForce[63] demonstrated that slow-wave frequency can also be altered by electric stimulation of the muscle layers). Gastrin does not affect the phase lags of the slow waves along the stomach. In addition, the incidence of slow waves accompanied by spike bursts is increased. Secretin inhibits contraction and lowers the incidence of spike potentials[60,64,65]. It has little effect on either the frequency or phase lag of the slow waves. The effects of cholecystokinin are unclear. Both inhibition and no effect have been reported[60,64,65]. Its effect on electrical activity appears slight[65]. The frequency and phase-lag pattern of the slow waves remain unchanged, and little change occurs in the incidence of spike bursts (the spike bursts might have led to contractions of lower amplitude after cholecystokinin). Recently, a new polypeptide has been isolated from the small intestine that enhances contractions of the stomach. This substance differs from gastrin structurally and physiologically, and has been named 'motilin' by Brown *et al.*[66]. Its effects on gastric electrical activity are unknown.

In summary, 'peristaltic' contractions of the caudad stomach can be influenced in their occurrence, force, frequency, direction and velocity. Whether contractions occur is influenced primarily by nervous (intrinsic and extrinsic) and hormonal mechanisms, although local distension of the smooth-muscle cells may also contribute. Apparently, the force of contraction also depends on nervous and hormonal interactions. The frequency of contractions, once contractions are initiated, is regulated primarily by the frequency of the gastric slow wave. This frequency is fairly constant, but it is altered by ingestion of food, administration of gastrin and vagal stimulation (the effect of vagal stimulation may be mediated by gastrin release). The direction and velocity of the 'peristaltic' contraction depends primarily on the phase-lag pattern of the slow wave. The phase-lag pattern is highly constant, apparently being altered only by vagotomy and gastric section.

5.4 GASTRIC EMPTYING

The rate at which material passes from the stomach into the duodenum depends on many factors, the physical and chemical composition of the material in the stomach being among the most important[67-69]. Solid material, material that contains lipid, or solutions with osmotic pressure deviating from near isotonic or containing acid, all empty at rates slower than the emptying rate of 200 mosmal saline.

Studies performed over the past century have demonstrated the presence of 'receptors' in the duodenum that respond to the chemical composition of the material bathing the duodenal mucosa. Hunt *et al.*[69] have identified three types of receptors: those responding to the osmotic pressure of solutions, those responding to acid, and those responding to lipid. Activation of these receptors slows gastric emptying. Neither the identity of the receptor nor the manner in which its activity delays emptying is known.

The organs responsible for control of gastric emptying are the stomach and proximal duodenum, which interact to regulate emptying[42]. The mechanism of their interaction is unknown. Several possibilities have been suggested:

(a) sphincteric activity at the gastroduodenal junction,

(b) co-ordinated activity cycles of the antrum and proximal duodenum, and

(c) activity of the gastric corpus.

The junction between the stomach and small bowel may have a sphincteric function (pyloric sphincter), as proposed by Cannon[70], to control flow of acid into the duodenum. Until recently, this was considered unlikely, since various procedures which obliterate the pylorus fail to alter emptying of various 'test meals'[68,71]. Also, several studies demonstrated that the pyloric region behaves as if it were merely a part of the antrum[35,41,55]. Indeed, many animals (notably the dog) have no anatomical region identifiable as a sphincter and the gastroduodenal junction is actually devoid of muscle[41,72].

Recently, however, several studies have indicated that this area may act as a functional sphincter. Dozois et al.[71] found that distal antrectomy (to remove the 'pyloric sphincter') does not influence the emptying of liquid meals but does accelerate the emptying of solids. A regulatory role of this area was also postulated by Isenberg and Csendes[73] and by Brink et al.[74], who found a zone of elevated pressure between the stomach and small bowel that might regulate emptying. They also found that infusion of the octapeptide of cholecystokinin (a hormone which delays gastric emptying) or acidification of the duodenum (which releases cholecystokinin and secretin) increases the pressure in this zone. Lipshutz and Cohen[33] isolated muscle from the antrum and pylorus of the opossum and plotted dose–response curves to gastrin and secretin. They reported that gastrin stimulated the antral muscle but not the pyloric muscle, and secretin had the opposite effects. Thus, the 'pyloric sphincter' may contribute to the regulation of emptying of solids and the regulation of emptying by the gastrointestinal hormones.

A second possible mechanism regulating emptying of the stomach is the contractile activity of the antrum relative to that of the duodenum. Weisbrodt et al.[75] found that liquid test meals which emptied rapidly caused increased antral contractions with little stimulation of duodenal activity, whereas liquid meals which emptied slowly had the opposite effect. They concluded that the gastric contents moved best from an active area to a relatively inactive area. Other studies have also correlated antral and duodenal activities[68]. Thomas and Crider[76] observed an association between contractions of the duodenum and stomach in the postprandial state. The duodenum contracted only after gastric contraction, whereas during the gastric contraction, duodenal contractions were inhibited.

The pathway for the co-ordination of antral and duodenal activity is unclear. Three have been postulated.

First, the slow wave rate of the antrum is much less than that of the duodenum (3–5 v. 12–18). In certain species, the gastric slow wave can be recorded from the proximal small bowel. The possibility exists that the superimposition of the gastric slow wave on the duodenal slow wave can modulate duodenal contractions[77,78]. This is supported by a demonstrable relationship between antral slow waves and duodenal contractions[79]. Transection of the gastroduodenal junction abolishes this relationship[80]. However, in the dog at least, antral slow-wave activity has not been recorded from the small bowel[41] and transection interrupts intrinsic nerve pathways as well as muscular connections.

Secondly, the correlation may be by way of either intrinsic or extrinsic nerve pathways. Since transection of the junction disrupts the co-ordination but probably leaves the extrinsic nerve uninjured, the latter are probably unimportant. Although the intrinsic nerves may play a role, their importance is unknown.

Thirdly, the co-ordination could be via the passage of chyme from the stomach to the duodenum. As long as the material does not excite duodenal receptors, no duodenal activity can occur, but if the chyme entering the duodenum ahead of the antral contraction does activate the duodenal receptors, the duodenum could contract rhythmically shortly after arrival of the chyme. This possibility is supported by the fact that 200 mosmol trisodium citrate solutions (which do not excite duodenal receptors) fail to stimulate duodenal contractions, whereas 10 mM oleic acid (which does excite receptors) elicits marked duodenal contractions[75]. However, Bedi and Code[80] found that transection of the gastroduodenal junction does not alter the emptying of a saline solution but does disrupt the co-ordination between the antrum and duodenum.

Possibly, too, neither the antrum nor the pyloric region is significant for control of gastric emptying. Gianturco[81] and Dozois et al.[71] have excised the antrum and found no differences in the emptying of liquids. Also, gastrin which enhances gastric antral contractions, does not hasten emptying but actually delays it[61,62]. If the antrum or 'pyloric sphincter' is unimportant, the activity of either the gastric body or of the duodenum must be able to regulate emptying. Gianturco[72] resected the body of the feline stomach and observed that a barium suspension emptied faster than before resection. This procedure also increased intragastric pressure upon instillation of the suspension. Thus, alterations of intragastric pressure by activity of the gastric body may influence emptying. A need exists for direct measurements of activity in the gastric corpus and intragastric pressure during emptying and in response to agents altering emptying. The role played by duodenal contraction has already been mentioned. In addition, Ludwick et al.[83] reported that after pyloroplasty (without vagotomy), both the antrum and duodenum contracted simultaneously and gastric emptying was markedly inhibited. Thus, duodenal contractions can alter gastric emptying.

The gastrointestinal hormones, gastrin[61,62], secretin[84,85] and cholecystokinin[84] inhibit gastric emptying in unknown ways. Both gastrin and cholecystokinin enhance gastric contractions, while secretin inhibits antral activity. Thus, these agents may operate via at least two different mechanisms. Further evidence of the dissociation between contractile activity and emptying is that both atropine and morphine delay emptying. Atropine decreases both antral and duodenal contractions, while morphine enhances contractions of both. In all of these cases, the relative contributions of the antrum, gastric body and duodenum may be the important factor. Further studies are needed.

In summary, gastric emptying depends partly upon the chemical and physical composition of ingested foods. Emptying appears to be partially regulated by receptors located in the duodenum. In addition to the action of the receptors, many hormones and drugs affect emptying. The nature of the receptors and how their activation or how drugs and hormones modulate emptying are unknown. Contractions of the stomach, pyloric region and duodenum have all been implicated in the control of gastric emptying in unknown ways.

5.5 SMALL INTESTINAL MOTILITY

Contractile activity of the small intestine must perform at least three functions:

(a) the mixing of ingested foodstuffs with digestive secretions,

(b) the circulation of all intestinal contents for maximal contact with the intestinal mucosa, and

(c) the propulsion of intestinal contents in a net aboral direction.

Anatomically, the small intestine has been divided into three areas: duodenum, jejunum and ileum. Most of the available data on contractile activity of the small intestine come from studies of the duodenum and proximal jejunum. This information is usually treated as though it applied to the whole intestine. However, a few investigations have uncovered differences in contractile activity between the proximal and distal areas of bowel. Thus, intestinal motility may not be a uniform phenomenon. In this review, then, unless otherwise specified, the discussion will concern the activities of the proximal small bowel.

5.5.1 Patterns of contraction

The small intestine is flaccid between periods of contraction. A pressure-sensing device placed in the lumen records a pressure of only 4–10 mmHg at these times. When the small intestine contracts, the lumen is partially or totally occluded. In the duodenum and proximal jejunum, Friedman et al.[86] found two main types of contractions:

(a) a localised eccentric contraction involving a segment of bowel less than 2 cm long and not occluding the lumen, and

(b) a concentric contraction involving a segment longer than 2 cm and usually occluding the lumen.

Pressure-sensing devices in the upper small intestine sense contractions appearing as peak-like curves. Most (>90%) of the pressure waves appear as symmetrical peaks of uniform shape with a mean duration (in man) of 5 s. These waves have been classified by some investigators as type I waves[87]. In the non-fasting human, these contractions are present 14–34% of the recorded time. At any given locus in the bowel, groups of one to three sequential contractions tend to occur, separated by periods of inactivity[88]. In the fasting human, the contractions tend to occur in larger groups, and a continuous group of contractions may last for several minutes[89]. Strain-gauge transducers sewn on the serosal surface of the upper small bowel of dogs also detect contractions of uniform shape and short duration. The temporal distribution of contractions recorded with gauges at any one locus also depends on the digestive state of the animal. In the unfed dog, Jacoby et al.[90] detected a pattern characterised further by Reinke et al.[91] and Carlson et al.[92]. For ca. 40 min, no contractions occur. This is followed by a period of 10–20 min during which groups of one to five sequential contractions are separated by periods of inactivity. Finally, during a period of 10–20 min, contractile activity is continuous. The continuous burst of contractions ends abruptly and the cycle repeats itself (Figure 5.7).

These three periods of activity have been called basal, intermediate (or pre-burst) and burst, respectively. Contractions in the fed dog are fairly evenly distributed over the entire recording period (Figure 5.7, intermediate). The general activity level depends on the amount, consistency and chemical composition of the ingested food.

These simple monophasic contractions (type I and II) not only have a temporal distribution at one locus, they have a spatial distribution along the small bowel. Multiple sensing devices (either pressure or strain-gauge

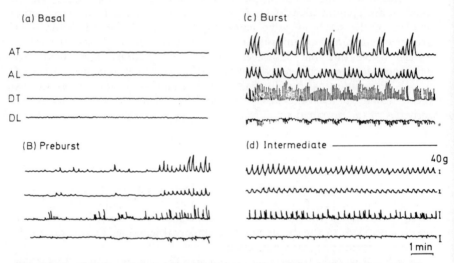

Figure 5.7 Gastric antral and duodenal contractile activity during fasting and after feeding. Recordings were made with strain-gauge transducers. AT, antrum transverse (circular); AL, antrum longitudinal; DT, duodenum transverse (circular); DL, duodenum longitudinal. (From Carlson *et al.*[92], by courtesy of Williams and Wilkins)

transducers) have been used, but the results are difficult to interpret. Apparently, the majority of contractions at one locus cannot be correlated readily with contractions at adjacent sites (Figure 5.8). However, some of the contractions do occur at adjacent sites with a sequential proximal-to-distal occurrence or phase lag[86,93].

A second type of pressure wave has been recorded from the upper small intestine of some species. This wave, consisting of an elevated basal pressure lasting from 10 s to 8 min, has been termed a type III wave. The amplitude of the rise in basal pressure varies greatly and is hard to assess, since monophasic (type I) waves are always superimposed on the increase in baseline pressure. The occurrence of these waves at a given locus is irregular, and the rate varies from 0 to 90 waves per hour[87]. Little is known of the spatial distribution of these waves along the upper small bowel. Strain-gauge recordings usually fail to show type III waves from the upper small bowel of dogs. Whether this represents a species difference or a variation in recording techniques is unknown. Possibly, in some species the response time of the smooth muscle is so short that during a series of large phasic contractions the muscle fails to relax completely between contractions. This would result in a partially occluded lumen and an increase in intraluminal pressure to resemble type III waves.

Contractions of the distal small intestine (ileum) tend to be more variable than those of the upper intestine. Phasic contractions (type I) occur in groups in the unfed animal, but their frequency and amplitude are usually less than those of the upper intestine. Little is known about the spatial relationships of contractions at adjacent sites of the lower intestine. Tonal

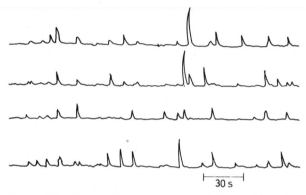

30 s

Figure 5.8 Intraluminal pressures recorded at multiple sites in the upper small intestine. From top to bottom, tracings are from progressively distal areas of bowel at 1 cm intervals. Pressures were recorded from healthy human subjects 15 min after the ingestion of 16 ounces of whole milk

contractions with superimposed phasic activity (type III) also occur here[87]. A contraction peculiar to this area has been called a *P*, or type IV, wave. This wave is tonal, though not accompanied by superimposed phasic activity; it is observed only rarely, being recorded just two to four times during continuous 12 h monitoring in dogs[91]. Little is known about the spatial relationships of type IV contractions.

5.5.2 Propulsion of intraluminal material

Movements of intestinal contents vary widely. For convenience, however, they can be classified as non-propulsive and propulsive. Non-propulsive movements probably mix and locally circulate the contents. Cannon[94] described these movements as a sectioning of intraluminal contents into a series of uniform segments, with the segments being further divided and joined with great rapidity. The contents are thereby mixed, circulated, and pushed to and fro, but no net propulsion occurs. These movements have been called rhythmic segmentation (probably the same as what was originally described as pendular movements). The contractions responsible for non-propulsive movements are probably phasic (types I and II) contractions which occur at multiple loci but have no sequential spatial relationship conducive to propulsion. Thus, type I contractile activity is also referred to as rhythmic segmentation.

Propulsive movements have been described by many investigators, most notably Bayliss and Starling[95]. They found that a piece of cotton, coated with petrolatum, was propelled along the extrinsically denervated small bowel of the anaesthetised dog. Others have described similar propulsion of barium or other radio-opaque material in the small bowel of intact unanaesthetised animals, including man. These movements propel the contents in an aboral direction over varying distances, but they cause little mixing. This propulsive activity has been called peristalsis.

(The term peristalsis has been used to describe many different phenomena. At one extreme, it is used as a general term to describe any type of contractile activity. At the other, it is used to describe a specific reflex movement elicited by isolated segments of small bowel, notably guinea-pig ileum. In this review, the term will be used as a synonym for propulsive movements.)

The type of contractions that produce propulsive movements are unclear. Some investigators found, under fluoroscopic examination with intraluminal balloon manometry, that propulsive movements were correlated with tonic, type III, pressure waves[87]. Friedman et al.[86], using a combination of fluoroscopy and manometry with opened-tipped catheters, found that propulsive movements correlated with phasic, type I, contractions, occurring with a proximal-to-distal sequence. Thus, both propulsive and non-propulsive movements can result from the same contractile activity: phasic, type I, contractions. Whether these contractions produce propulsion depends upon the temporal and spatial relationships of the contractions at adjacent sites of the bowel.

5.5.3 Control of contractile activity

Contractions of the small bowel are due to activities of smooth-muscle cells. These cells are arranged in two layers. In the outer layer, the long axis of the cells is arranged longitudinally. In the inner layer (closer to the lumen), the long axis of the cells is arranged circularly. In some species, the respective cells may not be regularly longitudinal and circular but may appear to be spiral. In most small-intestinal areas of most species, the circular muscle layer is thicker. In general, the musculature is most abundant in the proximal intestine, decreasing in thickness distally until the ileocecal sphincter[16].

As in the rest of the gastrointestinal tract, innervation of the gut can be divided into intrinsic and extrinsic nerves. There are many intrinsic neurones lying in several plexuses. The most prominent plexus, the myenteric or Auerbach's plexus, lies between the circular and longitudinal muscle layers. Nerves of this plexus probably constitute the major intrinsic neural influence on the bowel; subsequent discussion will deal with this plexus. Many of the cell bodies react positively to cholinesterase staining and are considered cholinergic nerves. Other cells exist which do not take up cholinesterase stains[16], the chemical mediator is unknown. They may be the cell bodies of the non-adrenergic inhibitory nervous system. Axons from the cell bodies of the myenteric plexus innervate the longitudinal and circular smooth-muscle cells. The synaptic junctions between nerve and muscle are diffuse; the separations range from 300 to 3000 Å. Thus, the diffusion paths between the nerve endings and the muscle cells are long, in contrast to the neuro-muscular junction of skeletal muscle. Despite this sizeable diffusion distance, acetylcholine is released from the nerves and acts on the muscle cells. The distribution of axons from the non-cholinergic cells of the myenteric plexus is unknown. But if these are the nerves of the non-adrenergic inhibitory system, the synaptic junctions may be narrower, and the transmitter may be ATP or another nucleotide[18]. The nerve-cell bodies of the plexus receive input from a wide variety of receptors in the mucosa and within the muscle wall itself, constituting local reflex arcs within the wall of the intestine. In addition to this input, axons from cells of the parasympathetic and sympathetic nervous system enter the myenteric plexus. Parasympathetic input comes from cell bodies located in the dorsal vagal nucleus via axons distributed in the vagal nerves. Every axon entering the myenteric plexus has been estimated to innervate several thousand nerve cell bodies. This implies that central vagal control may not be discrete. Most of the efferent vagal fibres appear to be preganglionic cholinergic. Inhibitory fibres have been reported to be present, as well, but the evidence is conflicting. Besides the efferent nerve fibres, the vagus contains many afferent fibres, coming from receptors in the intestinal wall. Sympathetic input originates from cell bodies located in the celiac and superior mesenteric ganglia. Axons from these cells pass to the intestine, accompanying branches of the celiac and superior mesenteric arteries (periarterial nerve fibres). These axons synapse with cells of the myenteric plexus and with smooth-muscle cells directly. In addition to the efferent axons, the periarterial nerves contain many afferent axons[16].

As in the stomach, small-bowel contractions are regulated by at least four mechanisms:
(a) inherent smooth-muscle cell activity,
(b) activity of the intrinsic nerves,
(c) activity of the extrinsic nerves, and
(d) circulating or locally released chemicals.
Most studies on control of small bowel motility have focused on the upper small bowel. The few studies of distal intestinal motility have not indicated significant qualitative differences between the two regions of the gut. Thus, control of the small bowel will be discussed as a whole.

Smooth-muscle cells of both muscle layers have a resting membrane potential resembling that of other smooth-muscle cells (*ca.* −60 mV). The membrane potential is unstable. Periodic depolarisations occur at a fairly regular frequency. Unfortunately, this phenomenon bears several synonyms: slow wave, basic electric rhythm (BER), pacesetter potential and electric-control activity. The slow wave is always in evidence regardless of the presence or absence of contractions. Its frequency depends upon the species and on the area of the small bowel. The frequency at any given locus is highly stable, changing only with metabolic rate or core temperature[96,97].

In a particular animal, Alvarez and Mahoney[53] found that slow-wave frequency decreases along the length of the small bowel. For example, the frequency in the dog is 17–22 cycles min^{-1} in the duodenum and 10–13 in the ileum. The decrease is not uniformly linear, however. Over the proximal quarter of the small bowel, the frequency is the same at all loci, and it decreases beyond this plateau to the ileocecal junction[98],[99] (Figure 5.9). Some investigators maintain that the decrease is stepwise with short frequency plateaux[100], while others hold that the decrease is linear after the initial plateau[101]. The ileal slow wave is more labile and variable in its amplitude than the proximal intestinal slow wave. Transection of the intestine at any level decreases slow-wave frequency below the incision. If the intestine is transected at progressively distal sites, the frequency beyond each section

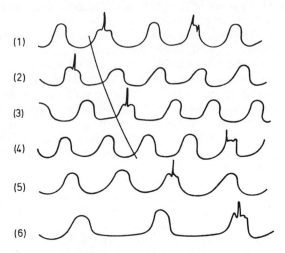

Figure 5.9 Slow waves and spike potentials recorded from multiple sites in the small intestine. Traces 1–6 represent progressively distal areas. Solid line connecting slow waves in tracings 1–4 indicates slow-wave coupling and phase-lag increase in the region of the frequency plateau. Traces 5 and 6 show decreases in slow-wave frequency at more distal areas. The rapid transients occurring on the peaks of some of the slow waves represent spike potential activity

decreases with each sectioning at a fairly linear rate from duodenum to ileum[99],[101],[102]. Thus, apparently each area of the intestine has an intrinsic frequency modulated by areas adjacent to it.

In the region of the frequency plateau (the proximal quarter of the gut), slow waves do not occur simultaneously at all points. Multiple electrodes detect a proximal-to-distal phase lag simulating a propagated slow wave (Figure 5.9). The degree of phase lag is usually expressed as an apparent velocity in cm s^{-1}. In the dog, the phase lag is stable, with an apparent velocity of 15–20 cm s^{-1} [96]. This stability is absent in other species. For example, Duthie et al. found that in man the phase lag between two sites in the duodenum was inconstant and varied both in value and direction[103]. Similar results have been reported in cats[104]. Although a change in the direction of phase lag is abnormal in the dog, it can be induced by local warming of a region in the frequency plateau. The warmed area develops a phase lead over areas both proximal and distal to it. The degree of phase lag is not uniform throughout the region of the frequency plateau (Figure 5.9). In the dog, the phase lag increases, causing a decline in apparent velocity from 15 cm s^{-1} in the proximal duodenum to 3 cm s^{-1} in the mid-jejunum[105].

Slow waves can be recorded from either muscle layer of the intact intestine. However, if the circular and longitudinal layers are separated, slow waves are recorded only from the longitudinal layer[106]. Bortoff and Sachs[107] found that slow waves are generated by cells of the longitudinal layer and spread electrotonically into the circular muscle layer. At any level of small bowel, slow waves occur simultaneously in both muscle layers. The pathways for co-ordination of slow-wave activity between the two layers may be via smooth muscle cells penetrating the myenteric plexus and directly connecting the two layers[108]. Although the circular layer is unnecessary for the generation of slow waves, Kobayashi et al.[108] reported that it may be necessary for the co-ordination of the waves at adjacent sites. Slow waves at adjacent gut segments lack a constant phase lag in the absence of the circular layer.

Generation of slow waves in the smooth-muscle cells of the longitudinal layer depends upon the cyclic bidirectional flux of sodium ions. During the depolarisation phase of the slow wave, a passive flux of sodium into the muscle cell occurs, followed by an active efflux of the ion during repolarisation[109]. The mechanism responsible for the initiation of the slow wave or for its frequency is unknown, but the process appears to depend upon ATP production by the mitochondria of the muscle cells. Job[110] has postulated that accumulation of ATP at the cell membrane leads to increased permeability to Na, giving depolarisation. This, in turn, activates a sodium pump that transports the ion out of the cell. The pump depletes the level of ATP at the membrane, thereby reducing membrane permeability to sodium and repolarisation of the membrane. After cessation of active sodium transport, ATP is regenerated and the cycle repeats itself.

The slow wave at one locus influences the slow waves at adjacent sites, especially in the region of the frequency plateau where the rate is stable but a phase lag attends the occurrence of slow waves at adjacent loci. The nature of slow-wave co-ordination in adjacent muscle cells is unclear. Originally, slow waves were thought to be propagated down the bowel via nexal contacts (nexal contacts being regions of fusion of the membranes of two adjacent smooth muscle cells). Recently, however, Daniel et al.[111] found that nexal contacts are absent in the longitudinal muscle layer. Close contacts of another type exist; these may be involved in the electrical interactions among the smooth-muscle cells of the longitudinal layer. Co-ordination of slow-wave activity in the longitudinal layer may involve the presence of the circular muscle layer (see later). Besides the unresolved pathways for slow-wave interaction, the relationship between the electrical and metabolic activities responsible for co-ordination of slow waves at adjacent sites is unknown. For example, if oscillations of membrane content of ATP cause generation of slow waves in a muscle cell, how are oscillations influenced by similar activities in adjacent cells?

Slow-wave activity of the small intestine has recently been modelled by Nelson and Becker[112], Diamont et al.[113] and Sarna et al.[101]. All have used relaxation oscillators as the basic slow-wave generators. In the modelling experiments, a computer can be programmed with the equations describing the oscillators so that the entire simulation can be produced on a computer.

Each oscillator would represent a smooth-muscle cell or a group of muscle cells in the longitudinal muscle layer which generate slow waves in unison. A chain of relaxation oscillators whose intrinsic frequencies decrease from one end to the other would mimic the multiple transected small intestine.

In addition to having its own intrinsic frequency, an oscillator can be influenced by other oscillators coupled to it. The interaction between two oscillators depends on the degree of coupling and is manifested by alterations in the frequencies of oscillation. If two oscillators with different frequencies (within limits) are coupled, the frequency of the slower oscillator would be 'pulled' toward the frequency of the faster one. If the coupling is strong enough, they will oscillate at the same frequency. Thus, a chain of tightly-coupled oscillators would mimic the frequency plateau existing in the proximal small bowel. More loosely coupled oscillators would mimic the distal areas of the small bowel. When two oscillators with different intrinsic frequencies are coupled, they oscillate at the same frequency, but not simultaneously. The oscillator with the higher intrinsic frequency has a phase lead over the slower one. Thus, the chain of tightly-coupled oscillators described above not only simulates the region of the frequency plateau, as far as frequency is concerned, it also models the phase-lag pattern of this region.

Slow waves are not the only electrical signals recorded from the small bowel. Spike potentials (also referred to as action potentials, action spikes, spikes and response activity), are rapid depolarisations of the membrane which are also recorded. Spike potentials occur primarily during the depolarisation phase of the slow wave and appear to be superimposed on the slow-wave recording (Figure 5.9). In the proximal small bowel of the dog, spike potentials occur during a particular phase of the slow wave, occupying *ca*. 20–40% of the slow-wave cycle[97].

Spike potentials do not occur with every slow wave, but when they do they are followed by contraction of the muscle which generated them. Unlike the slow wave, spike potentials are not coupled at adjacent loci and apparently do not spread in the longitudinal axis[97]. Muscle cells from both the longitudinal and circular layers generate spike activity. However, Bass and Wiley[114] found that spike potentials recorded from the intact intestine correlate with contractions of the circular muscle and not with contractions of the longitudinal muscle, perhaps because the circular layer is the larger muscle mass and is primarily responsible for contractile activity of the intestine.

Spike potentials occur almost simultaneously around the circumference of the bowel[115]. They appear to be propagated through the circular muscle. The pathway for this propagation may be via nexal contacts existing in this muscle layer but not in the longitudinal layer.

Spike potentials in the distal small bowel have not been studied thoroughly, nor has this activity been examined systematically in the dog. A few studies suggest that the period of the slow wave in which spikes can occur is longer in the lower small bowel and in other species. Also, in cats, periods of time pass when long bursts of spike potentials occur unassociated with slow-wave activity[104].

Slow waves, spike potentials, and contractions are inter-related. Spike potentials always precede a contraction, contractions do not normally occur without being preceded by spike potentials, and spike potentials occur during specific periods of a slow wave[97]. Thus, the slow wave determines the timing of contractions. Contractions occur at multiples of the slow-wave interval, and contractions do not occur at a rate greater than the slow-wave frequency. Since a gradient exists in the slow-wave frequency along the small bowel, there is also a gradient in the maximal frequency of contraction. In fact, Alvarez[116] demonstrated the gradient in the rate of contractions before the presence of slow waves was discovered. In addition to determining the temporal relationships of contractions at one locus in the bowel, slow waves also influence the spatial relationships of contractions at adjacent loci. The phase lag in the occurrence of slow waves at adjacent sites imposes a phase lag in the contractions at adjacent sites. Therefore, contractions occur at multiple loci with a proximal-to-distal phase lag. This could result in propulsive movements.

Although slow waves determine the temporal and spatial relationships of contractions occurring at loci along the bowel, they do not determine whether contractions will occur. The occurrence of contractions depends on other influences, such as nervous activity and the presence of circulating or local chemical agents.

Slow waves and spike potentials are generated by the muscle cells themselves, although they are altered by nervous and humoral factors. Several reflexes modify contractile activity and are disrupted by extrinsic nerve section[48]. For example, if a segment of intact bowel is distended, contractions in the rest of the bowel are inhibited (the so-called intestino-intestinal reflex, whose afferent and efferent pathways reside in the sympathetic nerves). Section of the nerves abolishes the reflex. The relaxation is presumably due to liberation of norepinephrine from the efferent nerves. In light of the adrenergic nature of this reflex, investigators have employed adrenergic receptor blocking agents in the treatment of reflex ileus with varying degrees of success[117]. Stimulation of the periarterial nerves can either elicit or suppress contractile activity. The response depends partly on the contractile state of the gut at the time of stimulation and upon the segment of the bowel being examined. Kewenter et al.[118] predicted that stimulation and inhibition of contractions are due to the presence of two sets of nerve fibres having different stimulus optima: inhibition is presumably due to activation of adrenergic nerves, and stimulation is due to activation of cholinergic nerves. (Other nerve types which cause stimulation have been implicated but their roles are unknown.) These authors found that stimulation of periarterial nerves causes inhibition in the ileum more often than in the upper small bowel, suggesting a difference in the relative distribution of the two nerve types to various regions of the bowel. Stimulation of vagal nerves usually increases the contractile activity of the small bowel, but vagal stimulation has been reported to produce inhibition[48].

The extrinsic nerves may exert a general control over the small bowel to modulate over-all contractile activity. Considering the relatively few efferent nerve fibres, one can hardly imagine a discrete control over small regions of the bowel. However, Carlson et al.[119] found that a discrete complex of electrical activity (the intestinal interdigestive myoelectric complex) apparently relies upon extrinsic innervation. This complex consists of a caudad moving band of high-amplitude spike potentials in the small bowel of fasting dogs, probably the electrical counterpart of the burst activity described above. In dogs prepared with Thiry–Vella loops with continuity of the bowel restored by end-to-end anastomosis, the complex was propagated along the bowel to the anastomosis, at which point it appeared on the gut loop and traversed it as if the segment were still in its natural place. Finally, the complex continued distal to the point of anastomosis and traversed the rest of the bowel. Since continuity of the intrinsic nerves and muscle was disrupted and intestinal contents did not flow through the loop, migration of the complex must have been controlled by extrinsic nerves in these experiments. In the absence of other factors, extrinsic nerves may have discrete control over small-bowel contractions.

The role of the intrinsic nerves in the control of intestinal contractility is difficult to assess. The extrinsically denervated small bowel still contracts, and several reflexes can be elicited. However, this could be a function of smooth muscle activity and properties as well as the effect of intrinsic nerves. Pharmacological agents that block nerve transmission have been used extensively to study the role of the intrinsic nerves. These studies have demonstrated that intrinsic nerves are unnecessary for intestinal contractility, but are needed for reflex activity[48]. Several investigators have attempted to destroy the intrinsic nerves selectively by perfusing segments of bowel with oxygen-free solutions[120,121]. Reflex activity is somewhat altered after anoxia, but the results are difficult to interpret. Some of the nerves apparently still function after anoxic perfusion. Anoxia reduces slow-wave frequency and amplitude, but this may reflect damage to the smooth-muscle cells themselves.

Stimulation of the intrinsic nerves leads to either contraction or relaxation. Usually contraction predominates, probably due to the release of acetyl-choline from nerve endings. Inhibition can also occur, sometimes in untreated preparations and invariably in atropine-treated preparations. The inhibition is not antagonised by adrenergic receptor blocking agents and is presumably mediated by the non-adrenergic inhibitory system. Burnstock et al.[18] have postulated that the transmitter in this system is ATP or another purine metabolite. In addition to these two nerves, other stimulating non-cholinergic nerves have been suggested[122].

Recently, recordings have been obtained from cells of the myenteric plexus. Wood[123] and Ohkawa and Prosser[124,125] found that neuronal activity was associated with inhibition of contractile activity. Agents which depressed neuronal activity (tetrodotoxin, lidocaine and hexamethonium) enhanced muscle spike potentials, while agents which stimulated neuronal activity (norepinephrine and epinephrine) depressed muscle activity. They also described several types of cells having different discharge characteristics. Some of the cells responded to distension of the gut. Interestingly, groups of neurones as close together as 0.5 mm had independent activities, suggesting that the myenteric plexus does not function as a 'nerve net'.

Contractile activity of the small intestine is altered by a number of gastro-intestinal hormones, by epinephrine from the adrenal glands, and by a variety of locally-released chemicals (serotonin, histamine, prostaglandins, etc.). Gastrin in large doses has been reported to increase contractility of the bowel[126]. Pentagastrin in low doses has little or no effect on the incidence of spike potentials in the canine duodenum, but it does increase the frequency of the slow wave[61]. Secretin decreases the incidence of contractions[127] and spike potentials[128], but fails to affect the frequency or apparent velocity of the slow wave. Cholecystokinin and caerulein stimulate bowel contractions slightly. The physiological role of the hormones on small intestinal contractile activity is uncertain.

Circulating epinephrine released from the adrenal glands inhibits contractile activity. Both in conscious dogs[92] and monkeys[129], nicotine depresses contractile activity of the stomach and small bowel; much of the response to nicotine is due to circulating epinephrine released from the adrenal glands. The effects of various circulating and locally-released substances have been thoroughly reviewed by others[130].

5.5.4 Summary

The small intestine mixes and propels the intestinal contents by at least three types of mechanical activity: phasic contractions not co-ordinated in a proximal-to-distal sequence, phasic contractions having a proximal-to-distal sequence and tonic contractions. The timing of phasic contractions at one locus and the spatial relationships of contractions at adjacent loci are regulated by the slow waves. The occurrence and force of contractions at a given locus depends on the inter-relationships among several factors: intrinsic and extrinsic nervous reflexes, activity of the autonomic nervous system and the presence of circulating and locally released chemical agents. The electrical events associated with tonic contractions (if, indeed, they are separate entities) are undefined.

5.6 COLONIC MOTILITY

Colonic motility is poorly understood. Its study is complicated by difficult access to the organ and by the wide anatomic variations among species. Anatomic differences are great enough to prevent development of a general view of contractile events in the colon. The discussion below will be concerned mainly with the results of studies performed on human subjects, although supplementary data from animal studies will be considered.

5.6.1 Patterns of contraction

On the basis of its contractile activity, the colon can be divided into three regions: the ileocaecal region, the main portion of the colon (ascending, traverse, descending, and sigmoid colon) and the anorectal region. Activity of these three regions serves several functions. The flow of intraluminal material into the colon is regulated by the ileocaecal junction. The colonic contents are mixed and propelled through the main portion of the colon where water and electrolytes are absorbed and secreted. Finally, the faecal contents are stored and evacuated during defaecation. In this discussion, the three areas will be discussed separately.

In man and certain other animals, the junction between the ileum and colon is occluded except when contents are moving from the ileum to the colon. If a pressure-sensing device is passed through this area, a zone of 1–4 cm is detected where pressures are *ca.* 20 mmHg higher than those on either side of the zone; this is called the ileocaecal sphincter[131]. Intermittently, the sphincter relaxes and contents from the ileum are discharged into the colon. The sphincter also acts as a valve to prevent movement of material from the colon into the small intestine. The structural arrangements of the sphincter probably permit this valvular action, since the function persists in the animal after death[132].

The main portion of the colon exhibits several types of contractile activity. At any instance, the colon is usually segmented, a pattern prominent in man and called 'haustrations'. Haustra are probably the result of structural as well as functional properties of the colon[133]. Points of concentration of muscular tissue and mucosal foldings contribute to their saccular appearance; the structural features persist after death. Haustra are more prominent in species having their longitudinal muscle arranged into bands of taenia coli; haustra and taenia appear during the same stages of colonic development[134]. These findings suggest that the taenia may contribute to haustral formation. Haustral contractions are not fixed. Ritchie has reported that segmental colonic contractions appear, disappear and re-form but that the loci of the rings of contraction are inconstant[135]. In those animals lacking taenia coli and muscular and mucosal sacculations, segmental contractions still occur[133].

Pressure-sensing devices placed in the colon detect phasic and tonic contractile activity. The phasic contractions (also called types I and II) have amplitudes of 10–50 mmHg and durations of 12–60 s. These waves occur at any one locus up to 50% of the recorded time, but the activity varies markedly[133]. At adjacent sites, segmenting contractions usually occur independently[133]. Occasionally they occur with either an oral-to-aboral or an aboral-to-oral phase lag. Tonic contractions of complex shape, lasting 1–15 min, occur less often. These waves are almost always accompanied by superimposed phasic activity. They have been grouped together as type III waves[133]. Perhaps the most striking pressure complex recorded from the colon is a large contraction lasting 20–60 s. These contractions usually occur with an oral-to-aboral phase lag and may be associated with the mass movements which will be described[136]. In normal individuals, these waves occur infrequently, but in certain diarrhoeal states (ulcerative colitis, and laxative-induced diarrhoea) they are more frequent. They have been called type IV waves. It should be apparent that colonic pressure waves are exceedingly complex and difficult to categorise. Many investigators have simply abandoned any fixed classification[137].

Strain-gauge transducers sewn on the serosal surface of the colon have been used to record activity of the circular muscle in cats and dogs[138,139]. Again, several types of contractions have been recorded, the most common being a phasic contraction lasting 12–15 s. These usually occur in groups of 5–10 but often occur singly. Tonal contractions (longer than 30 s) have been observed, as well; they vary in amplitude and are often accompanied by superimposed phasic activity. Recordings have also been made from the simian taenia coli (longitudinal muscle), in which both phasic and tonic contractions are found, with phasic activity predominating[129]. So far, strain-gauge units have not been used to study the spatial relationships of contractions at adjacent loci.

5.6.2 Propulsion of intraluminal contents

Material moves slowly through the large intestine, usually requiring 1–7 days. Movement is complex and not easily studied. In the ileocaecal region, chyme is discharged intermittently through the ileocaecal sphincter into the colon, an activity especially prominent after eating. Once in the colon, the contents are propelled to and fro. Cannon found that the contents frequently moved from the proximal colon back to the cecum[94]. In animals with a large caecum, Elliott and Barclay-Smith[140] also observed this retrograde motion. However, with each contraction of the proximal colon, some of its contents are propelled aborally.

In the main colon, various movements have been noted. Often contents are propelled bidirectionally from a point of contraction, and there is a mixing of contents among haustra. During this type of activity, little net aboral movement of contents takes place[133]. When propulsion does occur, it is usually a 'mass movement'. This type of movement was first described by Holznecht in 1909[141]. Since then, numerous other workers have observed it. In 'mass movement', phasic activity suddenly stops, with loss of haustration (not observed by all investigators). Then, a whole segment of intraluminal contents is swept rapidly in an aboral direction. This is followed by a return of haustration and phasic contractions. Mass movements are infrequent in healthy people and are estimated to occur only one to three times daily. Torsoli et al.[136] found they could induce events resembling 'mass movements' by introducing hyperosmolar solutions into the jejunum. These solutions induce sequential contractions of the colon with an oral-to-aboral phase lag. The pressure peaks recorded at each site last 20 s or longer and have amplitudes of 20–50 mmHg. Cineflurograms taken during this activity demonstrate a displacement of the colonic contents toward the rectum.

The rectum normally contains little or no material. Before defaecation, the rectum fills with faeces propelled by the sigmoid colon. When the rectum is distended, the internal anal sphincter relaxes. The combination of a distended rectum and a relaxed sphincter produces the sensation of a 'call to stool'. When the external anal sphincter is contracted voluntarily, the anal canal remains closed and the sensation remits. If the external anal sphincter is relaxed, defaecation occurs. During defaecation, the rectum empties partially or completely, with little or no movement of the contents in the rest of the colon[8]. Reinke et al.[91] recorded an increase in colonic activity shortly after the act of defaecation in the dog, but this may or may not be associated with movement of intraluminal contents.

5.6.3 Control of contractile activity

The smooth-muscle cells of the colon are arranged in layers: an outer layer where cells have their long axis orientated longitudinally and an inner layer whose cells are arranged in the circular axis. In the main portion of the human colon and certain other species, the cells of the longitudinal layer are arranged in three bands, the taenia coli. Between the bands, only a thin layer of longitudinal muscle is present. In the rectal area, the taenia diffuse out to form a uniform longitudinal layer. The circular muscle is continuous and fairly homogeneous throughout. In other species, notably dog and cat, the muscle is arranged in two complete layers, as in the human rectum[16]. The significance of this difference is unknown, except that true haustration exists in only those species possessing taenia coli. Differences in contractions between the two colon types have not been investigated.

The colon is innervated by intrinsic and extrinsic nerves. Many nerve cell bodies lie in several plexuses. The most prominent, the myenteric plexus, lies between the circular and longitudinal muscle layers of the colon. In those colons with taenia coli, the cell bodies are concentrated beneath the taenia[16]. Many of the cell bodies stain for cholinesterase and are probably cholinergic. Unlike the upper gastrointestinal tract, cell bodies containing catecholamines are present in certain areas of the colon[142]. In addition to these two types, other cell bodies are also present (perhaps non-adrenergic inhibitory). Axons from these cell bodies innervate the muscle cells in much the same way as in the small intestine (see above). The cells of the myenteric plexus receive input from a variety of receptors in the mucosa and muscle layers, as well as the extrinsic nerves. The parasympathetic innervation to the colon has two components[143]. The ileocaecal, ascending, and transverse parts of the colon are innervated by the vagi. The descending and sigmoid areas of the colon and the rectum are innervated by the sacral outflow via the pelvic nerves. These nerves consist of pre-ganglionic cholinergic fibres, although recent studies have demonstrated a large number of ganglion cells and post-ganglionic fibres within the nerves themselves. The nerves pass to the intrinsic plexuses and muscle along the blood vessels. Besides these efferent cholinergic fibres, the parasympathetic nerves contain many afferent fibres. These fibres form part of the reflex arcs (to be described). Sympathetic innervation is carried to the proximal regions of the colon by fibres arising from the superior mesenteric plexus[143]. The distal regions of the colon receive input from the inferior mesenteric plexus. In addition, the distal rectum and anal canal are innervated by sympathetic fibres from the hypogastric plexus. Most sympathetic nerves are post-ganglionic adrenergic fibres that accompany the parasympathetic fibres and the vascular supply passing to the intrinsic nerves and musculature of the colon. As with the parasympathetic nerves, many afferent fibres arise in the colon and flow to the sympathetic plexuses. These nerves form part of the reflex arcs influencing colonic motility. The significance of this complex innervation is not apparent.

Colonic contractile activity is influenced by at least four factors: intrinsic smooth-muscle cell properties, the intrinsic nerves, the extrinsic nerves, and circulating or locally released chemicals.

In contrast to the rest of the gastrointestinal tract, little is known about the temporal and spatial relationships of the electrical activities of colonic smooth muscle. This is paradoxical in view of the numerous, greatly detailed studies of the taenia coli of the guinea-pig (a muscle actually taken from the caecum). Nearly nothing is known of the activities of the smooth muscle of the ileocaecal sphincter. One wonders whether any electrical activity is present in this region which could account for its sphincteric activity.

Only recently has the activity of the main portion of the colon been investigated. Christensen *et al.*[144] reported that electrical activity could be recorded from isolated muscle of the proximal feline colon. This activity originated in cells of the circular muscle and consisted of three types.

First, a cyclic depolarisation and repolarisation of the membrane potential was observed, not associated with any contractile event and qualitatively resembling the slow waves of the stomach and small gut. The frequency of colonic slow wave at any one locus is fairly constant, but *in vitro* a gradient of frequency exists, the frequency in the proximal colon (2–3 cycles per min) being lower than in the distal colon (6–9 cycles per min). In the colon of the chronic unanaesthetised cat, however, the frequency is nearly the same throughout the colon (4–6 cycles per min)[145]. Thus, the gradient may be an artifact introduced by isolation of the colon. In either case, there is no descending oral-to-aboral gradient, as seen in the small bowel.

The second type of activity is spike activity, consisting of rapid fluctuations in membrane potential which precede and probably initiate contractions and usually occur during a specific period of the slow-wave cycle. Their presence also appears to alter the slow-wave cycle. When spike activity occurs, the duration of the slow wave is increased, and the larger the spike burst, the longer the slow-wave duration. At times, spike activity can be seen to continue over several slow-wave cycles. Thus, the duration of spike activity may vary over fairly long periods of time. Again, this contrasts with events in the small intestine.

In addition to slow waves and spikes, a third type of electrical activity consists of low-amplitude fluctuations of potential, with a frequency of 20–60 cycles per min. These potentials occur intermittently and can extend over the whole slow-wave cycle. Their significance is unknown, but occasionally they occur during periods of excessive contractile activity. Thus, the electrical activity of the colon is not as stereotyped as in the stomach and small bowel. Possibly, this wide range of electrical activity is related to the variety of mechanical activity in the colon.

At any one colonic locus, all three types of electrical activity can be recorded. The processes responsible for the generation of the activity have not been adequately studied. However, one study indicates that the ionic requirements of the slow waves resemble those of the stomach[146].

The spatial relationships of the electrical events have been studied only in the proximal colon of the cat, where it appears that the slow waves are phase-locked over short distances. Christensen and Hauser[147,148] found that these slow waves are coupled 60–90% of the time, and the slow waves spread in both the longitudinal and circular axes. The velocity of the apparent spread is much faster in the circular axis, perhaps because the long axis of the smooth-muscle cells is also in the circular axis. The direction of spread of the slow waves varies. The most common pattern in the proximal colon is for the slow waves to appear first at a site several cm from the ileocaecal junction and then to spread in both the oral and aboral directions. The significance of this pattern is unknown. However. if the spatial patterns of the slow wave determine the spatial pattern of colonic contractions (as is true for gastric slow waves and contractions), this electrical activity may be the basis for the contractile activity seen in the proximal colon (see earlier).

Presumably, the model of a matrix of relaxation oscillators could be used to simulate the slow-wave activity of the colon. However, more data will be needed before we know the applicability of this model.

Electrical activity has also been recorded from the anal canal of man. The activity can be divided into two distinct types. The first is a cyclic change in potential, with a frequency of 6–26 cycles per min. Schuster and his co-workers[149] have called this the basic electrical rhythm (BER) of the anal sphincter. This slow wave is generated by the smooth muscle of the internal anal sphincter and is associated with sphincteric contraction. Upon relaxation of the sphincter, the slow wave is usually inhibited. No spike activity is recorded from the internal sphincter. Thus, the slow wave differs from that seen in the rest of the gastrointestinal tract; i.e. in the anus, it is associated with a contractile event. The second type of activity recorded from the anal canal is a burst of rapid action potentials. Action potentials are recorded from the striated muscle of the external anal sphincter and are associated with its contraction. The external anal sphincter is under voluntary control and is innervated by motor neurones from the spinal cord.

The extrinsic nerves must exert a major influence on contractions of the colon, since emotional states are often reported to alter bowel activity[8]. However, few studies have been performed to investigate the control of the extrinsic nerves over colonic activity. Connell et al.[150] reported that interruption of the lumbar nerves (primarily sympathetic) to the colon results in an increased contractile activity of the sigmoid colon. This agrees with evidence from animal studies, which indicate an inhibitory influence of the sympathetic nerves on motility. Parasympathetic stimulation usually augments contractile activity, probably due to activation of cholinergic nerves[8].

A number of reflexes of the colon have their pathways in extrinsic nerves. The most prominent is an inhibition of contractions during colonic distention[8,48]. This resembles the intestine–intestinal reflex of the small bowel. The pathway of the reflex includes the inferior mesenteric ganglia and may also include the spinal cord. Recently, studies of the electrical activity of the cells of the inferior mesenteric ganglia demonstrated an increase in the activity of the cells with colonic distension[151]. Thus, inhibition is probably due to activation of inhibitory pathways to the colon. These pathways could either be adrenergic or non-adrenergic inhibitory.

The importance of the intrinsic nerves can be demonstrated by their absence or destruction. In an area devoid of the myenteric plexus (as in Hirchsprung's disease), the muscle contracts tonically. This usually leads to obstruction and the abnormal segment must be removed[8]. Studies on isolated strips of this aganglionic muscle indicate a loss of inhibitory mechanisms; the muscle fails to relax[48]. This would indicate that the intrinsic nerves are primarily inhibitory to muscle contractions. A similar situation exists for the oesophagus (see earlier).

Colonic contractions are also influenced by circulating hormones. Gastrin usually stimulates contractions, but the effect is not marked[8]. It does cause relaxation of the ileocaecal sphincter[152], allowing discharge of ileal contents into the colon. A few studies implicate gastrin release as the cause for increased colonic activity after eating (the gastro-colic reflex)[8,153]. A recent report questions this conclusion, however. The importance of the other hormones, secretin and cholecystokinin, has not been delineated. Epinephrine released from the adrenal gland can inhibit the main portion of the colon, but it may cause contraction of the distal areas[154]. The effects of other endogenous chemical agents on contractions of colonic musculature have been reviewed elsewhere[8].

In summary, contractions of the colon are complex and not fully understood. Qualitatively, the contractile mechanisms are apparently the same as those in the small bowel. However, the electrical activity of the colon has been studied so little that similarities and differences are hard to identify. A greater variety of contractile and electrical events apparently takes place in the colon, but the significance of this remains to be investigated.

5.7 MOTILITY OF THE BILIARY TRACT

Bile flow depends upon at least three mechanisms: the secretory pressure of the liver, the motor activity of the gall bladder and the motor activity of the bile duct. Elucidation of the exact role and importance of each of the mechanisms has been hampered by the inaccessibility of the structures and their small size. Moreover, the organisation of the bile tract varies widely among species[155], making wide variations in the mechanisms of bile flow possible.

5.7.1 Secretory pressure of the liver

The biliary tract differs from the rest of the gastrointestinal tract in that it is not open at both ends. The hepatic end is blind, being formed by the secretory cells of the liver. Thus, as fluid is secreted by these cells, pressures in the ducts rise. In animals whose gall bladders have been removed, biliary secretory pressures can reach 20–40 cm of bile[155]. Presumably, the maximal pressure that can be measured is limited by the escape of secretion through the liver and its lymphatics. Thus, the maximal secretory pressure of the hepatic cells may be even greater than the measured maximal pressure[155].

5.7.2 Gall bladder

The gall bladder is a distensible muscular organ that forms a blind out-pouching of the biliary tract of many species. It stores, concentrates and expels bile into the bile duct. The rate of biliary secretions varies in response to hormonal stimulation but is continuous. On the other hand, flow into the duodenum is intermittent, occurring primarily in response to eating. The gall bladder receives and stores bile during the interdigestive periods. It also concentrates bile by absorbing water and electrolytes. Because of this concentrating ability, it can hold large quantities of hepatic secretion[155].

Filling of the gall bladder depends upon a balance between its resistance to filling and the resistance to flow of bile through the terminal bile duct.

Whenever the resistance to filling is less than the resistance to flow, the gall bladder fills.

After the ingestion of food, especially lipids, the gall bladder contracts. The contractions normally empty the organ gradually. At least one report indicates that the contractions are rhythmic. Evacuation of the gall bladder depends primarily on the influence of hormones, especially cholecystokinin. Ivy and Oldberg[156] found that injection of small amounts of this substance caused powerful and prolonged gall bladder contractions. This effect is a direct hormonal action on the muscle cells, as it is not blocked by antagonists of the transmitters of the autonomic nervous system[157]. The gall bladder possesses nerve endings, and some evidence exists of a slight nervous influence on motor activity[155]. Cholinergic agents such as methacholine induce small rhythmic contractions[158] and atropine tends to delay evacuation. The effects of other agents on the motility of the gall bladder have been reviewed by Hallenbeck[155].

5.7.3 Bile duct

The bile duct consists of a fibromuscular tube and muscular sphincters. The exact structure and course of the duct varies markedly among species[155]. Some animals have very little muscle and a large portion of the duct is located in the duodenal wall. Others, including man, have quite a bit of smooth muscle. The main sphincteric mechanism, located at the terminal end of the common bile duct, is called the sphincter of Oddi. Although the muscle is embedded in the duodenal musculature, Schwegler and Boyden[159] presented evidence that the sphincter is derived *in situ* from the mesenchyme that envelops the bile duct. This occurs in the embryo about 4 weeks after the intestinal muscle has formed. Thus, it appears to be a separate entity. In certain species, sphincters may be present in other areas in the bile duct[160], but they will not be considered here.

The role of the bile duct and its sphincters in the propulsion of bile toward the duodenum is a controversial issue. Opinions range from the view that the sphincters are passive, with bile flow caused by the secretory pressure of the liver and motility of the duodenum, to the view that the duct transports bile by peristaltic contractions, with the sphincter of Oddi participating in the peristaltic sequence much the same as the lower oesophageal sphincter does during oesophageal peristalsis. Part of the discrepancy may be due to anatomic differences among the species studied or to differences in experimental techniques. For example, DuBois and Hunt [161] observed peristalsis in the common bile duct of the opossum. In the dog, no activity was seen[155]. Ludwick and Bass[158] placed strain gauges on the bile ducts of monkeys and recorded contractile activity. They concluded that the duct did contract, but not in a manner that could be considered peristaltic. In man, the results have been conflicting. Hopefully some of the techniques used to study oesophageal peristalsis can be applied to events in the bile duct.

Sphincteric activity of the terminal portion of the bile duct opposes the flow of fluid at pressures up to 30–80 cm of water[155]. This activity depends upon the musculature of the sphincter of Oddi and of the duodenum, whose relative contributions are difficult to assess. Several studies have shown that the sphincter of Oddi contracts independently of duodenal muscle activity[155,157,162]. In addition, this area can keep the bile duct closed despite pressures of 12–30 cm of water when the duodenum is relaxed. On the other hand, during duodenal contractile activity, pressure in the sphincter fluctuates with each contraction. This is not surprising, since the terminal bile duct courses through the thick duodenal musculature.

The effects of gastrointestinal hormones and pharmacological agents on the bile duct are uncertain. Ludwick and Bass[158] found that the simian bile-duct musculature did not respond to cholecystokinin either *in vivo* or *in vitro*, although the hormone did cause contraction of the gall bladder. Methacholine and epinephrine caused contraction of the common bile duct. Cholecystokinin elicited a decrease in the resistance of the sphincter of Oddi[157]. This action is sometimes masked by the fact that large doses of the hormone stimulate duodenal motility. Thus, the effect on the sphincteric mechanism varies. On isolated muscle from the sphincter of Oddi, only relaxation is seen. Andersson *et al.*[163] found that the relaxation is preceded by an increase in cyclic-AMP content of the tissue. The catecholamines cause muscle contraction by acting on a-adrenergic receptors and elicit relaxation by acting on β-adrenergic receptors[164]. The effects of other agents on sphincteric function have been determined by Menguy and reviewed by Hallenbeck[155].

In summary, bile is secreted by the liver under a pressure that can account for the flow of bile from the liver to the duodenum. Resistance to flow of bile into the duodenum is mainly due to sphincteric activity of the terminal bile duct. Many species have an organ (the gall bladder) associated with the biliary tract, which stores and concentrates the bile not flowing into the duodenum, while sphincteric pressures are high. The role of the bile duct in moving bile is unclear. It appears to act as more than a passive conduit. In some species, true peristalsis may occur.

After ingestion of a meal, especially one containing lipid, bile flow is enhanced. The gall bladder contracts, and the sphincter of Oddi relaxes. The action of cholecystokinin is primarily responsible, although nervous reflexes may play a minor role.

References

1. Code, C. F. and Heidal, W., (editors) (1968). *Handbook of Physiology, Sec. 6*, The Alimentary Canal, IV, Motility (Baltimore: Williams and Wilkins)
2. Bortoff, A. (1972). Digestion: Motility. *Ann. Rev. Physiol.*, **34**, 261
3. Christensen, J. (1971). The controls of gastrointestinal movements: Some old and new views. *N. Engl. J. Med.*, **285**, 85
4. Daniel, E. E. (1969). Digestion: Motor Function. *Ann. Rev. Physiol.*, **31**, 203
5. Farrar, J. T. (1963). Gastrointestinal smooth muscle function. *Amer. J. Dig. Dis.*, **8**, 103
6. Texter, E. C. (1964). The control of gastrointestinal motor activity. *Amer. J. Dig. Dis.*, **9**, 585
7. Ingelfinger, F. J. (1958). Esophageal motility. *Physiol. Rev.*, **38**, 533
8. Truelove, S. C. (1966). Movements of the large intestine. *Physiol. Rev.*, **46**, 457
9. Code, C. F. and Schlegel. (1968). Motor action of the esophagus and its sphincters. *Handbook of Physiology. Sec. 6*, The Alimentary Canal, Vol. 4, 1821 (C. F. Code, editor) (Baltimore: Williams and Wilkins)

GASTROINTESTINAL PHYSIOLOGY

10. Goyal, R. K., Sangree, M. H., Hersh, T. and Spiro, H. M. (1970). Pressure inversion point at the upper high pressure zone and its genesis. *Gastroenterology*, **59,** 754
11. Code, C. F., Kelley, M. L., Schlegel, J. F. and Olsen, A. M. (1962). Detection of hiatal hernia during esophageal motility tests. *Gastroenterology*, **43,** 521
12. Christensen, J. and Lund, G. F. (1969). Esophageal responses to distension and electrical stimulation. *J. Clin. Invest.*, **48,** 408
13. Pope, C. E. (1967). A dynamic test of sphincter strength: its application to the lower esophageal sphincter. *Gastroenterology*, **52,** 779
14. Doty, R. W. (1968). Neural organization of deglutition. *Handbook of Physiology*. Sec. 6 Vol. 4, 1861 (C. F. Code, editor) (Baltimore: Williams and Wilkins)
15. Levitt, M. N., Dede, H. H. and Ogura, J. H. (1965). The cricopharyngeus muscle, an electromyographic study in the dog. *Laryngoscope*, **75,** 122
16. Schofield, G. C. (1968). Anatomy of muscular and neural tissues in the alimentary canal. *Handbook of Physiology*, Sec. 6 Vol. 4, 1579 (C. F. Code, editor) (Baltimore: Williams and Wilkins)
17. Jacobowitz, D. (1969). The autonomic innervation of the esophagus of the dog. *J. Thorac. Cardio. Surg.*, **58,** 678
18. Burnstock, G., Campbell, G., Satchell, D. and Smythe, D. (1970). Evidence that adenosine triphosphate or a related nucleotide is the transmitter substance released by non-adrenergic inhibitory nerves in the gut. *Brit. J. Pharmacol.*, **40,** 668
19. Roman, C. (1966). Contrôle nerveux du péristaltisme oesophagien. *J. Physiol. Paris*, **58,** 79
20. Longhi, E. H. and Jordan, P. H., Jr (1971). Necessity of a bolus for propagation of primary peristalsis in the canine esophagus. *Amer. J. Physiol.*, **220,** 609
21. Meltzer, S. J. (1899). On the causes of the orderly progress of the peristaltic movements in the esophagus. *Amer. J. Physiol.*, **2,** 266
22. Jordan, P. H., Jr and Longhi, E. H. (1971). Relationship between size of bolus and the act of swallowing on esophageal peristalsis in dogs. *Proc. Soc. Exp. Biol. Med.*, **137,** 868
23. Weisbrodt, N. W. and Christensen, J. (1972). Gradients of contractions in the opossum esophagus. *Gastroenterology*, **62,** 1159
24. Lund, G. F. and Christensen, J. (1969). Electrical stimulation of esophageal smooth muscle and effects of antagonists. *Amer. J. Physiol.*, **217,** 1369
25. Castell, D. O. and Harris, L. D. (1970). Hormonal control of gastroesophageal sphincter strength. *N. Engl. J. Med.*, **282,** 886
26. Cohen, S. and Lipshutz, W. (1971). Hormonal regulation of human lower esophageal sphincter competence. *J. Clin. Invest.*, **50,** 449
27. Lipshutz, W., Hughes, W. and Cohen, S. (1972). The genesis of lower esophageal sphincter pressure: its identification through the use of gastrin antiserum. *J. Clin. Invest.*, **51,** 522
28. Lipshutz, W., Tuch, A. F. and Cohen, S. (1971). A comparison of the site of action of gastrin I on lower esophageal sphincter and antral circular smooth muscle. *Gastroenterology*, **61,** 454
29. Christensen, J. (1970). Pharmacologic identification of the lower esophageal sphincter. *J. Clin. Invest.*, **49,** 681
30. Lipshutz, W. and Cohen, S. (1971). Physiological determinants of lower esophageal sphincter function. *Gastroenterology*, **61,** 16
31. Arimori, M., Code, C. F., Schlegel, J. F. and Sturm, R. E. (1970). Electrical activity of the canine esophagus and gastroesophageal sphincter. *Amer. J. Dig. Dis.*, **15,** 191
32. Christensen, J., Freeman, B. W. and Miller, J. K. (1972). Local characteristics of lower esophageal sphincter muscle. *Clin. Res.*, **20,** 730
33. Lipshutz, W. and Cohen, S. (1972). Interaction of gastrin I and secretin on gastrointestinal circular muscle. *Amer. J. Physiol.*, **222,** 775
34. Sarna, S. K., Daniel, E. E. and Kingma, Y. J. (1972). Simulation of the electric-control activity of the stomach by an array of relaxation oscillators. *Amer. J. Dig. Dis.*, **17,** 299
35. Code, C. F. and Carlson, H. C. (1968). Motor activity of the stomach. *Handbook of Physiology*. Sec. 6, Vol. 4, 1903 (C. F. Code, editor) (Baltimore: Williams and Wilkins)

36. Lind, J. F., Duthie, H. L., Schlegel, J. F. and Code, C. F. (1960). Motility of the gastric fundus. *Amer. J. Physiol.*, **201**, 197
37. Davenport, H. W. (1971). *Physiology of the Digestive Tract*, 44 (Chicago: Year Book)
38. Cannon, W. B. and Lieb, C. W. (1911). The receptive relaxation of the stomach. *Amer. J. Physiol.*, **29**, 267
39. Anderson, J. J., Bolt, R. J., Ullman, B. M. and Bass, P. (1968). Differential response to various stimulants in the body and antrum of the canine stomach. *Amer. J. Dig. Dis.*, **13**, 147
40. Carlson, H. C., Code, C. F. and Nelson, R. A. (1966). Motor action of the canine gastroduodenal junction: a cine radiographic, pressure and electrical study. *Amer. J. Dig. Dis.*, **11**, 155
41. Bass, P. (1970). The electrical and mechanical activity of the gastroduodenal junction. *Jap. J. Smooth Muscle Res.*, **6**, 93
42. Edwards, D. A. W. and Rowlands, E. N. (1968). Physiology of the gastroduodenal junction. *Handbook of Physiology*, Sec. 6, Vol. 4, 1985 (Baltimore: Williams and Wilkins)
43. Thomas, J. E. and Baldwin, M. V. (1968). Pathways and mechanisms of regulation of gastric motility. *Handbook of Physiology*, Sec. 6, Vol. 4, 1937 (Baltimore: Williams and Wilkins)
44. Jansson, G. and Martinson, T. (1965). Some quantitative considerations on vagally induced relaxation of the gastric smooth muscle of the cat. *Acta. Physiol. Scand.*, **63**, 351
45. Martinson, J. (1965). Studies on the efferent vagal control of the stomach. *Acta. Physiol. Scand.*, 65, *Suppl. 1*, **255**, 1
46. Stadaas, J. and Aune, S. (1970). Intagastric pressure/volume relationship before and after vagotomy. *Acta Chir. Scand.*, **136**, 611
47. Chey, W. Y., Kosay, S., Hendricks, J., Brauerman, S. and Lorber, S. H. (1969). Effect of secretin on motor activity of stomach and Heidenhain pouch in dogs. *Amer. J. Physiol.*, **217**, 848
48. Kosterlitz, H. W. (1968). Intrinsic and extrinsic nervous control of motility of the stomach and the intestines. *Handbook of Physiology*, Sec. 6, Vol. 4, 2147 (Baltimore: Williams and Wilkins)
49. Beani, L., Blanchi, C. and Crema, A. (1970). Vagal non-adrenergic inhibition of guinea-pig stomach. *J. Physiol.*, **217**, 259
50. Kelly, K. A., Code, C. F. and Elveback, L. R. (1969). Patterns of canine gastric electrical activity. *Amer. J. Physiol.*, **217**, 461
51. Sugawara, K., Isaza, J. and Woodward, E. R. (1969). Effect of gastrin on gastric motor activity. *Gastroenterology*, **57**, 649
52. Johnson, L. P. and Magee, D. F. (1965). Cholecystokinin–pancreozymin extracts and gastric motor inhibition. *Surg. Gynecol. Obstet.*, **121**, 557
53. Alvarez, W. C. and Mahoney, L. J. (1922). Action currents in stomach and intestine. *Amer. J. Physiol.*, **58**, 476
54. Bozler, E. (1945). The action potentials of the stomach. *Amer. J. Physiol.*, **144**, 693
55. Daniel, E. E. and Irwin, J. (1968). Electrical activity of gastric musculature. *Handbook of Physiology*, Sec. 6, Vol. 4, 1969 (Baltimore: Williams and Wilkins)
56. Kelly, K. A. and Code, C. F. (1971). Canine gastric pacemaker. *Amer. J. Physiol.*, **220**, 112
57. Weber, J. and Kohatsu, S. (1970). Pacemaker localization and electrical conduction patterns in the canine stomach. *Gastroenterology*, **59**, 717
58. Kelly, K. (1971). Gastric motility and ulcer surgery. *Surg. Clin. N. Amer.*, **51**, 927
59. Kelly, K. A. and Code, C. F. (1969). Effect of transthoracic vagotomy on canine gastric electrical activity. *Gastroenterology*, **57**, 51
60. Kwong, N. K., Brown, B. H., Whittaker, G. E. and Duthie, H. L. (1972). Effects of gastrin I, secretin, and cholecystokinin–pancreozymin on the electrical activity, motor activity, and acid output of the stomach in man. *Scand. J. Gastroenterol.*, **7**, 161
61. Cooke, A. R., Chvasta, T. E. and Weisbrodt, N. W. (1972). Effect of pentagastrin on emptying and electrical and motor activity of the dog stomach. *Amer. J. Physiol.*, **223**, 934

62. Dozois, R. R. and Kelly, K. A. (1971). Effects of a gastrin pentapeptide on canine gastric emptying of liquids. *Amer. J. Physiol.*, **221**, 113

63. Kelly, K. A. and LaForce, R. C. (1972). Pacing the canine stomach with electric stimulation. *Amer. J. Physiol.*, **222**, 588

64. Sugawara, K., Isaza, J., Curt, J. and Woodward (1969). Effect of secretin and cholecystokinin on gastric motility. *Amer. J. Physiol.*, **217**, 1633

65. Kelly, K. A., Woodward, E. R. and Code, C. F. (1969). Effect of secretin and cholecystokinin on canine gastric electrical activity. *Proc. Soc. Expt. Biol. Med.*, **130**, 1060

66. Brown, J. C., Mutt, V. and Dryburgh, J. R. (1971). The further purification of motilin, a gastric motor activity stimulating polypeptide from the mucosa of the small intestine of hogs. *Can. J. Physiol. Pharmacol.*, **49**, 399

67. Hunt, J. N. (1959). Gastric emptying and secretion in man. *Physiol. Rev.*, **39**, 491

68. Thomas, J. E. (1957). Mechanism and regulation of gastric emptying. *Physiol. Rev.*, **37**, 453

69. Hunt, J. N. and Knox, M. T. (1968). Regulation of gastric emptying. *Handbook of Physiology*, Sec. 6, Vol. 4, 1917 (Baltimore: Williams and Wilkins)

70. Cannon, W. B. (1911). *Mechanical Factors of Digestion* (London: Arnold)

71. Dozois, R. R., Kelly, K. A. and Code, C. F. (1971). Effects of distal antrectomy on gastric emptying of liquids and solids. *Gastroenterology*, **61**, 675

72. Horton, B. T. (1928). Pyloric measurement with special reference to pyloric block. *Amer. J. Anat.*, **41**, 197

73. Isenberg, J. I. and Csendes, A. (1972). Effect of octapeptide of cholecystokinin on canine pyloric pressure. *Amer. J. Physiol.*, **222**, 428

74. Brink, B. M., Schlegel, J. F. and Code, C. F. (1965). The pressure profile of the gastroduodenal junctional zone in dogs. *Gut*, **6**, 163

75. Weisbrodt, N. W., Wiley, J. N., Overholt, B. F. and Bass, P. (1969). A relation between gastroduodenal muscle contractions and gastric emptying. *Gut*, **10**, 543

76. Thomas, J. E. and Crider. (1935). Rhythmic changes in duodenal motility associated with gastric peristalsis. *Amer. J. Physiol.*, **111**, 124

77. Bortoff, A. and Davies, R. (1968). Myogenic transmission of antral slow waves across the gastroduodenal junction *in situ*. *Amer. J. Physiol.*, **215**, 889

78. Brown, B. H., Ng, K. K., Kwong, K., Duthie, H. L., Whittaker, G. E. and Franks, C. I. (1971). Computer analysis and simulation of human gastroduodenal electrical activity. *Med. Biol. Eng.*, **9**, 305

79. Allen, G. L., Poole, E. W. and Code, C. F. (1964). Relationships between electrical activities of antrum and duodenum. *Amer. J. Physiol.*, **207**, 906

80. Bedi, B. and Code, C. F. (1972). Pathway of coordination of postprandial, antral and duodenal action potentials. *Amer. J. Physiol.*, **222**, 1295

81. Gianturco, C. (1934). Some mechanical factors of gastric physiology. *Amer. J. Roentgen.*, **31**, 745

82. Gianturco, C. (1934). Some mechanical factors of gastric physiology. *Amer. J. Roentgen.*, **31**, 735

83. Ludwick, J. R., Wiley, J. N. and Bass, P. (1969). Pyloroplasty and vagotomy: early effects on antral and duodenal contractile activity. *Arch. Surg.*, **99**, 553

84. Chey, W. Y., Hitanant, S., Hendricks, J. and Lorber, S. H. (1970). Effect of secretin and cholecystokinin on gastric emptying and gastric secretion in man. *Gastroenterology*, **58**, 820

85. Chvasta, T., Weisbrodt, N. W. and Cooke, A. R. (1971). The effect of pentagastrin and secretin on gastric emptying in the dog. *Clin. Res.*, **19**, 656

86. Friedman, G., Wolf, B. S., Waye, J. D. and Janowitz, H. D. (1965). Correlation of cineradiographic and intraluminal pressure changes in the human duodenum: an analysis of the functional significance of monophasic waves. *Gastroenterology*, **49**, 37

87. Hightower, N. C. (1968). Motor action of the small bowel. *Handbook of Physiology*, Sec. 6, Vol. 4, 2001 (C. F. Code, editor) (Baltimore: Williams and Wilkins)

88. Christensen, J., Glover, J. R., Macagno, E. O., Singerman, R. B. and Weisbrodt, N. W. (1971). Statistics of contractions at a point in the human duodenum. *Amer. J. Physiol.*, **221**, 1818

89. Foulk, W. T., Code, C. F., Morlock, C. G. and Bargen, J. A. (1954). A study of the motility patterns and the basic rhythm in the duodenum and upper part of the jejunum of human beings. *Gastroenterology*, **26**, 601

90. Jacoby, H. I., Bass, P. and Bennett, D. R. (1963). *In vivo* extraluminal contractile force transducer for gastrointestinal muscle. *J. Appl. Physiol.*, **18**, 658

91. Reinke, D. A., Rosenbaum, A. H. and Bennett, D. R. (1967). Patterns of dog gastrointestinal contractile activity monitored *in vivo* with extraluminal force transducers. *Amer. J. Dig. Dis.*, **12**, 113

92. Carlson, G. M., Ruddon, R. W., Hug, C. C. and Bass, P. (1970). Effects of nicotine on gastric antral and duodenal contractile activity in the dog. *J. Pharmacol. Exp. Theor.*, **172**, 367

93. Weisbrodt, N. W., Singerman, R. B., Macagno, E. O., Glover, J. R. and Christensen, J. (1970). Time and space correlations of human small bowel contractions: results of computer analysis. *The Physiologist*, **13**, 338

94. Cannon, W. B. (1902). The movements of the intestines studied by means of the Röntgen rays. *Amer. J. Physiol.*, **6**, 251

95. Bayliss, W. M. and Starling, E. H. (1899). The movements and innervation of the small intestine. *J. Physiol.*, **24**, 99

96. Prosser, C. L. and Bortoff, A. (1968). Electrical activity of intestinal muscle under *in vitro* conditions. *Handbook of Physiology*, Sec. 6, Vol. 4, 2025 (C. F. Code, editor) (Baltimore: Williams and Wilkins)

97. Bass, P. (1968). *In vivo* electrical activity of the small bowel. *Handbook of Physiology*, Sec. 6, Vol. 4, 2051 (C. F. Code, editor) (Baltimore: Williams and Wilkins)

98. Szurszewski, J. H., Elveback, L. R. and Code, C. F. (1970). Configuration and frequency gradient of electric slow wave over canine small bowel. *Amer. J. Physiol.*, **218**, 1468

99. Bunker, C. E., Johnson, L. P. and Nelsen, T. S. (1967). Chronic *in situ* studies of the electrical activity of the small intestine. *Arch. Surg.*, **95**, 259

100. Diamant, N. E. and Bortoff, A. (1966). Nature of the intestinal slow-wave frequency gradient. *Amer. J. Physiol.*, **216**, 301

101. Sarna, S. K., Daniel, E. E. and Kingma, Y. J. (1971). Simulation of slow-wave electrical activity of small intestine. *Amer. J. Physiol.*, **221**, 166

102. Diamant, N. E. and Bortoff, A. (1969). Effects of transection on the intestinal slow-wave frequency gradient. *Amer. J. Physiol.*, **216**, 734

103. Duthie, H. L., Brown, B. H., Robertson-Dunn, B., Kwong, K. K., Whittaker, G. E. and Waterfall, W. (1972). Electrical activity in the gastroduodenal area— slow waves in the proximal duodenum. A comparison of man and dog. *Amer. J. Dig. Dis.*, **17**, 344

104. Weisbrodt, N. W. and Christensen, J. (1972). Electrical activity of the cat duodenum in fasting and vomiting. *Gastroenterology*, **63**, 1004

105. McCoy, E. J. and Baker, R. D. (1969). Intestinal slow waves: decrease in propagation velocity along upper small intestine. *Amer. J. Dig. Dis.*, **14**, 9

106. Bortoff, A. (1965). Electrical transmission of slow waves from longitudinal to circular intestinal muscle. *Amer. J. Physiol.*, **209**, 1254

107. Bortoff, A. and Sachs, F. (1970). Electrotonic spread of slow waves in circular muscle of small intestine. *Amer. J. Physiol.*, **218**, 576

108. Kobayashi, M., Nagai, T. and Prosser, C. L. (1966). Electrical interaction between muscle layers of cat intestine. *Amer. J. Physiol.*, **211**, 1281

109. Lui, J., Prosser, C. L. and Job, D. D. (1969). Ionic requirements of slow waves and spikes. *Amer. J. Physiol.*, **217**, 1542.

110. Job, D. D. (1971). Effect of antibiotics and selective inhibitors of ATP on intestinal slow waves. *Amer. J. Physiol.*, **220**, 299

111. Daniel, E. E., Duchon, G. and Henderson, R. M. (1972). The ultrastructural bases for coordination of intestinal motility. *Amer. J. Dig. Dis.*, **17**, 289

112. Nelsen, T. S. and Becker, J. C. (1968). Simulation of the electrical and mechanical gradient of the small intestine. *Amer. J. Physiol.*, **214**, 749

113. Diamant, N. E., Rose, P. K. and Davison, E. J. (1970). Computer simulation of intestinal slow-wave frequency gradient. *Amer. J. Physiol.*, **219**, 1684

114. Bass, P. and Wiley, J. N. (1965). Electrical extraluminal contractile-force activity of the duodenum of the dog. *Amer. J. Dig. Dis.*, **10**, 183

115. Bass, P., Code, C. F. and Lambert, E. H. (1961). Motor and electric activity of the duodenum. *Amer. J. Physiol.*, **201**, 287
116. Alvarez, E. C. (1914). Functional variations in contractions of different parts of the small intestine. *Amer. J. Physiol.*, **35**, 177
117. Catchpole, B. N. (1969). Ileus: use of sympathetic blocking in its treatment. *Surgery*, **66**, 811
118. Kewenter, J., Pahlin, P. E. and Storm, B. (1970). The effect of periarterial nerve stimulation on the jejunal and ileal motility in cat. *Acta Physiol. Scand.*, **80**, 353
119. Carlson, G. M., Bedi, B. S. and Code, C. F. (1972). Mechanism of propagation of intestinal interdigestive myoelectric complex. *Amer. J. Physiol.*, **222**, 1027
120. Szurszewski, J. and Steggerda, F. R. (1968). The effect of hypoxia on the slow wave of the canine small intestine. *Amer. J. Dig. Dis.*, **13**, 168
121. Kyi, J. K. K. and Daniel, E. E. (1970). The effects of ischemia on intestinal nerves and electrical slow waves. *Amer. J. Dig. Dis.*, **15**, 959
122. Ambache, N., Verney, J. and Aboo Zar, M. (1970). Evidence for the release of two non-cholinergic spasmogens from the plexus-containing longitudinal muscle of the guinea-pig ileum. *J. Physiol.*, **207**, 8P
123. Wood, J. D. (1970). Electrical activity from single neurons in Auerbach's plexus. *Amer. J. Physiol.*, **219**, 159
124. Ohkawa, H. and Prosser, C. L. (1972). Electrical activity in myenteric and submucous plexuses of cat intestine. *Amer. J. Physiol.*, **222**, 1412
125. Ohkawa, H. and Prosser, C. L. (1972). Functions of neurons in enteric plexuses of cat intestine. *Amer. J. Physiol.* **222**, 1420
126. Smith, A. N. and Hogg, D. (1966). Effect of gastrin II on the motility of the gastrointestinal tract. *Lancet*, **1**, 403
127. Ramirez, M. and Farrar, J. T. (1960). The effect of secretin and cholecystokinin-pancreoxymin on the intraluminal pressure of the jejunum in the unanesthetized dog. *Amer. J. Dig. Dis.*, **15**, 539
128. Hermon-Taylor, J. and Code, C. F. (1970). Effect of secretin on small bowel myoelectric activity of conscious dogs. *Amer. J. Dig. Dis.*, **15**, 545
129. Weisbrodt, N. W., Hug, C. C., Wiley, J. N. and Bass, P. (1971). Contractile activity of gastric antrum and taenia coli in the unanesthetized monkey. *J. Appl. Physiol.*, **30**, 276
130. Bass, P. and Bennett, D. R. (1968). Local chemical regulation of motor action of the bowel-substance P and lipid-soluble acids. *Handbook of Physiology*, Sec. 6, Vol. 4, 2193 (C. F. Code, editor) (Baltimore: Williams and Wilkins)
131. Cohen, S., Harris, L. D. and Levitan, R. (1968). Manometric characteristics of the human ileocecal junctional zone. *Gastroenterology*, **54**, 72
132. Rendleman, D. F., Anthony, J. E., Davis, C., Buenger, R. E., Brooks, A. J. and Beattie, E. J. (1958). Reflux pressure studies in the ileocecal valves of dogs and humans. *Surgery*, **44**, 640
133. Connell, A. M. (1968). Motor action of the large bowel. *Handbook of Physiology*, Sec. 6, Vol. 4, 2075 (C. F. Code, editor) (Baltimore: Williams and Wilkins)
134. Pace, J. L. (1971). The age of appearance of the haustra of the human colon. *J. Anat.*, **109**, 75
135. Ritchie, J. A. (1971). Movement of segmental constrictions in the human colon. *Gut*, **12**, 350
136. Torsoli, A., Ramorino, M. L., Ammaturo, M. V., Capurso, L., Paoluzi, P. and Anzini, F. (1971). Mass movements and intracolonic pressures. *Amer. J. Dig. Dis.*, **16**, 693
137. Connell, A. M., Texter, E. C. and Vantrappen (1965). Classification and interpretation of motility records. *Amer. J. Dig. Dis.*, **10**, 481
138. Wienbeck, M., Weisbrodt, N. and Christenson, J. (1971). The electrical activity of the cat colon *in vivo*. *Gastroenterology*, **60**, 809
139. Rinaldo, J. A., Orinion, E. O., Simpelo, R. V., Check, F. E. and Beauregard, W. (1971). Differential response of longitudinal and circular muscles of intact canine colon to morphine and bethanechol. *Gastroenterology*, **60**, 438
140. Elliott, T. R. and Barclay-Smith, E. (1904). Antiperistalsis and other muscular activities of the colon. *J. Physiol.*, **31**, 272
141. Holzknecht, G. (1969). The normal peristalsis of the colon. *Amer. J. Dig. Dis.*, **14**, 57

142. Costa, M. and Furness, J. B. (1971). Catecholamine containing nerve cells in the mammalian myenteric plexus. *Histochemie*, **25**, 103

143. Youmans, W. B. (1968). Innervation of the gastrointestinal tract. *Handbook of Physiology*, Sec. 6, Vol. 4, 1655 (C. F. Code, editor) (Baltimore, Williams and Wilkins)

144. Christensen, J., Caprilli, R. and Lund, G. F. (1969). Electric slow waves in circular muscle of cat colon. *Amer. J. Physiol.*, **217**, 771

145. Wienbeck, M., Christensen, J. and Weisbrodt, N. W. (1972). Electromyography of the colon in the unanesthetized cat. *Amer. J. Dig. Dis.*, **17**, 356

146. Wienbeck, M. and Christensen, J. (1971). Cationic requirements of colon slow waves in the cat. *Amer. J. Physiol.*, **220**, 513

147. Christensen, J. and Hauser, R. L. (1971). Longitudinal axial coupling of slow waves in proximal cat colon. *Amer. J. Physiol.*, **221**, 246

148. Christensen, J. and Hauser, R. L. (1971). Circumferential coupling of electric slow waves in circular muscle of cat colon. *Amer. J. Physiol.*, **221**, 1033

149. Ustach, T. J., Tobon, F., Hambrecht, T., Bass, D. D. and Schuster, M. M. (1970). Electrophysiological aspects of human sphincter function. *J. Clin. Invest.*, **49**, 41

150. Connell, A. M., Frankel, H. and Guttmann, L. (1963). The motility of the pelvic colon following complete lesions of the spinal cord. *Paraplegia*, **1**, 98

151. Crowcroft, P. J., Holman, M. E. and Szurszewski, J. H. (1970). Excitatory input from the colon to the inferior mesenteric ganglion. *J. Physiol.*, **208**, 19P

152. Castell, D. O., Cohen, S. and Harris, L. D. (1970). Response of human ileocaecal sphincter to gastrin. *Amer. J. Physiol.*, **219**, 712

153. Connell, A. M. and Logan, C. J. H. (1967). The role of gastrin in gastroileocolic responses. *Amer. J. Dig. Dis.*, **12**, 277

154. Weisbrodt, N. W., Hug, C. C., Schmiege, S. K. and Bass, P. (1970). Effects of nicotine and tyramine on contractile activity of the colon. *Europ. J. Pharmacol.*, **12**, 310

155. Hallenbeck, G. A. (1968). Biliary and pancreatic intraductal pressures. *Handbook of Physiology*, Sec. 6, Vol. 2, 1007. (C. F. Code, editor) (Baltimore: Williams and Wilkins)

156. Ivy, A. C. and Oldberg, E. (1928). A hormone mechanism for gallbladder contraction and evacuation. *Amer. J. Physiol.*, **86**, 599

157. Hedner, P. and Rorsman, G. (1969). On the mechanism of action for the effect of cholecystokinin on the choledocho duodenal junction in the cat. *Acta Physiol. Scand.*, **76**, 248

158. Ludwick, J. R. and Bass, P. (1967). Contractile and electrical activity of the extahepatic biliary tract and duodenum. *Surg. Gynecol. Obstet.*, **124**, 536

159. Schwegler, R. A., Jr and Boyden, E. A. (1937). The development of the pars intestinalis of the common bile duct in the human fetus, with special reference to the origin of the ampulla of vater and sphincter of Oddi. *Anat. Record.*, **68**, 17

160. Shelhamer, J. and Goyal, R. K. (1973). Physiology of the bile transport: manometric studies of common bile duct and sphincter of Oddi. *Gastroenterology*, **64**, 686

161. DuBois, F. S. and Hunt, E. A. (1933). Peristalsis of the common bile duct in the opossum. *Anat. Record.*, **53**, 387

162. Hauge, C. W. and Mark, J. B. D. (1965). Common bile duct motility and sphincter mechanism. *Ann. Surg.*, **162**, 1028

163. Andersson, K. E., Andersson, R., Hedner, P. and Persson, C. G. A. (1972). Effect of cholecystokinin on the level of cyclic AMP and on mechanical activity in the isolated sphincter of Oddi. *Life. Sci.*, **11**, 723

164. Persson, C. G. A. (1971). Adrenoceptor functions in the cat cholecdocho duodenal junction *in vitro*. *Brit. J. Pharmacol.*, **42**, 447

6
Salivary Secretion

L. H. SCHNEYER
University of Alabama Medical Center
and
N. EMMELIN
University of Lund

6.1 INTRODUCTION

In mammals, the salivary glands provide the digestive fluid for the first segment of the alimentary canal, the mouth. The saliva is important in alimentary function, principally because of its solvent, demulcent and dispersive actions. For example, during mastication these actions help form the semi-solid bolus of food. Over a longer period of time, they protect the masticatory apparatus. Saliva plays a role in mediating taste and in facilitating deglutition. Moreover, its amylase promotes digestion of starch and glycogen.

The importance of the various alimentary functions of saliva becomes evident when salivary flow is stopped or severely impeded for long. The digestion of starch is not greatly affected, because of pancreatic amylase. However, the health and even the integrity of the oral tissues are disturbed. Inflammation of the oral mucosa and dissolution of tooth crowns have been noted frequently in xerostomia[1-3]. Hence, the most important contribution of saliva to alimentary function is undoubtedly to protect the teeth and buccal mucosa.

Mammalian saliva is notable for its diverse composition and production rate. Saliva may differ widely from homologous glands of different species, and even in different glands of the same species. In fact, salivary composition as well as flow rate differ widely in the same gland when different degrees or modes of stimulation are employed. None the less, one can make several generalisations when describing salivary composition and flow[3-12]. First, secretomotor autonomic nerves invariably control flow in the normal animal. In most instances, no saliva is secreted in the absence of secretomotor activity. However, even when 'spontaneous' secretion is present (i.e. secretion occurring without stimulation of the secreto–motor innervation), the flow is basal and can be accelerated by superimposition of secretomotor stimulation. Secondly, the total osmolality of final saliva is either isotonic to that of serum, or, more often, hypotonic. Thirdly, the osmolality of hypotonic saliva rises and tends to approach isotonicity when flow rate increases. Fourth, saliva often contains a strikingly high concentration of potassium. In many salivas, potassium concentration $[K^+]$ is 2–10 times greater than that of serum, and, under special stimulatory conditions, may reach levels 30 times those of serum. Such levels, closely approaching the $[K^+]$ of intracellular water, are rare in extracellular fluids. Finally, the saliva in many mammals contains appreciable levels of the digestive enzyme, amylase, as well as other macromolecules. Alternating periods of stimulation and rest establish a cycle of discharge and accumulation (secretory cycle) in cells of the gland.

The glands that produce most of the total saliva consist of three main pairs: parotid, submaxillary (or submandibular) and sublingual. In addition to the major gland pairs, numerous smaller glands lie just beneath the oral mucous membrane covering the lips (labial glands), palate (palatine glands), tongue (lingual glands) and cheek (buccal glands). These major and minor glands are located some distance from where their secretions are finally discharged. However, for each gland, at least one excretory duct leads from the parenchyma of the gland and carries salivary fluid to the oral cavity. Hence, all salivary glands are exocrine. In many ways, salivary glands resemble other exocrine glands, which together constitute one of the major effector systems of the body[3-12]. All are non-excitable organs and display no propagated action potential, even though electrical changes in the gland cells may accompany secretory activity. The secretory responses, possibly including the accompanying electrical changes, are not all-or-none phenomena, but can be graded. Secretory cells of exocrine glands are functionally as well as anatomically asymmetrical, i.e. the luminal and serosal membranes are identical neither in behaviour nor in form. Moreover, secretion by exocrine glands is controlled by autonomic secretomotor nerves, not by motor fibres arising directly from the central nervous system.

Nerves contribute to the regulation of the activity and even the morphology of salivary glands. Control by parasympathetic fibres is particularly striking, since they can evoke a broad range of secretory flow. Parasympathetic innervation also regulates glandular structure and size[13]. In many glands, secretomotor fibres are present in the sympathetic innervation. Although these may not affect salivary flow or regulate glandular structure markedly, they do affect salivary composition[3-13]. Moreover, both branches of the autonomic nervous system contain fibres which influence vascular smooth muscle in the gland, and thus are important regulators of glandular blood flow[4,5,8].

Since the major alimentary function of salivary glands is to provide an important bathing fluid, let us consider the mechanisms by which this fluid is formed and regulated. We shall discuss and analyse the processes of salivary secretion and regulation as they are understood currently.

6.2 THE SECRETORY UNIT

6.2.1 Development and morphology

Salivary glands develop early in prenatal life from thickenings of the oral epithelium[14-16]. These thickenings represent accumulations of presumptive glandular epithelial cells and soon begin to show sprouts. The sprouts grow inward from the oral epithelium and develop into branching cords, which still retain contiguity with the oral lining. With the later appearance of central cavities in the epithelial cords, the gland anlagen become tubular. The tubule cells differentiate further to form acini and ducts. The appearance of completely differentiated acini and of at least one variety of ductal element, the granular duct, is delayed generally until the early stages of postnatal life[16-18]. At birth, however, the secretory unit of the salivary gland has already attained its general form as a racemose structure. The main execretory duct has become the stem, and the acinus or its precursor, the terminal tubule, is the most proximal unit. The entire secretory unit contains a central lumen, continuous with the oral cavity itself. The general form of the secretory unit as it appears in the submaxillary gland of the mature

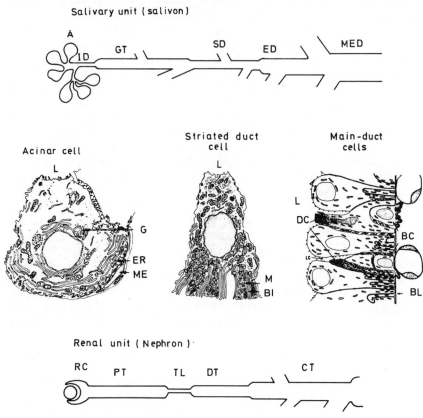

Figure 6.1 Representation of a salivary unit, salivary cell types, and, for comparison, a kidney unit. Symbols: Salivon, A=acinus; ID=intercalated duct; GT=granular tubule, S=striated duct; ED=excretory duct; MED=main excretory duct. Cell types, L=lumen; G=golgi; ER=endoplasmic reticulum; ME=myoepithelial cell; M= mitochondrion; BI=basal infoldings; DC=dark cell; LC=light cell; BC=basal cell; BL=basal lamina. Nephron, RC=renal corpuscle; PT=proximal tubule; TL=thin loop; DT=distal tubule; CT=collecting tubule. (Cellular representations are from Tamarin and Sreebny[21], by courtesy of *J. Morphology* and Shackleford and Schneyer[96], by courtesy of *Anat. Rec.*)

rat is shown schematically in Figure 6.1. For brevity, the salivary secretory unit will be referred to as the 'salivon' (like the analogous term, 'nephron', denoting the morphological and functional unit of kidney).

The salivon of the salivary gland in some ways resembles but in other ways differs from the nephron in the kidney. For example, salivon is a converging system, while the elements in the renal tubule are arranged more linearly (Figure 6.1). Thus, from proximal to distal (following the direction of salivary flow) in the salivary secretory unit, several acini (or terminal tubules) converge on each intercalated duct. Numerous intercalated ducts are drained by each striated duct, or directly into its granular segment, if present. And numerous striated ducts empty into fewer excretory ducts, which, in turn, all converge to form the main excretory duct. Generally, a single main excretory duct leads from each gland and ends at the oral mucosa.

In the salivary gland, as in the kidney, blood vessels enter the organ mainly at the hilus. In the kidney, these vessels form a portal system, with the primary arterioles leading to the capillary system of the renal corpuscle. In salivary glands, a portal system may also be present, but arterial blood seems to supply distal structures first and acini later[19]. In the extraparenchymal main excretory duct, flow of blood also occurs in a direction opposite that of saliva[20]. Thus, in salivary glands much of the arterial supply to the entire secretory unit may be countercurrent. In further contrast to the kidney, the salivon apparently possesses no looped segment comparable to the thin loop of Henle in the nephron.

The various elements of the salivon show characteristic differences from one another in cell size and number, and in cytoarchitecture[16,21-24] (Figure 6.1). Acinar cells account for most of the total mass of the salivon, are its largest cells, and are generally arranged in groups to form ovoid acini. Granules usually fill the apical cytoplasm of acinar cells; the basal and lateral cytoplasm is well provided with endoplasmic reticulum. Intercalated ducts are comprised of cells much smaller than acinar cells. In striated ducts, the cells are also large and are distinguished by parallel infoldings of the basal membrane. These infoldings and the columns of mitochondria enclosed in the cytoplasm between the membrane folds give the cells their striated appearance. In some glands (e.g. rodent submaxillary), the proximal segment of the striated duct consists of cells containing many round granules. The segment is then separately designated as the granular duct.

Excretory ducts contain three main epithelial cell types. Of these, light cells (called this because of their electronlucency) are most common. The second type, also columnar, is the dark cell. The electron-dense nature of its cytoplasm is evidently due to close spacing of numerous microfilaments. Often, the lateral junction between adjacent light and dark cells is displaced basally by a deep luminal cleft. The third cell type in the excretory duct is the basal cell. Of the three cell types, only basal cells fail to contact the duct lumen. In general, the epithelial cells of the salivon constitute a single layer with no true stratification.

One other type of cell in the salivary gland must be mentioned, the myoepithelial cell. Myoepithelial cells appear close to acini and intercalated ducts, which they encompass with tentacle-like extensions from the cell body. The cytoplasm of myoepithelial cells contains bundles of parallel filaments possessing contractile properties.

Nerves also enter the gland at the hilus and travel in the stroma. The nerve fibres lose their myelin sheaths before penetrating close to parenchymal cells[23-27]. Most aspects of neural regulation will be discussed in later sections of this chapter. We should mention here, however, that the structure and size of the salivary glands, in both mature and immature animals, is affected by the level of neural stimulation[13]. This relationship seems to be mainly mediated by the secretory activity evoked by neural stimulation.

The parasympathetic nerves are particularly effective in evoking salivary flow and are also the main nerves influencing gland structure. While sympathetic fibres to the glands may also be secretomotor, they do little to regulate gland size. The separate roles of the two autonomic branches in affecting glandular morphology can be demonstrated by severing selectively the nerves. Marked atrophy occurs in response to parasympathetic, but not to sympathetic, neurectomy[13]. Acinar cells are particularly affected and undergo pronounced regressive changes after parasympathectomy. In immature animals, where growth and differentiation of the salivon are incomplete, changes in glandular activity can also affect development[13,28,29]. Here, too, acini are mainly affected. However, both autonomic branches play a significant role in regulating postnatal glandular development. Thus, after parasympathectomy, morphological differentiation is notably retarded, and acinar cells fail to attain their normal size or number[28]. Effects of parasympathectomy on cell number, as reflected by the glandular content of DNA, are

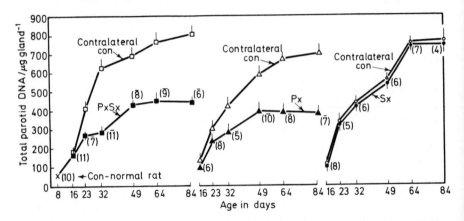

Figure 6.2 Relationship between total DNA of rat parotid gland and postnatal age. Surgical interruption of the parasympathetic and sympathetic innervation (PxSx) or of the parasympathetics alone (Px) decreases postnatal parotid growth in relation to control (con). Sympathectomy alone (Sx) is ineffective. (From Schneyer and Hall[28], by courtesy of the American Physiology Society.)

shown in Figure 6.2. Sympathectomy, on the other hand, results in significantly inhibited biochemical development of the gland; normal high levels of amylase do not develop in cells of the sympathectomised growing gland[29].

6.2.2 Summary

The secretory units of the salivary gland are derived embryologically from the oral epithelium with which they remain continuous throughout life. Each mature secretory unit consists of acini and ducts. Three or four main segments of the duct system can be distinguished. From proximal to distal (following the flow of saliva), these are: intercalated ducts, striated ducts (sometimes with a separately distinguishable granular duct segment) and excretory ducts. Myoepithelial cells, believed to perform a contractile rather than a secretory function, are frequently present around acini and intercalated ducts. The entire secretory unit (salivon) shows a progressive reduction, from proximal to distal, in the number of elements (convergence). The arterial supply to the salivon runs countercurrent to the salivary flow. The secretory activity of the salivon is controlled by the autonomic secretomotor innervation, which also influences the morphological and biochemical characteristics of the whole gland.

6.3 SECRETION OF FLUID AND ELECTROLYTES

Salivary glands are relatively small organs, accounting for only a small fraction of total body weight ($<1\%$ in most animals). Relative to their weight, however, the glands are capable of secreting at remarkably high flow rates[3]. In humans, for example, the submaxillary or parotid gland can secrete its weight in saliva within 20 min. The dog is capable of even more copious secretion than man, and with sustained stimulation a brisk salivary flow can continue for hours.

Because secretion of saliva occurs primarily as a consequence of trans-epithelial transport of inorganic electrolytes, it is important to discuss:

(a) the inorganic composition of saliva;

(b) the relationship between salivary flow rate and saliva composition;

(c) ionic and electrical changes associated with the stimulated state; and

(d) the sites and mechanisms of glandular transport of electrolytes and water.

6.3.1 Inorganic composition of saliva

Generalisations about the inorganic composition of saliva are difficult, because composition varies widely among species, among salivas from different gland pairs of the same species, and even in saliva from the same gland when the mode or intensity of stimulation is changed. For the sake of clarity then, the discussion in this section will focus upon the composition of saliva evoked by parasympathetic or parasympathomimetic stimulation of maximal intensity. Effects of changing intensity and mode of stimulation will be considered in a later section.

6.3.1.1 Isotonic salivas

Saliva which is isotonic to plasma is obtained from the parotid glands of sheep[30] and sublingual glands of the cat[31] and dog[32], as well as the parotid gland of the rat[33]. Sheep parotid saliva is isotonic at all flow rates[30]. This is probably also true for cat or dog sublingual saliva[31,32]. In rat parotid saliva, isotonicity is attained only with stimulation of near-maximal intensity[33].

As in plasma, the major cations in these salivas are Na^+ and K^+. Cl^- and HCO_3^- are the major anions. The concentrations of the osmotically important ions are not necessarily always the same in isotonic saliva as in an ultra-filtrate of plasma, however. Thus, in rat parotid saliva during isotonic secretion, $[K^+]$ is relatively high in comparison with that in plasma[33]. In sheep parotid saliva, the concentration of HCO_3^- is appreciably higher than plasma levels[30,34]. This has functional significance in sheep, because maintenance of an alkaline pH is important for ruminal digestion[34].

6.3.1.2 Hypotonic salivas

In hypotonic salivas, Na^+ and K^+ are the osmotically important cations, and Cl^- and HCO_3^- are the main anions. In these salivas, sodium concentration $[Na^+]$ may be as low as 20 mequiv l^{-1}, as in rat submaxillary saliva[33,35], or as high as 100 mequiv l^{-1}, as in parotid or submaxillary saliva from the human[36,37] or dog[38,39]. $[K^+]$ is generally high in these salivas, at least compared with plasma levels. In rat submaxillary saliva, $[K^+]$ is usually 40–50 mequiv l^{-1} [33,35] in other hypotonic salivas, it usually ranges between 10 and 20 mequiv l^{-1} [33,36–39] during near-maximal parasympathetic stimulation. The bicarbonate concentration $[HCO_3^-]$ in saliva from strongly stimulated parotid glands of the human[36] and dog[32] is higher than plasma levels, while chloride concentration $[Cl^-]$ is lower. Total osmolality may be one-half to two-thirds that of plasma in these cases.

Other inorganic substances are, of course, present in saliva, and they may be important, but not osmotically. Calcium, for example, is present in low concentration—usually *ca.* 2–4 mequiv l^{-1} in human saliva[40], lower than its plasma concentration. The concentration of ionised Ca^{2+} in saliva is also lower than in the plasma[41]. Phosphate, on the other hand, is ordinarily present in higher concentration in saliva than in plasma[40]. Thus, in man at least, the ratio of calcium to phosphate is <1.0 in saliva, but exceeds 1.0 in plasma.

6.3.2 Relationship between salivary flow rate and saliva composition

In 1878, Heidenhain[42] first noted that the percentage of total salts in saliva increases and levels off as the strength of stimulation and hence salivary flow rates progressively increase above resting values. Langley and Fletcher[43] later referred to this relationship as Heidenhain's law. Heidenhain's law has general application to salivary secretion of electrolytes and now appears to represent the final expression of a balance of several basic secretory processes.

The particular inorganic constituents of saliva that rise in concentration when flow rates increase are the sodium, chloride and bicarbonate ions[36–38,44]. Potassium responds differently[38]. Salivary $[K^+]$ usually remains remarkably constant when salivary flow rate changes, even over a wide range. (At extremely low flow rates, however, $[K^+]$ may be elevated in the saliva, and decrease over a brief span of increasing flow rates[36].)

In an early kinetic study, Thaysen *et al.*[36] examined the effects of changing salivary flow on rates of appearance of the osmotically important ions. They found that, with Na$^+$, salivary output increases (expressed as μequiv min^{-1} [36], or μg min^{-1} g^{-1} of gland[9]), first non-linearly. Later, as salivary flow continues to increase progressively, the change in Na$^+$ output approaches linearity. From these effects (Figure 6.3), these workers deduced[9,36] that

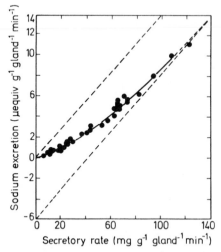

Figure 6.3 Rate of secretion of sodium relative to the rate of parotid flow. The upper line predicts the rate of secretion of sodium in the absence of reabsorption. The lower line predicts the rate of sodium secretion if precursor fluid contains [Na$^+$] at 140 mequiv l^{-1} and the amount of sodium reabsorbed each minute is constant. The middle line shows that a line drawn from observed values[36] approaches the bottom line as an asymptote when flow rate increases. (From Thaysen[9], by courtesy of Springer-Verlag.)

Na$^+$ may be transferred at a constant rate into a precursor saliva and later be partially reabsorbed by a transport process of limited capacity (low T_M). They further suggested[9,36] that the [Na$^+$] of the precursor fluid is close to plasma levels.

Thaysen *et al.*[36] found that K$^+$ output changed linearly with flow rate over virtually the entire range estimated. One would expect this, since salivary [K$^+$] is practically independent of the rate of salivary flow. Thaysen suggested that K$^+$ like Na$^+$ is transferred into the precursor solution at a constant rate, but that, unlike Na$^+$, K$^+$ is not re-absorbed[36]. He thought that K$^+$ might be secreted in the ducts[9]. He also proposed that [K$^+$] in precursor fluid is low, in some cases at plasma levels and that precursor fluid is essentially isotonic to plasma. Implicit in Thaysen's hypothesis is the assumption that the ionic composition of precursor fluid is unchanged by alterations in stimulation intensity and that water that enters precursor fluid during its formation is not exchanged significantly later in the duct system[9].

Recently, it became possible to test Thaysen's analysis directly using the techniques of micropuncture and microperfusion. These experiments and their implications will be discussed in detail in Section 6.3.4. Many of Thaysen's speculations now appear to be substantiated by direct evidence. Precursor fluid has been found to contain Na^+ and K^+ levels, which, in many glands, generally resemble those of plasma. Na^+ is re-absorbed effectively in the salivary duct system, but the duct system is relatively impermeable to water. In fact, salivary hypotonicity evidently results from ductal net re-absorption of sodium, exceeding net ductal secretion of other ions, and a net movement of water from the duct system which remains small. However, several aspects of Thaysen's hypothesis require modifications. Ductal secretion of K^+ not only occurs, as Thaysen suspected, but sometimes is surprisingly pronounced. Moreover, Thaysen's hypothesis provides no adequate explanation for certain other phenomena, particularly (as Thaysen recognised[9]) salivary transients.

6.3.3　Ion transients and electrical correlates

When saliva is collected over a period of at least several minutes (the *usual* time taken to collect samples for analysis), the resultant values for the concentration of salivary constituents represent averages for the whole sample and give no clue concerning rapid transient changes. Even the early literature[36,45] indicates that such changes do occur in potassium concentration, for example.

It remained for Burgen[46] to show that a transiently high $[K^+]$ in saliva is found characteristically in samples collected within the first few minutes after the start of stimulation. Burgen called this transient elevation a rest-transient and convincingly showed that this extra K^+ is derived from an intracellular pool, mainly in acinar cells[19]. Thus, during the rest-transient, tissue K^+ levels fall and venous as well as salivary $[K^+]$ is high. Balance studies[46] showed that the extra K^+ in the saliva and venous blood, during the transient, closely matches the amount of K^+ lost by the gland tissue in the same time period (Figure 6.4). Glandular K^+ loss and the elevation of salivary and venous $[K^+]$ subside within 3 min, even though stimulation continues (Figure 6.4). Upon cessation of stimulation another rate-change transient appears. Glandular K^+ rises slowly in concentration and venous $[K^+]$ falls below the arterial level. Within 15 min this rate-change transient subsides and glandular and venous $[K^+]$ return to steady-state resting values.

Rate-change transients for K^+ have been found in other glands, including dog parotid[46], sheep parotid[47,48] and cat submaxillary glands[49]. Intracellular ions other than potassium (Na^+, I^-, and Ca^{2+})[49-52] also show rate-change transients when glandular stimulation is started and when it is stopped. The rest-transient for K^+ and other intracellular ions is altered by changes in the strength of stimulation, but in this case the relationship between salivary concentration and strength of stimulation, or flow rate, seems to have a different basis from that observed during steady-state secretion[8,46,50].

Ion transients of saliva are important signals of cellular changes accompanying initiation of the stimulated state, or its resolution and return to the resting condition. Another sign of the link between stimulus and secretion is a change in transmembrane potential, starting immediately after application of the stimulus and lasting as long as stimulation continues.

This change has been most extensively studied in acinar cells. There, the resting transmembrane potential is distinctly low compared to the levels in

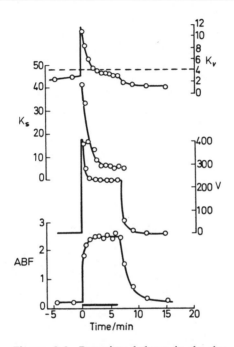

Figure 6.4 Potassium balance in the dog submaxillary gland relative to a period of stimulation. Ordinates: K_v, venous potassium concentration in mequiv l^{-1} (broken line shows arterial potassium); K_s, salivary potassium concentration in mequiv l^{-1}; V, salivary flow rate in mg g^{-1} min^{-1}; ABF, arterial blood flow in ml g^{-1} min^{-1}. The heavy solid line along the abscissa shows the period of stimulation. (From Burgen[46], by courtesy of the Physiological Society.)

most excitable cells. Lundberg, who first measured acinar transmembrane potentials, recorded values in cat submaxillary[53] and sublingual glands[54,55] of 20–35 mV (inside negative) across the contraluminal or luminal membrane of resting acinar cells. Generally similar values for resting membrane potentials in acinar cells have been found in the submaxillary and parotid glands of the rat[56], the submaxillary gland of the dog[57] and the cat parotid gland[58]. After the start of parasympathetic stimulation of a gland or administration of cholinergic drugs, the membrane potential of acinar cells usually changes. In cat submaxillary and sublingual glands, the change involves a pronounced hyperpolarisation; e.g. acinar cytoplasmic negativity increases[53-55]. Lundberg called this change in transmembrane potential the 'secretory potential'[53]. Secretory potentials have been found in acinar cells of all salivary glands, but their magnitude and direction are not the same in all glands. In cat submaxillary and sublingual glands, the secretory potential starts after a latent period, often several hundred milliseconds long[55,59]. Even when liberal allotments are made for conduction time along the pre- and post-ganglionic fibres, delay at the parasympathetic ganglion and time for release and diffusion of neural mediator at the receptor sites, much of the latent period remains unexplained (60 ms)[59]. It would be important in future work to identify the events transpiring during the 60 ms 'silent' period before the secretory potential appears.

The acinar secretory potential may be as large as -35 mV in a hyperpolarising direction (cat submaxillary or sublingual)[55], or as small as -6 mV (cat parotid gland)[60] or less and reversed in sign, as in rat submaxillary gland[61]. The hyperpolarising electrical response has been designated type I by Lundberg[55]. Interestingly, this response is not 'all or none', but can be graded[53], as shown in Figure 6.5. Duct cells also show an electrical response

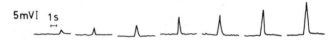

Figure 6.5 The secretory potential (type I) from a single cell relative to stimulus strength. Single shocks of varying strength provided minimal (at left), submaximal, and maximal (at right) stimuli to the chorda nerve. (From Lundberg[53], by courtesy of *Acta Physiol. Scand.*)

to stimulation, but here membrane depolarisation (type III response)[55] is the prevalent change. The resting membrane potential of duct cells seems to be generally higher (35–90 mV) than in acinar cells. However, the identity of the duct cells involved in the type III response to cholinergic stimulation has not been established.

Although unstimulated acinar cells characteristically show low membrane potentials, intracellular [K$^+$] is high—as high, in fact, as in excitable cells (*ca.* 140–150 mequiv l^{-1} of cell water)[55,62]. Hence, the membrane potential of unstimulated acinar cells is far from its equilibrium value; if K$^+$ is the major permeating ion, the value should be *ca.* -90 mV (inside of cell, negative). This value is readily calculated from the Nernst equation: $E_{K^+}=$ 60 log [K$^+$]$_o$ [K$^+$]$_o^{-1}$ where E_{K^+} is the potassium equilibrium potential, and [K$^+$]$_o$ and [K$^+$]$_i$ are the molar concentrations of potassium outside (in interstitial fluid) and inside (in cell water) the cell, respectively. Thus, [K$^+$]$_i$ of the resting cell must be maintained against a gradient of *ca.* 65 mV by energy-yielding processes linked to active transport. The acinar transmembrane potential also is not near the sodium equilibrium potential, which, for a [Na$^+$]$_i$ value of *ca.* 20 mequiv l^{-1} of cell water and the usual [Na$^+$]$_o$ values, is *ca.* $+110$ mV. Therefore, the low cellular levels of sodium must also be maintained by energy-linked transport, in this case involving net extrusion of intracellular ion. Chloride ion is, however, distributed generally in accord with the electrical forces acting across the cell membrane. Its distribution seems to require no expenditure of energy by the cell.

Why is the membrane potential of the acinar cell so much lower than the K^+ equilibrium potential and the membrane potential in excitable cells? The answer is not that acinar cells are impermeable to K^+ and that the distribution of Cl^- sets the value of the potential, since changing $[Cl^-]_o$ does not significantly alter the membrane potential[63-66] but changing $[K^+]_o$ does[63-68]. However, changing $[K^+]_o$ does alter the membrane potential by less than the predicted value of 60 mV/10-fold change in $[K^+]_o$.[64,66-68] (Figure 6.6). Moreover, the alteration in membrane potential occurring in

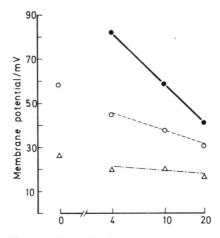

Figure 6.6 Membrane potential of acinar cells relative to $[K^+]$ of the external fluid. The upper line is based on values calculated from the potassium equilibrium potential at three different values of external $[K^+]$. Observed changes in the secretory and resting potentials are shown by the middle and lowest lines, respectively. (From Petersen[67], by courtesy of the Royal Society.)

response to a change in $[K^+]_o$ in some glands can be increased by substituting a bulky impermeant cation for Na^+ outside the cell[68]. Apparently, then, in acinar cells the permeability of the membrane to ions other than K^+ and Cl^- provides the main difference from excitable cells and accounts for the low resting membrane potentials of the secretory cells.

When acinar cells are stimulated, the permeability to K^+ and to Na^+, as well as to other ions, is increased. This has been shown *in vitro* in slices of rat submaxillary gland[69,70] and *in vivo* in cat submaxillary gland[71,72]. The increase in permeability to K^+ mainly accounts for the appearance of the secretory potential[67]. The hyperpolarisation characterising the secretory potential is evidently the result of a tendency of the membrane potential to approach an equilibrium value far exceeding the resting value (see Figure

6.6). Moreover, E_{K^+} is approached more closely during stimulation when extracellular [Na$^+$] is low[72]. This has been accomplished by reducing [Na$^+$] in the vascular supply of a perfused gland. In contrast, reduction of extra-cellular [Cl$^-$] lacks effect on the secretory potential[64,73]. Therefore, the acinar secretory potential, like the resting potential, is essentially a K$^+$ diffusion potential. However, the outward K$^+$ current associated with the secretory potential is to some extent short-circuited by a simultaneous inward movement of Na$^+$ (Figure 6.6). This concept of the basis for the acinar secretory potential, due mainly to the work of Imai and Yoshimura, and Petersen and Poulsen, differs from that originally proposed by Lundberg[31,55]. Lundberg suggested that electrogenic transport of chloride across the contraluminal membrane of acinar cells into the cytoplasm provides the mechanism for hyperpolarisation. One of Lundberg's experi-ments[31], in which hyperpolarisation could still be demonstrated across acinar membranes subjected to a voltage difference at values up to and even exceeding 100 mV (inside negative), is not easily explained by the potassium diffusion concept. However, most data support this concept, and it is now widely accepted.

The increase in ionic permeability generating the secretory potential also leads to the appearance of the rest-transients for K$^+$ and other ions. Hence, the secretory potential and the rest-transients are related events. In essence, the permeability change occurring at the onset of stimulation disturbs the steady state that prevails in the resting condition. [K$^+$]$_i$ is higher than the equilibrium value, remaining high even after the transmembrane potential increases from 25 to 50 or 60 mV. Hence, K$^+$ leaves the acinar cell and enters interstitial fluid and the acinar lumen. This provides the rest-transient. When intra cellular [K$^+$] reaches a new steady state, usually within several minutes, the rest-transient is completed and steady-state secretion has become estab-lished. When stimulation is stopped, the ionic permeability of the acinar membranes decreases. K$^+$ re-accumulates in cell water until a new steady state, characteristic of the rest condition, is again reached.

6.3.4 Transfer of electrolytes and water at acini and ducts

During the rest-transient, when salivary electrolytes are released from cytoplasmic pools, all cells of the salivon may well be involved in this release. In the preceding section, transients of particular ions (e.g. Na$^+$ and K$^+$) known to involve acinar cells were emphasised especially, because correla-tions between the transients and accompanying changes in potential are best delineated in acinar cells. However, ion transients also occur in duct cells[50,51]. None the less, the role of the ducts in elaboration of the final saliva is now better understood for the steady state rather than the transient phase of secretion. Most saliva is, of course, secreted during steady-state secretion, when stimulation has been maintained for some time. This section will concern the separate functions of the ducts and the acini in forming saliva during steady-state secretion.

Direct evidence concerning the separate secretory functions of the acini and the ducts comes largely from recent work in which micropuncture, microcatheterisation and microperfusion techniques were applied to the salivary gland. The technical difficulties have been considerable, owing mainly to the small luminal diameter of these glands (often no more than 4 μm in the proximal segments of the salivon[21]) and to their heterogeneity. Micropuncture samples obtained from proximal segments of the salivon were not, in fact, from acini but from intercalated ducts[74], and perhaps sometimes even from granular ducts[10]. Still, data from micropuncture analysis have provided valuable information about the osmolality and composition of proximal, or precursor, fluid, as well as some information about the composition of fluid in the distal ducts, particularly the excretory ducts. The functional characteristics of excretory ducts have been studied more effectively by microcatheterisation and by microperfusion. Microperfusion involves cannulation of the proximal and distal ends of a segment of the main excretory duct and passing of fluid of known composition through the lumen[75].

Even before the advent of micropuncture sampling of precursor fluid, indirect evidence suggested that a sodium-rich potassium-poor isotonic fluid is formed in the proximal segment of the salivon and that most salivary water is produced by transfer to the lumen in that segment[39,76,77]. However, the experimental methods used in earlier studies were dubious and the interpretations of the data controversial. In the middle 1960s, first Martinez et al.[74], and then Young and Schögel[35] and Mangos et al.[78] (working in Karl Ullrich's laboratory), succeeded in obtaining fluid samples by micropuncture directly from intercalated ducts in rat submaxillary and parotid gland. These samples were analysed for Na^+, K^+, Cl^- and total osmolality. The micropuncture samples generally resembled serum in total osmolality and in molar concentration of osmotically important ions. Thus, direct evidence was at last found from two different glands that fluid from a proximal part of the salivon, probably the intercalated ducts, is essentially plasma-like in composition, at least with respect to osmolality and Na^+ and K^+ concentrations. An earlier, isolated attempt by Yoshimura[65] to obtain micropuncture samples may also have been successful, but it depended upon multiple punctures with each pipette to obtain pooled samples. The data from that preliminary study also indicated that $[Na^+]$ is high in proximal fluid. Young and Schögel[35] found that the composition of the intercalated duct fluid was essentially unchanged by stimulation, although its rate of formation could be altered.

The mechanism of formation of precursor fluid remains unclear, and even the relationships between known events in the stimulus–secretion chain need clarification. For example, secretion seems not to be an obligatory sequel to establishment of the secretory potential[67]. Hence, the ionic changes causing membrane hyperpolarisation during stimulation are only indirectly linked to secretion. Workers have suggested that Ca^{2+} may be involved in the linkage between stimulation and secretion[79]. Omission of Ca^{2+} from the vascular supply to a perfused gland results in a slow reduction, and finally cessation, of cholinergically-evoked secretion[79]. Here, too, the secretory potential is hardly affected[80], and the electrolyte composition of any remaining secretory fluid is little changed[79]. Thus, the role of Ca^{2+} in secretion of fluid and electrolytes during cholinergic stimulation is unclear. Ca^{2+} and cyclic-AMP seem to be more important to secretion of protein, especially in response to adrenergic, rather than cholinergic, stimulation.

The transfer of fluid across the luminal border of the acinar cells may depend on active Na^+ transfer. One report[81] indicates that micropuncture samples from intercalated ducts tend to be slightly hypertonic in some cases, suggesting that transport of electrolytes precedes water transport across the luminal border of acini and intercalated ducts. In addition, Petersen[82] has recently reported that ethacrynic acid blocks salivary secretion, but not the uptake of K^+ by the gland. By extension of the analysis of Whittembury and Proverbio[83] of the effects of ethacrynic acid on kidney slices, Petersen suggested that the inhibitory effect of this agent on salivary secretion is attributable to an inhibition of Na^+ efflux from acinar cells to the lumen. Thus, the evidence only suggests a role for active Na^+ transport in the formation of acinar fluid. Procurement of fluid samples from striated ducts has proved technically even more difficult than from intercalated ducts. Consequently, evidence concerning the secretory functions of the striated ducts has been largely indirect. However, collection of fluid samples from excretory ducts has been feasible at various levels. From analysis of these samples and micropuncture samples from intercalated ducts, the secretory functions of much of the distal duct system have recently been clarified. In rat submaxillary gland, for example, the concentration of Na^+ and the total osmolality of the luminal fluid have been shown to decrease; the concentration of K^+ increases, as the saliva flows distally from intercalated ducts to the termination of the main excretory duct in the mouth[35,74]. The changes in the composition of saliva as it passes through the duct system of the gland are evidently progressive. In rat submaxillary gland, at least, they involve virtually the entire duct system, including the main excretory duct[35,74] (Figure 6.7). In some ductal regions, however, re-equilibration can apparently occur between the luminal and interstitial fluids[35]. In rat submaxillary[35] and parotid[78] glands, partial re-equilibration is thought to occur in a section of the striated duct, since $[Na^+]$ and osmolality of fluid from small excretory ducts are actually lower when the gland is strongly stimulated than when it is nearly at rest[35,78] (Figure 6.7). In the strongly stimulated gland, the saliva is presumed to pass equilibration sites too rapidly to permit appreciable changes in its composition.

In the main excretory duct of rat submaxillary gland, absorption of Na^+ (and Cl^-) and secretion of K^+ (and HCO_3^-) are certainly evident, but they are too slow to effect appreciable changes in the saliva, unless the flow rate is very low. However, the main excretory duct can be perfused through its lumen (a feat first performed by Young and his co-workers[75]) and can thus be used to provide important information concerning the cellular basis for ductal transport. Recently, this valuable approach has been further refined by Knauf[84] and by Field and Young[85] to permit perfusion *in vitro* as well as *in situ*.

In the adult rat, the main excretory duct is *ca.* 27 mm long from gland hilus to oral opening[20]. The duct contains a single layer of epithelial cells, heavily invested by connective tissue, and is well supplied by blood vessels. The lumen of the duct often assumes an irregular shape and tapers from hilus to mouth end. For these reasons, exchange rates across the duct are often cited for the whole duct, or for a specified length, rather than for a unit area of the luminal surface.

When a main excretory duct from rat submaxillary gland is perfused *in situ* with isotonic NaCl, Na^+ is absorbed from the perfusate and K^+ is secreted into it[20,75]. Transfer rates average *ca.* 37 and 20 nl min^{-1} for the whole duct for Na^+ and K^+, respectively, when the perfusion rate is 0.5 μl min^{-1}, or greater. During perfusion, a difference in potential of *ca.* -70 mV (lumen negative) can be measured across the duct at the tip of the hilar catheter[20,75]. Thus, Na^+, at least, is transferred against an electrochemical gradient, and energy must be expended by the ductal epithelial cells to effect the transfer. Moreover, when the perfusion rate is decreased to zero, the transductal potential drops drastically (to -11 mV), and zero rates of

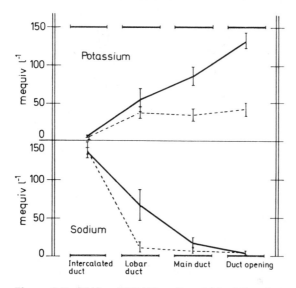

Figure 6.7 $[K^+]$ and $[Na^+]$ in saliva obtained from four loci of the duct system of the rat submaxillary gland. Solid lines connect points from unstimulated glands, and broken lines denote stimulated glands. (From Young and Schögel[35], by courtesy of *Arch. Ges. Physiol.*)

Na^+ and K^+ transport are approached[75]. At steady state, virtually all of the Na^+ is absorbed from the luminal solution ($[Na^+]$ is *ca.* 2 mequiv 1^{-1}) and K^+ is elevated significantly ($[K^+]$ is *ca.* 130 mequiv 1^{-1}). These events, first reported by Young *et al.*[75], indicate that transport of K^+ as well as Na^+ must require energy expenditure and therefore involve active processes. Evidence for active transport in mediating efflux of Na^+ from the duct lumen and for influx of K^+ has also emerged from the comparison of one-way flux ratios with ratios calculated by the Ussing equation. Schneyer[86] showed that the observed ratios are inconsistent with solely passive mechanisms for Na^+ transport from the duct lumen or K^+ transport to the lumen. An interesting observation from that work concerns the small back-flux of K^+ to the blood. This, and the observation that transductal potential difference (p.d.) does not depend on luminal $[K^+]$ (Figure 6.8), as it assuredly does on luminal $[Na^+]$, suggest that the luminal membrane is relatively impermeable to K^+ and that secretion of that ion across the luminal membrane is probably carrier-mediated[86]. Similarly, Knauf and Frömter[87] found that the conductance of the luminal membrane to K^+ is low in the submaxillary main excretory duct of man. Knauf and Frömter suggested that exchange for H^+ of the luminal fluid is the basis for secretion of K^+; Schneyer[88]

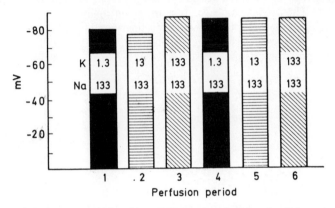

Figure 6.8 Relationship of the transepithelial p.d. of the rat main excretory duct to $[K^+]$ in luminal fluid. In these experiments, the lumen was perfused with an isotonic solution containing Na_2SO_4, K_2SO_4 and mannitol. (From Schneyer[86], by courtesy of the American Physiology Society)

has provided some evidence that the main ion exchanging with K^+ is Na^+. In either event, the exchange must be non-electrogenic, since no p.d. is generated in the process.

The transductal potential difference is, however, affected by the concentration of K^+ at the contraluminal membrane. Knauf[89] has shown that when K^+ is omitted from the solution bathing the serosal (nutrient) side of an isolated perfused duct, the transductal p.d. is lowered considerably (Figure 6.9). In its response to changes in luminal $[Na^+]$ and serosal $[K^+]$, the salivary duct evidently behaves much like other secretory epithelial layers.

Na^+ absorption and K^+ secretion in the duct system of the rat submaxillary gland are accompanied by net movements of the osmotically important anions, Cl^- and HCO_3^-. Net absorption of Cl^- occurs along the salivary duct[20,90], while HCO_3^- is secreted[91]. In the perfused main excretory duct, Cl^- conductance is low, virtually as low as it is for sulphate[20]. If perfusion rate is reduced sufficiently and adequate time is allowed for attainment of a steady state, $[Cl^-]$ in the perfusate stabilises at *ca.* 80 mequiv l^{-1} [90]. Since, at the same time, the transductal potential reaches a value of *ca.* -10 mV, luminal $[Cl^-]$ is in approximate equilibrium with $[Cl^-]$ of plasma water and thus appears to be distributed in accord with electrical forces, i.e. passively[90]. In other glands, Cl^- conductance in the main excretory duct may be higher than in rat. This is true in the submaxillary duct of man[87].

Secretion of HCO_3^- by the cells of the main excretory duct of rat submaxillary gland cannot, like absorption of Cl^-, be accounted for by passive processes[91]. HCO_3^- accumulates in the luminal fluid of the perfused duct, reaching concentrations exceeding those in plasma. While active processes must be invoked to explain the distribution of HCO_3^- between luminal fluid and interstitium at steady state, whether these processes are primarily involved in HCO_3^- transport *per se*, or whether they are indirectly involved by mediating the transport of H^+ from the lumen, remains unknown.

Net movement of water between luminal fluid and the interstitium of the perfused main excretory duct of the rat is notably slow, even in response to high osmotic gradients[75]. This resistance to water movement probably characterises most or all of the duct system and largely explains the development of hypotonicity in the saliva[74,75]. In the duct system, absorption of osmotically active ions exceeds secretion[20,74,75]. If water does not equilibrate across the epithelial cells, luminal fluid must become hypotonic. One factor which could contribute to the low osmotic permeability of the ductal epithelium is the form of the junctions between lateral membranes of adjacent cells.

Diamond and his co-workers[92,93] have emphasised that in epithelial layers, the lateral intercellular membranes can be important sites of net transport of water, a movement which would occur in response to osmotic

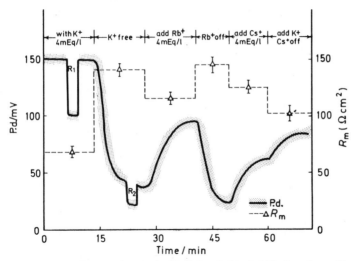

Figure 6.9 Changes in transepithelial p.d. (shaded line) and specific resistance (broken line) of isolated rabbit main excretory duct, relative to $[K^+]$ in the nutrient solution. At R_2 and R_2, $[Na^+]$ in the luminal perfusate was reduced from 150 to 15 mequiv l^{-1}. (From Knauf[89], by courtesy of *Pflügers Arch.*)

gradients between cytoplasmic water and the fluid in lateral intercellular space[92]. The osmotic gradients would result from active ion transport across the contraluminal epithelial membrane, including the lateral membrane, basal to the tight junctions[92]. Diamond's analysis bears a relationship to earlier models suggested by Curran[94] and Durbin[95] for water movement across epithelial cells.

In many epithelial secreting tissues, the lateral intercellular spaces form long channels, as, for example, in the gall bladder[92]. In that tissue, the length of the channel and the permeability of the lateral membranes to water suffice to provide osmotic equilibration and the absorbed fluid is isotonic[92,93]. In the salivary duct, the lateral intercellular channels are often short. Shackleford and Schneyer[96] found that luminal clefts frequently exist between lateral membranes of adjacent cells in the rat submaxillary main excretory duct (Figure 6.1). These clefts extend into the epithelial layer to a depth of about one-third the height of the cells. Basal to the clefts, lateral membranes of adjacent cells are joined by tight junctions. Thus, the lateral intercellular channels are foreshortened wherever a luminal cleft appears. The shortness of these channels may help retard net water movement from the cells into the channels and contribute to the development of hypotonicity in the saliva.

6.3.5 Summary

Salivary glands can secrete large quantities of fluid relative to their weight. The fluid secreted may be hypotonic or isotonic to plasma. In either event, Na^+ and K^+ are osmotically the most important cations. Cl^+ and HCO_3^- are the major anions. High $[K^+]$ and $[HCO_3^-]$, relative to serum levels, represent a frequent and distinctive feature of saliva. Hypotonic salivas tend to approach isotonicity at high flow rates (Heidenhain's law), due mainly to an increase in the content of Na^+, Cl^- and, sometimes, HCO_3^-. Saliva formed in the first part of salivon can be plasma-like in its $[Na^+]$, $[K^+]$, $[Cl^-]$, and total osmolality. More distally, in the ducts, Na^+ and Cl^- are partially reabsorbed, and K^+ and HCO_3^- are secreted. Net movement of water is unimpressive across the duct epithelium, and hypotonicity may, therefore, develop in ductal saliva. When stimulation of a gland is started or drastically altered, transient events occur in the gland. An increase in K^+ release from the gland cells is the best-documented transient change. This K^+ transient is related to an increase in membrane permeability, which is associated with stimulation and leads to elevated $[K^+]$ in the saliva and in the venous drainage from the gland. The rising permeability that marks the onset of stimulation is also often accompanied by a change in membrane potential (secretory potential), since intracellular K^+ in the resting cell is not in electrochemical equilibrium with K^+ in interstitial fluid. Relationships between the secretory potential and frank secretion are unclear. Ca^{2+} may play some role as an intermediary. The final composition of the saliva is attained in the ducts, by re-absorptive and secretory mechanisms. Active transport is involved in re-absorption of Na^+ but not Cl^-, and in secretion of K^+ and probably HCO_3^-. Despite recent advances in our understanding of secretory processes in the salivary gland, informational gaps remain. The mechanisms of formation of the precursor fluid by the acini, secretion of K^+ and HCO_3^- and transfer of water by the ducts and stimulus–secretion coupling require clarification.

6.4 SECRETION OF PROTEIN

Generally, saliva is a more dilute fluid than serum, not only in its concentration of inorganic salts but in its total protein content. For example, in human submaxillary or parotid saliva, the total protein may be *ca.* 0.1 or

0.5 g (100 ml)$^{-1}$, respectively[97], compared to approximately 6 g (100 ml)$^{-1}$ in serum. In the rat, too, the total protein in saliva is much less than that in serum, especially in submaxillary and sublingual fluids[98]. Moreover, the proportions of the total represented by specific proteins often differ strikingly in saliva and serum, and some proteins may be present in a higher concentration than in saliva, e.g. amylase. The activity of this enzyme is low in serum, but high in saliva. Proportionately, amylase may account for as much as 25 % of the total salivary protein, as it does in mixed saliva of man[97,99]. Salivary amylase is derived from acini[100,101] and cells of granular ducts[101], where it is synthesised and accumulated. The enzyme is relatively stable and its activity is readily measured. It can be separated in pure form from tissue or secretory fluid[102]. For these reasons, studies of protein secretion from the salivary gland (as in the pancreas) have usually focused on amylase as the test protein. Therefore, in this discussion we will emphasise secretion of amylase.

6.4.1 The secretory cycle

The secretory cycle refers to the sequence of accumulation, intracellular translocation and release of secretory products by the gland cells[11]. Secretory products are released during stimulation. During stimulation, intracellular glandular stores are depleted to some extent and eventually a new intracellular steady-state level of the secretory product is established. Cessation of stimulation leads to re-accumulation of the product and an approach to steady-state levels characteristic of the resting state. The extent to which these cyclic changes become apparent depends upon the strength, duration and synchrony of cellular stimulation. A secretory cycle can be delineated even with electrolytes, since stimulation leads to a disturbance (rest-transient) of the steady-state which had been established for intracellular ion levels at rest. During continued stimulation, a new steady-state is ultimately reached, and this in turn is disturbed when stimulation ceases (rate-change transient). Historically and conventionally, however, the term 'secretory cycle' is reserved for events related to the accumulation–discharge–accumulation sequence for protein secretory products.

Events in the glandular secretory cycle have been elucidated in the past decade. Synthesis of digestive enzymes is now known to be initiated at ribosomes attached to endoplasmic reticulum (i.e. at 'rough' endoplasmic reticulum), which is located basally in the cells[103,104]. Newly-synthesised enzyme is released by the ribosomes and enters the cisternae of the endoplasmic reticulum[104,105]. Within the cisternae, the enzyme molecules drift in an apical direction toward the Golgi complex[104]. The mechanism of intracisternal transport of the enzyme solution is unknown. When the enzyme reaches the Golgi complex, it becomes localised in vacuoles[104]. A membrane is formed surrounding these vacuoles and the enclosed enzyme solution is condensed progressively[104,106,107]. The vacuoles migrate toward the cell apex and, with further condensation of their contents, become recognisable as zymogen granules. The zymogen granules are discharged across the luminal membrane when the cells are stimulated.

This sequence of intracellular events was primarily delineated for the pancreas but has been essentially confirmed for the salivary gland as well[12,108–110]. The original work, mainly by Palade and Siekevitz and their co-workers, used ingenious combinations of tracer studies, cell fractionation, autoradiography, and electron microscopy. For example, in one set of experiments[104] groups of guinea-pigs were given intravenous injections of [^{3}H]-leucine at selected intervals after pancreatic secretion was induced by feeding. The pancreas was removed and prepared for autoradiographic examination with the electron microscope. Examination showed that radio-activity appeared first in the endoplasmic reticulum at the base of acinar cells and later in the Golgi region. Later still, radioactivity was mainly limited to zymogen granules. Other experiments[105,106] with pulse labelling (administration of tagged compound in a single dose, followed by a 'chaser' of untagged compound) revealed the same sequence: synthesis on rough endoplasmic reticulum, appearance at the Golgi complex and inclusion in zymogen granules. Use of these techniques in studies of the parotid gland has established that this secretory sequence is characteristic for salivary glands, too[12,108–110] (Figure 6.10).

6.4.2 Stimulus–secretion coupling

Several problems in protein secretion remain to be considered. For example, how is a message transferred from the autonomic receptor site, at the basal membrane of the cell, to the luminal membrane where secretory protein is released? How is secretory protein transferred from zymogen granules to the acinar lumen? What are the effects of the release of secretory protein upon other cellular processes?

The entire pattern of neural control of secretion is complicated by the fact that in many glands secretomotor impulses are derived from both branches of the autonomic nervous system and that cellular responses to adrenergic and cholinergic stimuli differ. When a gland responds to adrenergic stimuli, these stimuli are generally more effective than cholinergic stimuli in producing high salivary concentrations of the electrolytes, K^+ [111,112], HCO_3^- [113,114] and Ca^{2+} [115] and the protein amylase[116,117]. This is especially true for β-adrenergic stimuli[116]. Transmission of a 'message' from the adrenergic receptor site probably involves cyclic adenosine 3',5'-mono-phosphate (cAMP), and Ca^{2+}, at least when β-adrenergic receptors are involved[118,119]. Recently, direct evidence has indicated that parotid gland cAMP increases distinctly during stimulation by epinephrine or isopro-terenol[118,119]. The increase in cAMP induced by isoproterenol is more pro-nounced when theophylline is also given[118]. Earlier, Bdolah and Schramm[120] showed that administration of the dibutyryl derivative of cAMP, or theo-phylline, caused secretion of amylase by incubated slices of rat parotid gland. cAMP serves as a mediator of the effects of various hormones, including catecholamines, in other systems besides salivary glands[118]. According to Sutherland and his co-workers[118], the external stimulus (or 'first messenger') acts to enhance the activity of adenyl cyclase at the cell membrane and thus promotes conversion of ATP to cAMP. cAMP then acts as a 'second messenger' to initiate succeeding events in the sequence between stimulus and final response. The cellular level of cAMP is partially regulated by a cytoplasmic phosphodiesterase which can promote cAMP degradation[118]. The enhancing effect of theophylline on cellular cAMP levels depends upon its ability to inhibit cytoplasmic phosphodiesterase. No evidence exists that cAMP mediates the stimulatory effect of cholinergic agents on secretion. During adrenergic stimulation, however, cAMP probably provides one link in the coupling between stimulation and secretion.

Calcium ion probably also plays a role in linking stimulus to secretion. Douglas and Poisner[79] found that when Ca^{2+} is omitted from the fluid perfusing the cat submaxillary gland, protein secretion is inhibited. This inhibitory effect of calcium deficit could be demonstrated when either

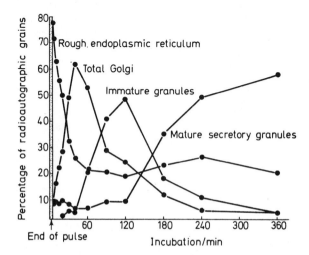

Figure 6.10 Sequence of appearance of label in cell structures of parotid slices, after pulse labelling with [³H]-leucine. (From Castle *et al.*[110], by courtesy of *J. Cell. Biol.*)

epinephrine or acetylcholine was used to stimulate secretion. Omission of Ca^{2+} from the medium bathing slices of salivary gland resulted in a marked interference with secretion of amylase in response to epinephrine or dibutyryl cAMP in the medium[119,121]. The mode of action of Ca^{2+} in promoting protein secretion is unknown[122]. Some evidence[123] suggests that Ca^{2+} is involved in release of the enzyme from zymogen granules. Possibly, then, Ca^{2+} is necessary for the final step in protein secretion. This would be consistent with the absence of any marked effect of lowered Ca^{2+} on the secretory potential and also with the fact that exogenous Ca^{2+} is not needed to enhance the oxygen consumption accompanying stimulation[124]. Probably, however, Ca^{2+} plays a more extensive role in the secretory process than can presently be demonstrated.

The entire process of enzyme release from cells is not well understood. Some evidence[125] suggests that fusion of the membrane of the zymogen granule with the intracellular surface of the luminal membrane is involved in the secretory process. This may be followed by localised dissolution of the fused membranes and release of enzyme to the exterior. However, it is also possible that dissolution of the zymogen membrane alone occurs, resulting in release of zymogen protein to the cytoplasm. Transfer of protein across the cell membrane to the lumen may then occur separately from any fusion. This sequence would explain the presence of dissolved enzyme in the cytoplasm, apart from that contained in zymogen granules[12].

The linkage between stimulus and secretion could have even wider ramifications than is generally realised. For example, the stimulus evoking secretion may act indirectly to induce formation of new DNA[13]. This effect is thought to depend upon depletion of glandular stores of secretory protein, which occurs as a sequel to stimulation. A correlation between secretion of protein and ensuing DNA synthesis has been noted by Radley[126], Kirby *et al.*[127] and Schneyer[13]. Future work should explore the possibility that a stimulus–secretion, DNA-synthesis chain could be the basis for a number of growth phenomena in secretory tissues[128–131].

6.4.3 Summary

Total protein of saliva is generally lower than that of serum, but selected proteins, such as amylase, may be present in considerably higher concentration in saliva. Glandular processes of protein secretion have, therefore, often been studied using àmylase as the test protein. Amylase levels of the salivary gland normally pass through cyclic changes corresponding to periods of stimulation and rest. During stimulation, glandular amylase is discharged and tissue levels fall. During rest, newly-synthesised amylase accumulates in the gland. These changes comprise a secretory cycle. The cytologic sequence of events during the secretory cycle includes transfer of amylase from zymogen granules to lumen across the luminal membrane, synthesis of new enzyme on the ribosomes of the basally-placed rough endoplasmic reticulum, intracisternal transport to the Golgi region (where the protein becomes encapsulated), and apical accumulation of fully-formed zymogen granules. The physiological sequence of events is less clear, but probably involves a role for the secretory potential, Ca^{2+}, and, with adrenergic stimulation, cAMP. Events in the secretory cycle may have wider implications than heretofore realised, since growth phenomena may also be affected by secretion of cell proteins.

6.5 REGULATION

Those who lecture on secretion in the digestive tract often point out that nervous control mechanisms are particularly important in the rostral glands and hormones are more important in glands lower down in the tract. This rule certainly applies to the salivary glands. There seems to be no hormone which, under physiological conditions, evokes salivation. Secretory nerves, on the other hand, abound and may even be supplied from both divisions of the autonomic nervous system. The glands are, in fact, highly dependent on these connections with the central nervous system. A salivary gland may be as profoundly affected structurally and functionally by section of its preganglionic parasympathetic nerve, for instance, as skeletal muscle is by destruction of its motor innervation. Salivary secretion ceases (for all practical purposes) and marked atrophy ensues with denervation. One can still evoke secretion by injecting drugs, and the gland cells can be shown to gradually acquire an increased sensitivity to chemical stimuli, in agreement with Cannon's 'law of denervation'.

Thus, the regulatory function of the nerves has two aspects. One, the subject of this section, concerns the immediate effect of the nerves and results in flow of saliva. The other is a long-term effect on the structure, chemical composition and function of the glands. Obviously, the nerves affect processes responsible for synthesis, growth, and sensitivity of the glandular cells (see Refs. 8, 13 and 132). These effects are at least partly due to the repeated action of the secretory impulse and its neurotransmitter. For example, supersensitivity resembling that caused by parasympathetic denervation can be produced by prolonged treatment with agents that specifically abolish the release or action of acetylcholine (botulinum toxin or parasympatholytics, respectively)[132]. The possibility of a 'trophic' effect of the nerves, independent of the neurotransmitter, may also have to be considered. A long-term regulatory function of hormones must also be taken into account. Thus, hypophysectomy is known to cause atrophy, reduced sensitivity to secretory agents and diminished secretory capacity in salivary glands[133].

6.5.1 Variations in flow rate and composition of saliva

One of the functions of the saliva is to moisten and protect the oral mucosa and the teeth; a slow sustained 'resting secretion' helps ensure this. During a meal, the demands on the glands greatly increase. Saliva, then, must fulfil its manifold digestive functions and simultaneously protect the oral structures against mechanical, chemical and thermal damage from the food. Hence, the function of the salivary gland system is characterised by a background of continuous secretion (which can be very slow during sleep), upon which intermittent increases occur (often to high levels, as during meals).

These variations involve not only the volume of saliva but also its organic and inorganic constituents. According to Pavlov and some later investigators[134,135], the saliva varies in a seemingly purposeful way, adapted to the various digestive and protective functions of the saliva. The concept of the wide variation in the composition of the mixed saliva emptied into the mouth is easy to accept. A great number of different salivary glands produce salivas of different composition and the proportions of the contributions of the glands which together form the mixed saliva may vary considerably. Furthermore, the saliva discharged from a single gland is highly variable, being the product of activity in a complex system of effector cells. Different secretory cells in the first part of the salivon add the products of their synthetic work to the primary acinar fluid. The cells lining the duct system modify this fluid to a varying extent. Activity in the smooth muscles of the glandular vessels may alter the composition of the saliva by varying the amounts of blood offered to the secretory cells. The myoepithelial cells, assumed to contribute to salivary flow, may also contribute, for example by changing the time of contact between luminal fluid and duct cells. The ensuing discussion concerns the regulatory mechanisms known or suspected to act on these various effectors.

A continual basal flow is provided by glands endowed with the ability to secrete 'spontaneously'. This term was used by Babkin[11] to describe secretion going on incessantly even in the absence of extraneous stimuli. Most glands do not discharge saliva unless stimulated. Their secretion ceases in deep anaesthesia, after denervation, or after administration of ganglionic blocking or parasympatholytic drugs. However, some glands continue to secrete under these conditions, e.g., the sublingual glands of cats, dogs, and rats, the submaxillary glands of rabbits, and the parotid glands of ruminants[136-142]. Humoral factors to the gland are unlikely causes of the secretion; the sublingual gland of the cat secretes even when isolated in Tyrode's solution in a bath[136]. The resting membrane potential of acinar cells is higher, according to Lundberg[55], in sublingual than in submaxillary glands of cats and also in parotid glands[58] and perhaps does not really represent a 'resting' potential[4]. Apart from this, no differences between a spontaneously-active and a resting gland have been noted which could be related to the different states of the glands. The spontaneous secretion is impressive in ruminants but small in other species; it cannot account for more than a minor part of even the 'resting secretion' of mixed saliva, except during sleep. Usually the 'resting' flow is evoked largely by extra glandular stimuli. This is even more true with the brisk salivation during a meal.

6.5.2 Control of acinar secretion

Some salivary glands respond to sympathetic nerve stimulation with secretion and they also secrete if epinephrine or norepinephrine is injected. The doses must be large, however, and catecholamines circulating in the blood under reasonably physiological conditions cannot excite the glands unless the secretory cells are exceptionally sensitive. This may occur after parasympathetic decentralisation or denervation when 'paralytic salivary secretion' may appear[143]. No other hormones are known to evoke secretion of saliva. Nor is there any indication that a local hormonal mechanism controls salivary secretion, analogous to that by which polypeptides are assumed to control the glandular blood vessels, although some polypeptides exist in the body which, on injection, cause secretion of saliva (e.g. substance P, see Ref. 144). True hormones or local hormones may have a modulating or permissive influence on the glandular response to secretory nerve impulses, but this remains speculative as far as acute effects are concerned. Undoubtedly the main control of acinar secretion is affected by the parasympathetic and sympathetic nerves.

6.5.3 Parasympathetic nerves

6.5.3.1 The course of the nerves

Parasympathetic secretory nerves seem to be distributed to all salivary glands: the large pairs and the small mucosal glands in the mouth and pharynx[136,145]. Parasympathetic impulses evoke the highest flow rates obtainable from the glands[146]. Secretion from the parotid gland of the dog may proceed faster when elicited reflexly from the mouth than when produced by electrical stimulation of the auriculotemporal nerve at an optimal frequency. However, this merely reflects the fact that the gland receives additional parasympathetic secretory nerves by other routes[147,148]. After section of the auriculotemporal nerve, the secretory response of the gland to reflex stimulation is diminished but by no means abolished[11,149]. Recently, new secretory fibres have been detected that leave the mandibular nerve, join the internal maxillary artery and travel with a branch of this artery to the gland; some fibres may also reach the gland from the facial nerve. After section of these sets of nerves, together with the auriculotemporal nerve, the parotid gland usually fails to respond to the stimulus of citric acid poured into the mouth[150]. The new nerves are obviously cholinergic, for their stimulation increases the yield of acetylcholine in a perfusate of the gland during simultaneous auriculotemporal excitation and atropine abolishes the secretory effect of nervous stimulation[150,151]. Generally, the parasympathetic innervation of the parotid gland can be said to be complex. The arrangement of the nerves varies from one species to another. Cats may resemble dogs in this respect (Ekstrom and Emmelin, unpublished observations). In man, secretory fibres are supplied not only by the auriculotemporal nerve but also by the chorda tympani[152,153]. In cattle, the main innervation reaches the gland with the salivary duct, as Moussu's nerve[154]. The paraysmpathetic secretory nerves for the submaxillary gland are contained mainly in the chorda tympani, but nerves may reach the gland by other routes, at least in some species (e.g. man[155] and dog[156,157]).

6.5.3.2 Intraglandular arrangement of nerves

To attain maximal salivation, the parasympathetic nerves must be excited electrically at a frequency of 10–20 shocks s^{-1} [147,158–160]. When the secretory responses of submaxillary glands of dogs to feeding are compared (in the same dogs) with the responses to electrical stimulation of the chorda-lingual nerve (Figure 6.11), the highest flow rates during a meal correspond to an impulse frequency of 4–8 s^{-1} in the efferent nerve. The frequency-response curve rises steeply up to *ca.* 8 s^{-1}. At 4 s^{-1} the flow is already half the maximal rate. When secretion is elicited reflexly for protective rather than digestive purposes by putting some rejectable substance into the mouth, the impulse frequency may exceed 8 s^{-1}[147]. When frequency is varied to the lowest level able to evoke secretion, this level differs widely in different glands, apparently depending partly on the type of neuroeffector contact present. The common *en passant* contact of 'interstitial' or 'indirect' type, with a distance between axon and effector cell of *ca.* 1000 Å, was described in salivary glands of cats by Garrett[161]. Some glands (e.g. parotid glands of rats or submaxillary glands of cats and monkeys) also possess a more intimate 'intra-acinar' or 'direct' type of contact, with a distance below 200 Å (see Garrett[27]). In the cat, the submaxillary gland differs from the parotid in the content of intra-acinar axons[27,59]. Also it has a much denser supply of parasympathetic nerves[162]. Interestingly, repetitive stimulation is required to produce secretion from the parotid[60,163], whereas in the submaxillary gland a single shock causes secretion in all cats[164] or at least in some[158,163].

If the 'secretory potential' is taken as an indicator of secretory cell activity produced by the nerve, a single shock applied to the parasympathetic nerve appears to affect the submaxillary[53,59] but not the parotid gland[60] of the cat. The finding that in a few submaxillary glands no potentials are evoked by the single shock[53] can be reasonably connected with the observation that in occasional glands intra-acinar axons are difficult to detect[27]. These findings imply that the minute amount of acetylcholine released by the single shock

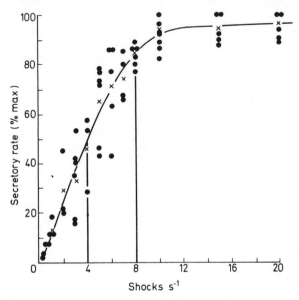

Figure 6.11 Secretory rate of flow from the dog submaxillary relative to the frequency of electrical stimulation of the chorda-lingual nerve. Vertical lines show the range of secretory rates when the glands were maximally activated by feeding. (From Emmelin and Holmberg[147], by courtesy of Physiological Society.)

is sufficient to affect the glandular cell, provided a close contact exists between axon and effector. Larger quantities of acetylcholine, released during repetitive stimulation, are required for the transmitter to reach the gland cell from a more distant axon in a concentration high enough to activate the cell. At stimulation frequencies of 10–20 s^{-1} all acinar cells are fully activated. Labile acetylcholine is unlikely to convey the message for more than a short distance.

Nexuses have been demonstrated between gland cells, and possibly activation can spread across the nexus from one cell to another within an acinus[7,165]. On the other hand, in at least some glands, each acinar cell seems to have its own parasympathetic nerve supply. Creed and Wilson[59] calculated, from electron microscopy studies, that two to five nerve junctions are associated with each secretory cell in the submaxillary gland of the cat. An even more marked convergence in this gland is suggested in physiological observation. Whether spread of activation through tight junctions between the cells contributes to this is unknown. Thus, Lundberg[53] discovered that the secretory potential recorded from an acinar cell increased stepwise when the intensity of the shocks applied to preganglionic parasympathetic fibres was gradually raised (see Figure 6.5). He concluded that at least five to ten axons converge on the acinar cell in the submaxillary gland of the cat. In this gland, convergence can also be demonstrated in the following ways[166]. The chorda-lingual nerve is cut and its peripheral end sewn to both the central end of the same nerve and that of the cut hypoglossal nerve. After regeneration for a few months, a preparation is available in which secretion can be evoked by electrical stimulation both of the hypoglossal and the chorda-lingual nerve central to the suture. The secretion is abolished both by ganglion blocking and by parasympatholytic drugs, indicating that axons in the severed nerves have re-innervated the parasympathetic ganglion cells. At simultaneous stimulation of the two nerves using frequencies of stimulation just below the secretory threshold for each nerve, saliva fails to flow. Similarly, when one nerve is stimulated at a frequency causing a small secretory response, the effect is not augmented by excitation of the other nerve at a subliminal frequency. Hence, no facilitation is obtained in this type of experiment, implying that little overlap occurs between the fields of distribution of the preganglionic axons in the ganglion.

Quite a different picture is obtained when both nerves are excited at frequencies causing secretion. Pronounced facilitation can be observed; if each nerve evokes a barely perceptible flow, the combined stimulation of the nerves causes rapid salivation, indicating marked convergence of the post-ganglionic parasympathetic axons on to the glandular cells. If the frequency of stimulation is increased until each nerve elicits its maximal secretory response, in many preparations this maximum is about the same for each nerve and the same as that of the contralateral normal gland, activated through its chorda-lingual nerve. Simultaneous stimulation of both nerves now causes a flow *not* larger than when each nerve is stimulated separately. The morphological basis of this observation may be that the single axon forms *en passant* contacts with many glandular cells[161]. Spread of activation from cell to cell within an acinus may also have to be considered. The discovery that dog parotid gland is supplied by numerous secretory fibres outside the auriculotemporal nerve has made possible similar experiments with separate and simultaneous stimulation of two different sets of nerves; convergence at the postganglionic level has been demonstrated in this gland, as well[149].

6.5.3.3   *Chemical transmission of the parasympathetic impulses*

In the early 1930s, numerous investigators demonstrated that acetylcholine is released in the submaxillary gland of the cat when the chorda tympani is stimulated[167–173]. Perfusion of this gland includes the parasympathetic ganglia and acetylcholine released when the chorda is stimulated has been shown to originate partly from the ganglionic synapses and partly from the postganglionic nerves contacting the secretory cells[174]. Recently, liberation of acetylcholine was studied in the parotid gland of the dog during stimulation of most of the parasympathetic nerves; this is one of the few preparations in which one can collect perfusion fluid when postganglionic parasympathetic nerves are stimulated. The yield of acetylcholine was considerably smaller than in the submaxillary gland of the dog[151], partly because only the post-ganglionic junctions and not the synapses delivered transmitter into the perfusate. However, the observation probably also reflects the fact that the parotid is less richly supplied with parasympathetic fibres than the sub-maxillary gland[150].

Even when no impulses travel from the central nervous system through the parasympathetic pathway, a small continuous 'leakage' of acetylcholine occurs from the postganglionic axons[175-177]. The amounts released are ordinarily too small to evoke secretion, but they may have a facilitatory effect[176] and, over the long term, modify the sensitivity of the gland cells[177]. Under certain conditions, the leaking acetylcholine may suffice to cause salivation. This happens when a cholinesterase inhibitor has been adminis-tered. It also happens as a transient phenomenon a day or two after secretion of the postganglionic nerves. This 'degeneration secretion' is due to a tempor-ary increase in the leakage of acetylcholine from degenerating axons[178,179]. In his microelectrode recordings from acinar cells, Lundberg[53] occasionally saw small, spontaneously appearing potentials; he regarded them as due to injury to the neurones[55]. One wonders whether such potentials are affected by cholinesterase inhibitors and atropine, particularly since Dean and Matthews[180] recently observed miniature potentials in pancreatic acinar cells which they attributed to acetylcholine. During 'degeneration secretion' after parasympathetic denervation, the membrane of the acinar cells is hyperpolarised[181], a finding compatible with the view that it is exposed to acetylcholine.

All salivary glands investigated are able to synthesise acetylcholine[182]. The activity of choline acetyltransferase in the glands varies among species and also among different glands in the same species; in the latter case the activity is higher as the parasympathetic innervation becomes more dense. In general, activity is high and has a great safety factor for manufacture of acetylcholine, even in amounts needed for intense and prolonged secretory activity (see Nordenfelt[183]). The transmitter-hydrolysing enzyme, acetyl-cholinesterase, is present in the glands and seems, similarly, to operate with a wide margin of safety[5]. For example, the activity of acetylcholinesterase has been reduced by pharmacological means to two-thirds of its original level before an increased secretory effect of acetylcholine becomes notice-able[184].

Interference with the synthesis of acetylcholine by injection of hemi-cholinium, or with release by administration of botulinum toxin, abolishes salivary secretion elicited by parasympathetic stimulation[185,186]. Secretion is more commonly abolished, however, with the aid of drugs preventing the action of acetylcholine (e.g. atropine or, more efficiently, methylscopo-lamine; see Refs. 6 and 8).

6.5.4 Sympathetic nerves

6.5.4.1 Effects of nerve stimulation

Electrical stimulation of the cervical sympathetic trunk causes secretion in some but not all glands. In cats, the response from the submaxillary gland is usually large, but it is small from the parotid glands. In dogs, some secretion is obtained from the submaxillary glands but none from the parotid glands. In rabbits, the opposite is true. In rats, both glands respond with secretion. The variability also applies to the single gland of the same species. In the feline submaxillary gland, secretion is usually abundant, although seldom as large as during parasympathetic stimulation but in some cats, secretion is scanty and in a few it is lacking altogether.

Repetitive stimulation is always necessary for sympathetic secretion, occasionally at a frequency as low as 0.2 s^{-1} but more often 1–5 s^{-1} [187]. The response tends to diminish or even cease despite continued stimulation, particularly when high-frequency stimulation is used. Intra-acinar sympathetic axons have been described in some glands, but generally they seem rare[27], and the glandular cells mainly depend on interstitial neuro-effector sites. No secretory potentials can be evoked by single-shock stimulation[53,59]. Even if the sympathetic transmitter is more stable than acetylcholine, concentrations high enough to activate the acinar cells can obviously be reached only by repetitive stimulation. Moreover, the secretory cells are far more sensitive to acetylcholine than to norepinephrine when the drug is administered intravenously.

Whether the sympathetic nerves act on the same glandular cells as the parasympathetic nerves, or whether the two nerves control different cells, has been disputed for a century (see Refs. 4 and 5). The sympathetic nerves have generally been assumed to affect cells with a parasympathetic innervation. Two arguments favour this view. During intracellular recording from a single acinar cell, a secretory potential can be evoked by both sympathetic and parasympathetic stimulation[53]; a condition for the validity of this argument is that activation or the electrical change does not spread from one cell to another. Moreover, when parasympathetic stimulation causes its maximal secretory response, additional sympathetic stimulation cannot accelerate the salivary flow even if the sympathetic stimulation has, in itself, a marked secretory effect[146,147,188].

Histochemical investigations show that glands in which sympathetic stimulation causes salivation are supplied with adrenergic nerves in the acinar region. On the other hand, the sublingual gland of the rat, in which no sympathetic secretion is obtained, is almost devoid of such nerves[189]. However, such a consistency between morphological and physiological findings seems to be exceptional. Other glands not responding with secretion to sympathetic stimulation receive numerous adrenergic fibres apart from those of the vessels—for example, the submaxillary gland of the rabbit[190,191] or the parotid gland of the dog[192]. Some, but not all, fibres may innervate myoepithelial cells. When one considers this along with the fact that even when sympathetic stimulation does cause salivation the response is highly variable, one is tempted to assume that the sympathetic innervation of acinar cells has some other, more important function than producing acinar primary secretion. When Heidenhain[42] used the term 'trophic' to describe some nerves of salivary glands, the implication was that such nerves operate to add organic material elaborated by the gland cells to the saliva; 'trophic' fibres were assumed to be present particularly in sympathetic nerves. Saliva collected from the main duct is known to have a different composition after sympathetic than after parasympathetic stimulation. This applies not only to inorganic material but to organic constituents[4]. With regard to components such as electrolytes, the primary saliva produced in the acini probably has the same composition whether secreted in response to sympathetic or parasympathetic impulses[193]. Probably, however, differences in protein content found in the final saliva[194,195] are present when the primary saliva is formed. The chief function of sympathetic innervation at the acinar level may be to add specific organic constituents to the fluid produced by simultaneous parasympathetic activity; the dual innervation of the acinar cells favours this.

6.5.4.2 Chemical transmission of the sympathetic impulses

Norepinephrine is present in salivary glands and apparently in the post-ganglionic sympathetic neurone. Little or no norepinephrine can be detected when this neurone has degenerated[196-198]. Release of catecholamines on stimulation of the sympathetic fibres of salivary glands has been demonstrated by bioassay[199]. The norepinephrine found and liberated is derived mostly from sympathetic vasoconstrictor nerves and probably also from motor nerves of myoepithelial cells. However, for glands with sympathetic nerves causing secretion of fluid, several arguments support the concept that these secretory fibres are adrenergic. In these glands (as in many other salivary glands), fluorescent fibres surround the acini and in these glands catecholamines evoke salivation. The secretory effect of injected catecholamines is enhanced when the axonal re-uptake mechanism for the sympathetic transmitter is blocked with cocaine[199-201]. Secretion caused by sympathetic nerve stimulation is abolished by drugs interfering with the synthesis (a-methyltyrosine), storage (reserpine)[202], or release (bretylium, guanethidine)[203-205] of norepinephrine. It is also abolished by sympatholytic agents[206,207].

Experiments with various sympathomimetic and sympatholytic agents have revealed that both a- and β-adrenoreceptors may be engaged in mediating the secretory effect. In certain salivary glands, the a-receptors are solely involved in sympathetic secretion, e.g. the submaxillary gland of the cat. In other glands, only β-receptors are used (the submaxillary gland of the dog). Both receptors may be present in some glands, for example the submaxillary gland of the rat or the parotid gland of the rabbit. Whether a-receptors in one gland exist in the same or different cells, or whether they participate in production of fluids of different composition remains uncertain. The β-receptors of salivary glands seem to be of the β_1 type, since the β_2-receptor-stimulating Salbutamol has little secretory effect compared with isoproterenol, which activates both kinds of β-receptors[208]. Furthermore,

Practolol, a drug with selective blocking action on β_1-receptors, antagonises the secretory effects of isoproterenol and epinephrine[209]. The effects referred to thus far are mainly those on fluid secretion. β-Receptors seem to be more significant than a-receptors in the action of sympathetics on the composition of the saliva and biosynthesis and growth.

6.5.5   Control of the ducts

The secretory and absorptive processes in the ducts that transform the primary saliva into the final product expelled into the mouth have long been suspected to be under control of the glandular nerves. Nerves surrounding the ducts have been described[161,162,210]. Some glands have both cholinergic and adrenergic fibres[191,192]. Species differences seem to exist in this respect; thus, no adrenergic nerves were found around the ducts in the salivary glands of rats[189] but were in the submaxillary gland of the rabbit[190,191]. In the submaxillary gland of the cat, secretory potentials could be recorded from cells assumed to be duct cells during both sympathetic and para-sympathetic stimulation, suggesting a dual innervation of these cells[53]. Since both carbachol and isoproterenol can modify the composition of the primary saliva during its passage through the ducts of the rat submaxillary gland, workers have concluded that the duct cells are supplied with cholinergic and β-adrenoreceptors[114,211,212].

As to hormonal control mechanisms, whether β-receptors of the ducts are sensitive enough to be activated by epinephrine circulating in the blood in physiological concentrations remains to be seen. The adrenal cortex may be of greater interest; aldosterone is important for sodium and potassium transport in the ducts[213]. Antidiuretic hormone reduces the sodium concentration in saliva produced by the submaxillary gland of the dog, suggesting that it stimulates the absorption of sodium in the duct system[214].

6.5.6   Myoepithelial cells and salivary secretion

Morphological investigations show that myoepithelial cells surround the acini; such cells have also been found around intercalary and striated ducts. Axons partly bare of their Schwann cell investments have been detected in contact with the cells and electron-microscopic observations suggest that both sympathetic and parasympathetic nerves may contribute[161,215]. Physiological experiments indicate that impulses in sympathetic nerves contract the myoepithelial cells. According to some authors, the cells receive para-sympathetic motor nerves as well (see Refs. 6, 163, 164 and 216).

The role of the myoepithelial cells in salivary secretion is uncertain. A reasonable assumption is that these cells expel saliva from the glands. In the submaxillary gland of the dog, sympathetic nerve stimulation causes secretion mediated by β-receptors and contraction of myoepithelial cells elicited via a-receptors[217,218]. Injecting the β-receptor stimulant isoproterenol or stimulating the sympathetic nerve after administration of an a-receptor blocking agent causes saliva to flow from the gland even in the absence of myoepithelial contraction. When secretion is combined with such contraction, however, saliva is more quickly expelled into the mouth, which may be important for the digestive and protective functions of the gland[219]. One can further show (Figure 6.12) that secretion can continue against a much

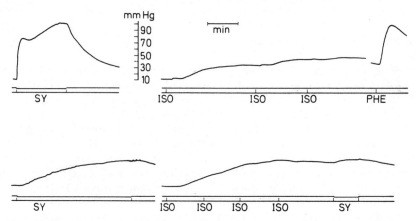

Figure 6.12 Pressure in the submaxillary duct system (mmHg). SY: stimulation of the vagosympathetic nerve at 20 shocks s^{-1}. ISO: intravenous injection of isoproterenol, 50 μg kg^{-1}. PHE: intravenous injection of phenylephrine, 50 μg kg^{-1}. The lower panel shows the effects after intravenous injection of dihydroergotamine, 0.4 mg kg^{-1}. (From Emmelin and Gjorstrup[220], by courtesy of the Physiological Society.)

higher pressure when supported by contracted myoepithelial cells than when these cells are relaxed[220]. This may be of particular value when the saliva is highly viscous, as in the submaxillary gland of the dog during sympathetic activity.

6.5.7 Control of the blood vessels of the glands

Catecholamine-fluorescent nerves have been demonstrated in contact with glandular vessels[221] and electrical stimulation of the cervical sympathetic trunk causes glandular vasoconstriction which is abolished by α-receptor blocking drugs[207]. Of more interest for the special function of salivary glands is the vasodilator mechanism. This must be extremely efficient when one considers that a gland may secrete a volume of saliva equal to the weight of the gland within a few minutes. Claude Bernard[222], impressed by the intense vasodilation he discovered when a gland is activated by stimulation of its parasympathetic nerves, attributed the vasodilation to a new type of nerve. Later investigators introduced the idea of a functional hyperaemia due to vasodilator 'metabolites' from the active secretory cells. Eventually the potent vasodilator peptides kallidin and bradykinin were considered as likely agents responsible for the vasodilation. The important question of the vasodilator mechanism has been debated for years by opposing groups of investigators, most recently between Schachter and his colleagues[223],[224] (who emphasised the role played by vasodilator nerves) and Hilton and Lewis[225,226] (who champion the kinin mechanism). Gautvik[227] has produced experimental evidence to show that the vasodilation has an early phase caused by activity in vasodilator nerves, followed by a phase during which kininogenase is released from active secretory cells to form the vasodilator kinin.

Interestingly, kinins have been implicated in the functional hyperaemia of various exocrine glands, but not in skeletal muscle. In glands, the powerful permeability-increasing effect of the kinins may be of particular value, apart from the vasodilator effect. Whether chemical agents other than kinins contribute to the vasodilation in active salivary glands is unknown. Perhaps other factors that have been implicated in the functional hyperaemia in skeletal muscle must be considered, e.g. hyperosmolality[228,229] and potassium ions[230]. Potassium is released from secreting gland cells[46]. Most salivary glands produce hypotonic saliva from plasma; in the ducts the isotonic primary saliva becomes hypotonic, and possibly the blood passing the ducts has become sufficiently hypertonic to dilate the vessels near the acini, to which it then passes. Recent experiments do not support the idea that potassium ions are responsible for functional hyperaemia in salivary glands[231].

6.5.8 Summary

In some salivary glands, the secretory machinery is continuously active ('spontaneous secretion'), but most glands discharge saliva only when acted upon by external stimuli, which are mainly of nervous origin (particularly parasympathetic). Increasing evidence suggests that the processes by which the primary acinar saliva is modified in the more distal part of the salivon are also controlled by the parasympathetic and sympathetic nerves. Hormones such as aldosterone and the antidiuretic hormone may impose additional regulatory effects. Impulses in glandular nerves also cause contraction of myoepithelial cells, promoting the flow of saliva. The greatly increased flow of blood through the secreting gland probably results from activity in parasympathetic vasodilator nerves in co-operation with potent vasodilator and permeability-increasing kinins formed during secretion.

Acknowledgement

Acknowledgement is made for support to scholarly activities of Dr Schneyer under terms of U.S.P.H.S. Research Career Award (SK6-DE 03341).

References

1. Faber, M. (1943). The causes of xerostomia. *Acta Med. Scand.*, **113**, 69
2. Bertram, U. (1967). Xerostomia. Clinical aspects, pathology and pathogenesis. *Acta Odontol. Scand.*, **25**, Suppl. 49

3. Schneyer, L. H. and Schneyer, C. A. (1967). Inorganic composition of saliva. *Handbook of Physiology. Alimentary Canal*, Sect. 6, Vol. 2, 497 (C. F. Code, editor) (Washington, D.C.: Amer. Physiol. Soc.)
4. Burgen, A. S. V. and Emmelin, N. G. (1961). *Physiology of the Salivary Glands* (London: Arnold)
5. Emmelin, N. (1967). Nervous control of salivary glands. *Handbook of Physiology. Alimentary Canal*, Sect. 6, Vol. 2, 595 (C. F. Code, editor) (Washington, D.C.: Amer. Physiol. Soc.)
6. Emmelin, N. (1967). Pharmacology of salivary glands. *Handbook of Physiology. Alimentary Canal*, Sect. 6, Vol. 2, 665 (C. F. Code, editor) (Washington, D.C.: Amer. Physiol. Soc.)
7. Burgen, A. S. V. (1967). Secretory processes in salivary glands. *Handbook of Physiology. Alimentary Canal*, Sect. 6, Vol. 2, 561 (C. F. Code, editor) (Washington, D.C.: Amer. Physiol. Soc.)
8. Emmelin, N., Schneyer, C. A. and Schneyer, L. H. (1972). The pharmacology of salivary secretion. *The International Encyclopedia of Pharmacology and Therapeutics*, Sect. 39, in the press (Oxford: Pergamon Press)
9. Thaysen, J. H. (1960). Handling of alkali metals by exocrine glands other than kidney. *Handbuch der Experimentellen Pharmakologie*, Part 2, Vol. 13, 424 (Berlin: Springer)
10. Schneyer, L. H., Young, J. A. and Schneyer, C. A. (1972). Salivary secretion of electrolytes. *Physiol. Rev.*, **52**, 720
11. Babkin, B. P. (1950). *Secretory Mechanism of the Digestive Glands*, 23 (New York: Hoeber)
12. Schramm, M. (1967). Secretion of enzymes and other macromolecules. *Ann. Rev. Biochem.*, **36**, 307
13. Schneyer, C. A. (1972). Regulation of salivary gland size. *Regulation of Organ and Tissue Growth*, 211 (R. Goss, editor) (New York: Academic Press)
14. Thoma, K. H. (1919). A contribution to the knowledge of the development of the submaxillary and sublingual salivary glands in human embryos. *J. Dental Res.*, **1**, 95
15. Gasser, R. F. (1970). The early development of the parotid gland around the facial nerve and its branches in man. *Anat. Rec.*, **167**, 63
16. Leeson, C. R. (1967). Structure of salivary glands. *Handbook of Physiology. Alimentary Canal*, Sect. 6, Vol. 2, 463 (C. F. Code, editor) (Washington, D.C.: Amer. Physiol. Soc.)
17. Jacoby, F. and Leeson, C. R. (1959). The postnatal development of the rat submaxillary gland. *J. Anat.*, **93**, 201
18. Schneyer, C. A. and Schneyer, L. H. (1961). Secretion by salivary glands deficient in acini. *Amer. J. Physiol.*, **201**, 939
19. Burgen, A. S. V. and Seeman, P. (1958). The role of the salivary duct system in the formation of the saliva. *Can. J. Biochem. Physiol.*, **36**, 119
20. Schneyer, L. H. (1968). Secretory processes in perfused excretory duct of rat submaxillary gland. *Amer. J. Physiol.*, **215**, 664
21. Tamarin, A. and Screebny, L. M. (1965). The rat submaxillary salivary gland. A correlative study by light and electron microscopy. *J. Morphol.*, **117**, 295
22. Shackleford, J. M. and Wilborn, W. H. (1968). Structural and histochemical diversity in mammalian salivary glands. *Ala. J. Med. Sci.*, **5**, 180
23. Scott, B. L. and Pease, D. C. (1959). Electron microscopy of the salivary and lacrimal glands of the rat. *Amer. J. Anat.*, **104**, 115
24. Shackleford, J. M. and Schneyer, C. A. (1964). Structural and functional aspects of rodent salivary glands including two desert species. *Amer. J. Anat.*, **115**, 279
25. Tandler, B. and Ross, L. L. (1969). Observations of nerve terminals in human labial salivary glands. *J. Cell Biol.*, **42**, 339
26. Hand, A. R. (1970). Nerve-acinar cell relationships in the rat parotid gland. *J. Cell Biol.*, **47**, 540
27. Garrett, J. R. (1972). Neuro-effector sites in salivary glands. *Oral Physiology*, 83 (N. Emmelin and Y. Zotterman, editors) (Oxford: Pergamon Press)
28. Schneyer, C. A. and Hall, H. D. (1970). Autonomic regulation of postnatal changes in cell number and size of rat parotid. *Amer. J. Physiol.*, **219**, 1268

29. Schneyer, C. A. and Hall, H. D. (1972). Effects of removal of superior cervical ganglion or auriculotemporal nerve on course of postnatal change in rat parotid amylase. *Proc. Soc. Exp. Biol. Med.*, **140**, 911

30. Kay, R. N. B. (1960). The rate of flow and composition of various salivary secretions in sheep and calves. *J. Physiol.* (*London*), **150**, 515

31. Lundberg, A. (1957). The mechanism of establishment of secretory potentials in sublingual gland cells. *Acta Physiol. Scand.*, **40**, 35

32. Yoshimura, H., Iwasaki, H., Nishikawa, T. and Matsumoto, S. (1959). Role of carbonic anhydrase in the bicarbonate secretion from salivary glands and mechanism of ionic excretion. *Jap. J. Physiol.*, **9**, 106

33. Schneyer, C. A. and Schneyer, L. H. (1960). Electrolyte levels of rat salivary secretions in relation to fluid-flow rate. *Amer. J. Physiol.*, **199**, 55

34. McDougall, E. I. (1948). Studies on ruminant saliva. 1. The composition and output of sheep's saliva. *Biochem. J.*, **43**, 99

35. Young, J. A. and Schögel, E. (1966). Micropuncture investigation of sodium and potassium excretion in rat submaxillary saliva. *Arch. Ges. Physiol.*, **291**, 85

36. Thaysen, J. H., Thorn, N. A. and Schwartz, I. L. (1954). Excretion of sodium, potassium, chloride and carbon dioxide in human parotid saliva. *Amer. J. Physiol.*, **178**, 155

37. Knauf, H. and Fromter, E. (1970). Die Kationenausscheidung der grossen Speicheldrusen des Menschen. *Pflügers Arch.*, **316**, 213

38. Gregersen, M. I. and Ingalls, E. N. (1931). The influence of rate of secretion on the concentrations of potassium and sodium in dog's submaxillary saliva. *Amer. J. Physiol.*, **98**, 441

39. Brusilow, S. W. and Cooke, R. E. (1959). Role of parotid ducts in secretion of hypotonic saliva. *Amer. J. Physiol.*, **196**, 831

40. Chauncey, H. H., Feller, R. P. and Henriques, B. L. (1966). Comparative electrolyte composition of parotid, submandibular and sublingual secretions. *J. Dental Res.*, **45**, 1230

41. Dreisbach, R. H. (1960). Calcium binding by normal human saliva. *J. Dental Res.*, **39**, 1133

42. Heidenhain, R. (1878). Ueber secretorische und tropische Drusennerven. *Arch. Ges. Physiol.*, **17**, 1

43. Langley, J. N. and Fletcher, H. M. (1889). On the secretion of saliva, chiefly on the secretion of salts in it. *Phil. Trans. Roy. Soc. London, B*, **180**, 109

44. Werther, M. (1886), Einige Beobachtungen uber die absonderung der Salze im Speichel. *Arch. Ges. Physiol.*, **38**, 293

45. Wills, J. H. and Fenn, W. O. (1938). Potassium changes in submaxillary glands during stimulation. *Amer. J. Physiol.*, **124**, 72

46. Burgen, A. S. V. (1956). The secretion of potassium in saliva. *J. Physiol.* (*London*), **132**, 20

47. Coats, D. A. and Wright, R. D. (1957). Secretion by the parotid gland of the sheep: the relationship between salivary flow and composition. *J. Physiol.* (*London*), **135**, 611

48. Coats, D. A., Denton, D. A. and Wright, R. D. (1958). The ionic balances and transferences of the sheep's parotid gland during maximal stimulation. *J. Physiol.* (*London*), **144**, 108

49. Petersen, O. H. and Poulsen, J. H. (1968). The secretion of sodium and potassium in cat submandibular saliva during the first period after start of stimulation. *Acta Physiol. Scand.*, **73**, 93

50. Burgen, A. S. V. and Terroux, K. G. (1962). The effect of changes in the rate of flow of the saliva on the concentration of iodide in parotid saliva. *J. Physiol.* (*London*), **163**, 239

51. Burgen, A. S. V. (1964). Kinetic methods for the study of salivary secretions: their scope and limitations. *Salivary Glands and Their Secretions*, 197 (L. M. Sreebny and J. Meyer, editors) (Oxford: Pergamon Press)

52. Dreisbach, R. H. (1959). Secretion of calcium by rat submandibular gland. *Amer. J. Physiol.*, **196**, 645

53. Lundberg, A. (1955). The electrophysiology of the submaxillary gland of the cat. *Acta Physiol. Scand.*, **35**, 1

54. Lundberg, A. (1957). Secretory potentials in the sublingual gland of the cat. *Acta Physiol. Scand.*, **40**, 21

55. Lundberg, A. (1958). Electrophysiology of salivary glands. *Physiol. Rev.*, **38**, 21

56. Schneyer, L. H. and Schneyer, C. A. (1965). Membrane potentials of salivary gland cells of rat. *Amer. J. Physiol.*, **209**, 1304

57. Imai, Y. (1965). Studies on the secretory mechanism of the submaxillary gland of dog. Part 1. Electrophysiological studies with microelectrode. *J. Physiol. Soc. Jap.*, **27**, 304

58. Fritz, M. E. and Botelho, S. Y. (1969). Membrane potentials in unstimulated parotid gland of the cat. *Amer. J. Physiol.*, **216**, 1180

59. Creed, K. E. and Wilson, J. A. F. (1969). The latency of response of secretory acinar cells to nerve stimulation in the submandibular gland of the cat. *Aust. J. Exp. Biol. Med. Sci.*, **47**, 135

60. Fritz, M. E. and Botelho, S. Y. (1969). Role of autonomic nerve impulses in secretion by the parotid gland of the cat. *Amer. J. Physiol.*, **216**, 1392

61. Schneyer, L. H. (1969). Observations on secretory potentials in rat submaxillary gland. *The Exocrine Glands*, 30 (S. Y. Botelho, F. P. Brooks and W. B. Shelley, editors) (Philadelphia: University of Pennsylvania Press)

62. Schneyer, L. H. and Schneyer, C. A. (1960). Electrolyte and inulin spaces of rat salivary glands and pancreas. *Amer. J. Physiol.*, **199**, 649

63. Imai, Y. (1965). Study of the secretion mechanism of submaxillary gland of dog. Part 2. Effect of exchanging ions in the perfusate on salivary secretion and secretory potential, with special reference to the ionic distribution in gland tissue. *J. Physiol. Soc. Jap.*, **27**, 313

64. Yoshimura, H. and Imai, Y. (1967). Studies on the secretory potential of acinal cell of dog's submaxillary gland and the ionic dependency of it. *Jap. J. Physiol.*, **17**, 280

65. Yoshimura, H. (1967). Secretory mechanism of saliva and nervous control of its ionic composition. *Secretory Mechanisms of Salivary Glands*, 56 (L. H. Schneyer and C. A. Schneyer, editors) (New York: Academic Press)

66. Petersen, O. H. and Poulsen, J. H. (1967). The effects of varying the extracellular potassium concentration on the secretory rate and on resting and secretory potentials in the perfused cat submandibular gland. *Acta Physiol. Scand.*, **70**, 293

67. Petersen, O. H. (1971). Initiation of salt and water transport in mammalian salivary glands by acetylcholine. *Phil. Trans. Roy. Soc. London*, B, **262**, 307

68. Fritz, M. E. (1972). Cationic dependence of resting membrane potentials of parotid acinar cells. *Amer. J. Physiol.*, **223**, 644

69. Schneyer, L. H. and Schneyer, C. A. (1964). Effects of pilocarpine on exchange of K^{42} in slices of submaxillary gland. *Proc. Soc. Exp. Biol. Med.*, **116**, 813

70. Schneyer, L. H. (1967). Exchange of potassium in rat submaxillary gland. *Secretory Mechanisms of Salivary Glands*, 32 (L. H. Schneyer and C. A. Schneyer, editors) (New York: Academic Press)

71. Petersen, O. H. (1970). Some factors influencing stimulation-induced release of potassium from the cat submandibular gland to fluid perfused through the gland. *J. Physiol. (London)*, **208**, 431

72. Petersen, O. H. (1970). The dependence of the transmembrane salivary secretory potential on the external potassium and sodium concentration. *J. Physiol. (London)*, **210**, 205

73. Petersen, O. H. (1971). Secretory transmembrane potentials in acinar cells from the cat submandibular gland during perfusion with a chloride-free sucrose solution. *Pflügers Arch.*, **323**, 91

74. Martinez, J. R., Holzgreve, H. and Frick, A. (1966). Micropuncture study of submaxillary glands of adult rats. *Arch. Ges. Physiol.*, **290**, 124

75. Young, J. A., Frömter, E., Schögel, E. and Hamann, K. F. (1967). A micro-perfusion investigation of sodium resorption and potassium secretion by the main excretory duct of the rat submaxillary gland. *Arch. Ges. Physiol.*, **295**, 157

76. Langley, L. L. and Brown, R. S. (1960). Stop-flow analysis of ionic transfer in the dog parotid gland. *Amer. J. Physiol.*, **199**, 59

77. Henriques, B. L. (1961). Acinar-duct transport sites for Na^+ and K^+ in dog submaxillary salivary gland. *Amer. J. Physiol.*, **201**, 935

78. Mangos, J. A., Braun, G. and Hamann, K. F. (1966). Micropuncture study of sodium and potassium excretion in the rat parotid saliva. *Arch. Ges. Physiol.*, **291**, 99

79. Douglas, W. W. and Poisner, A. M. (1963). The influence of calcium on the secretory response of the submaxillary gland to acetylcholine or to noradrenaline. *J. Physiol. (London)*, **165**, 528

80. Petersen, O. H., Poulsen, J. H. and Thorn, N. A. (1967). Secretory potentials, secretory rates and water permeability of the duct system in the cat submandibular gland during perfusion with calcium free Locke's solution. *Acta Physiol. Scand.*, **71**, 203

81. Holzgreve, H., Martinez, J. R. and Vogel, A. (1966). Micropuncture and histologic study of submaxillary glands of young rats. *Arch. Ges. Physiol.*, **290**, 134

82. Petersen, O. H. (1971). Formation of saliva and potassium transport in the perfused cat submandibular gland. *J. Physiol. (London)*, **216**, 129

83. Whittembury, G. and Proverbio, F. (1970). Two modes of Na extrusion in cells from guinea pig kidney cortex slices. *Pflügers Arch.*, **316**, 1

84. Knauf, H. (1972). The isolated salivary duct as a model for electrolyte transport studies. *Pflügers Arch.*, **333**, 82

85. Field, M. J. and Young, J. A. (1972). Sodium and potassium transport by the rat submaxillary main duct perfused *in vitro*. *Proc. Aust. Physiol. Pharmacol. Soc.*, **3**, 159

86. Schneyer, L. H. (1969). Secretion of potassium by perfused excretory duct of rat submaxillary gland. *Amer. J. Physiol.*, **217**, 1324

87. Knauf, H. and Frömter, E. (1970). Elektrische Untersuchungen am Hauptausfuhrungsgang der Speicheldrusen des Menschen. I. Potentialmessung. *Pflügers Arch.*, **316**, 238

88. Schneyer, L. H. (1970). Amiloride inhibition of ion transport in perfused excretory duct of rat submaxillary gland. *Amer. J. Physiol.*, **219**, 1050

89. Knauf, H. (1972). The minimum requirements for the maintenance of active sodium transport across the isolated salivary duct epithelium of the rabbit. *Pflügers Arch.*, **333**, 326

90. Young, J. A. (1968). Microperfusion investigation of chloride fluxes across the epithelium of the main excretory duct of the rat submaxillary gland. *Pflügers Arch.*, **303**, 366

91. Young, J. A., Martin, C. J., Asz, M. and Weber, F. D. (1970). A microperfusion investigation of bicarbonate secretion by the rat submaxillary gland. The action of a parasympathomimetic drug on electrolyte transport. *Pflügers Arch.*, **319**, 185

92. Diamond, J. M. and Tormey, J. McD. (1966). Studies on the structural basis of water transport across epithelial membranes. *Fed. Proc. (Fed. Amer. Soc. Exp. Biol.)*, **25**, 1458

93. Diamond, J. M. and Bossert, W. H. (1967). Standing-gradient osmotic flow. A mechanism for coupling of water and solute transport in epithelia. *J. Gen. Physiol.*, **50**, 2061

94. Curran, P. F. (1960). Na, Cl and water transport by rat ileum *in vitro*. *J. Gen. Physiol.*, **43**, 1137

95. Durbin, R. P. (1960). Osmotic flow of water across permeable cellulose membranes. *J. Gen. Physiol.*, **44**, 315

96. Shackleford, J. M. and Schneyer, L. H. (1971). Ultrastructural aspects of the main excretory duct of rat submandibular gland. *Anat. Rec.*, **169**, 679

97. Hall, H. D., Merig, J. J. and Schneyer, C. A. (1967). Metrecal induced changes in human saliva. *Proc. Soc. Exp. Biol. Med.*, **124**, 532

98. Hall, H. D. and Schneyer, C. A. (1964). Paper electrophoresis of rat salivary secretions. *Proc. Soc. Exp. Biol. Med.*, **115**, 1001

99. Schneyer, L. H. (1956). Amylase content of separate salivary gland secretions of man. *J. Appl. Physiol.*, **9**, 453

100. Flatland, R. F., Schneyer, L. H. and Schneyer, C. A. (1969). Amylase activity of acinar cells separated from guinea pig submaxillary gland. *Proc. Soc. Exp. Biol. Med.*, **131**, 243

101. Shear, M. (1972). Substrate film techniques for the histochemical demonstration of amylase and protease in salivary glands. *J. Dental Res.*, **51**, 368

102. Loyter, A. and Schramm, M. (1962). The glycogen–amylase complex as a means of obtaining highly purified α-amylases. *Biochim. Biophys. Acta*, **65**, 200

103. Siekevitz, P. and Palade, G. E. (1960). A cytochemical study on the pancreas of the guinea pig. V. *In vivo* incorporation of leucine-1-^{14}C into the chymotrypsinogen of various cell fractions. *J. Biophys. Biochem. Cytol.*, **7**, 619

104. Caro, L. G. and Palade, G. E. (1964). Protein synthesis, storage and discharge in the pancreatic exocrine cell: an autoradiographic study. *J. Cell Biol.*, **20**, 473

105. Jamieson, J. D. and Palade, G. E. (1967). Intracellular transport of secretory proteins in the pancreatic exocrine cell: I. Role of the peripheral elements of the golgi complex. *J. Cell Biol.*, **34**, 577

106. Jamieson, J. D. and Palade, G. E. (1967). Intracellular transport of secretory proteins in the pancreatic exocrine cell. II. Transport to condensing vacuoles and zymogen granules. *J. Cell Biol.*, **34**, 597

107. Redman, C. M., Siekevitz, P. and Palade, G. E. (1966). Synthesis and transfer of amylase in pigeon pancreatic microsomes. *J. Biol. Chem.*, **241**, 1150

108. Schramm, M. and Bdolah, A. (1964). The mechanism of enzyme secretion by the cell. III. Intermediate stages in amylase transport as revealed by pulse labelling of slices of parotid gland. *Arch. Biochem. Biophys.*, **104**, 67

109. Gromet-Elhanan, Z. and Winnick, T. (1963). Microsomes as sites of α-amylase synthesis in the rat parotid gland. *Biochim. Biophys. Acta*, **69**, 85

110. Castle, J. D., Jamieson, J. D. and Palade, G. E. (1972). Radioautographic analysis of the secretory processes in the parotid acinar cell of the rabbit. *J. Cell Biol.*, **53**, 290

111. Kesztyus, L. and Martin, J. (1937). Uber den Einfluss von Chorda und Sympathicusreizung auf die Zusammensetzung des Submaxillarspeichels. *Arch. Ges. Physiol.*, **239**, 408

112. Schneyer, C. A. (1962). Salivary gland changes after isoproterenol-induced enlargement. *Amer. J. Physiol.*, **203**, 232

113. Yoshida, Y., Sprecher, R. L., Schneyer, C. A. and Schneyer, L. H. (1967). Role of β-receptors in sympathetic regulation of electrolytes in rat submaxillary saliva. *Proc. Soc. Exp. Biol. Med.*, **126**, 912

114. Young, J. A. and Martin, C. J. (1971). The effect of a sympatho- and a parasympatho-mimetic drug on the electrolyte concentrations of primary and final saliva in the rat submaxillary gland. *Pflügers Arch.*, **327**, 285

115. Dreisbach, R. H. (1964). Effect of isoproterenol on calcium metabolism in rat salivary gland. *Proc. Soc. Exp. Biol. Med.*, **116**, 953

116. Schneyer, C. A. and Hall, H. D. (1966). Autonomic pathways involved in a sympathetic-like action of pilocarpine on salivary composition. *Proc. Soc. Exp. Biol. Med.*, **121**, 96

117. Pohto, P. (1968). Effect of isoprenaline, pilocarpine and prenylamine on amylase secretion in rat parotid saliva. *J. Oral Therap. Pharmacol.*, **4**, 467

118. Robison, G. A., Butcher, R. W. and Sutherland, E. W. (1968). Cyclic AMP. *Ann. Rev. Biochem.*, **37**, 149

119. Rasmussen, H. and Tenenhouse, A. (1968). Cyclic adenosine monophosphate, Ca^{2+}, and membranes. *Proc. Nat. Acad. Sci. USA*, **59**, 1364

120. Bdolah, A. and Schramm, M. (1965). The function of 3'5'-cyclic AMP in enzyme secretion. *Biochem. Biophys. Res. Commun.*, **18**, 452

121. Selinger, Z. and Naim, E. (1970). The effect of calcium on amylase secretion by rat parotid slices. *Biochim. Biophys. Acta*, **203**, 335

122. Rubin, R. P. (1970). The role of calcium in the release of neurotransmitter substances and hormones. *Pharmacol. Rev.*, **22**, 389

123. Yoshida, H., Miki, N., Ishida, H. and Yamamoto, I. (1968). Release of amylase from zymogen granules by ATPase and a low concentration of Ca^{2+}. *Biochim. Biophys. Acta*, **158**, 489

124. Lindsay, R. H., Ueha, T. and Hanson, R. W. (1970). Enzyme secretion *in vitro* in the absence of alterations in oxidation. *Biochem. Biophys. Res. Commun.*, **39**, 616

125. Parks, H. F. (1962). Morphological study of the extrusion of secretory materials by the parotid glands of mouse and rat. *J. Ultrastruct. Res.*, **6**, 449

126. Radley, J. M. (1969). Ultrastructural changes in the rat submaxillary gland following isoprenaline. *Z. Zellforsch. Mikrosk. Anat.*, **97**, 196

127. Kirby, K. C., Jr., Swern, D. and Baserga, R. (1969). The effect of structural modification of the isoproterenol molecule on the stimulation of deoxyribonucleic acid synthesis in mouse salivary glands. *Molec. Pharmacol.*, **5**, 572

128. Barka, T. (1965). Stimulation of DNA synthesis by isoproterenol in the salivary gland. *Exp. Cell Res.*, **39**, 355
129. Pohto, P. (1966). Catecholamine induced salivary gland enlargement in rats. *Acta Odontol. Scand.*, Suppl. **24**, 6
130. Baserga, R., Sasaki, T. and Whitlock, J. P., Jr. (1969). The pre-replicative phase of isoproterenol stimulated DNA synthesis. *Biochemistry of Cell Division*, 77 (Springfield, Illinois: Thomas)
131. Schneyer, C. A. (1970). Mitosis induced in adult rat parotid following normal activity of the gland. *Proc. Soc. Exp. Biol. Med.*, **134**, 98
132. Emmelin, N. (1965). Action of transmitters on the responsiveness of effector cells. *Experientia*, **21**, 57
133. Ohlin, P. (1966). *Nervous and Hormonal Control of Salivary Glands in Rats.* (Thesis). *Acta Univ. Lund.*, Sect. II, No. 7, 1
134. Baxter, H. (1933). Variations in the inorganic constituents of mixed and parotid gland saliva activated by reflex stimulation in the dog. *J. Biol. Chem.*, **102**, 203
135. Montgomery, M. F. and Stuart, J. S. (1936). Studies upon the secretion of oral and pharyngeal mucus. *Amer. J. Physiol.*, **115**, 497
136. Emmelin, N. (1953). On spontaneous secretion of saliva. *Acta Physiol. Scand.*, **30**, *Suppl.* **111**, 34
137. Nordenfelt, I. and Ohlin, P. (1957). Supersensitivity of salivary glands of rabbits. *Acta Physiol. Scand.*, **41**, 12
138. Ohlin, P. and Perec, C. (1965). Salivary secretion of the major sublingual gland of rats. *Experientia*, **21**, 408
139. Eckhard, C. (1893). Noch einmal die Parotis des Schafes. *Centr. Physiol.*, **7**, 365
140. Moussu, M. (1890). De l'innervation des glandes parotides chez les animaux domestiques. *Arch. Physiol. Norm. Pathol.*, **5**, 68
141. Coats, D. A., Denton, D. A., Goding, J. R. and Wright, R. D. (1956). Secretion by the parotid gland of the sheep. *J. Physiol.* (*London*), **131**, 13
142. Kay, R. N. (1958). Continuous and reflex secretion by the parotid gland in ruminants. *J. Physiol.* (*London*), **144**, 463
143. Emmelin, N. (1952). 'Paralytic secretion' of saliva. An example of supersensitivity after denervation. *Physiol. Rev.*, **32**, 21
144. Emmelin, N. (1972). Control of salivary glands. *Oral Physiology*, 1 (N. Emmelin and Y. Zotterman, editors) (Oxford: Pergamon Press)
145. Montgomery, M. F. (1934). Studies upon secretory activity of glands of the oral and pharyngeal mucous membranes. *Proc. Soc. Exp. Biol. Med.*, **31**, 717
146. Emmelin, N. (1955). On the innervation of the submaxillary gland cells in cats. *Acta Physiol. Scand.*, **34**, 11
147. Emmelin, N. and Holmberg, J. (1967). Impulse frequency in secretory nerves of salivary glands. *J. Physiol.* (*London*), **191**, 205
148. Emmelin, N., Garrett, J. R. and Holmberg, J. (1968). Uncharted secretory nerves in the parotid gland of the dog. *Experientia*, **24**, 460
149. Holmberg, J. (1971). The secretory nerves of the parotid gland of the dog. *J. Physiol.* (*London*), **219**, 463
150. Holmberg, J. (1972). *The Secretory Innervation of the Dog's Parotid Gland.* (Thesis). (Lund: Studentlitteratur)
151. Holmberg, J. (1972). Release of acetylcholine in the parotid gland of the dog during stimulation of postganglionic nerves. *Acta Physiol. Scand.*, **86**, 115
152. Reichert, F. L. and Poth, E. J. (1933). Pathways for the secretory fibres of the salivary glands in man. *Proc. Soc. Exp. Biol. Med.*, **30**, 973
153. Diamant, H. and Wiberg, A. (1965). Does the chorda tympani in man contain secretory fibres for the parotid gland? *Acta Oto-Laryngol.*, **60**, 255
154. Moussu, M. (1888). Nerf moteur ou secreteur de la glande parotide chez le boeuf. *Compt. Rend. Soc. Biol.*, **40**, 280
155. Laage-Hellman, J.-E. and Stromblad, B. C. R. (1960). Secretion from human submaxillary gland after section of the chorda tympani. *J. Appl. Physiol.*, **15**, 295
156. Seo, M. (1934). Observations on the salivary secretion from the denervated submaxillary gland. *Tohoku J. Exp. Med.*, **22**, 563
157. Emmelin, N. and Stromblad, R. (1953). Salivary secretion after section of the chorda tympani in non-anaesthetized dogs. *Acta Physiol. Scand.*, **30**, 65

158. Beznak, M. and Farkas, E. (1936–1937). The interpretation of some phenomena of salivary secretion caused by direct electrical stimulation of the effector nerve, in terms of the present knowledge of the nervous impulse and of its chemical transmission. *Quart. J. Exp. Physiol.*, **26**, 265

159. Wills, J. H. (1941). Some factors in secretion by submaxillary glands of the cat. *Amer. J. Physiol.*, **134**, 441

160. Diamant, H., Enfors, B. and Holmstedt, B. (1959). Salivary secretion in man elicited by means of stimulation of the chorda tympani. *Acta Physiol. Scand.*, **45**, 293

161. Garrett, J. R. (1966). The innervation of salivary glands. I. Cholinesterase-positive nerves in normal glands of the cat. *J. Roy. Microscop. Soc.*, **85**, 135

162. Garrett, J. R. (1966). The innervation of salivary glands. II. The ultrastructure of nerves in normal glands of the cat. *J. Roy. Microscop. Soc.*, **85**, 149

163. Emmelin, N., Garrett, J. R. and Ohlin, P. (1968). Neural control of salivary myoepithelial cells. *J. Physiol. (London)*, **196**, 381

164. Darke, A. C. and Smaje, L. H. (1971). Myoepithelial cell activation in the submaxillary salivary gland. *J. Physiol. (London)*, **219**, 89

165. Dewey, M. M. and Barr, L. (1964). A study of the structure and distribution of the nexus. *J. Cell Biol.*, **23**, 553

166. Ekstrom, J. and Emmelin, N. (1971). The functional organization of the parasympathetic secretory innervation of the submandibular gland. *J. Physiol. (London)*, **213**, 727

167. Babkin, B. P., Alley, A. and Stavraky, G. W. (1932). Humoral transmission of chorda tympani effect. *Trans. Roy. Soc. Can.*, Sect. V., **26**, 89

168. Babkin, B. P., Gibbs, O. S. and Wolff, H. G. (1932). Die humorale Uebertragung der Chorda-tympani-Reizung. 1. Mitt. *Arch. Exptl. Pathol. Pharmakol.*, **168**, 32

169. Feldberg, W. (1933). Die blutdrucksenkende Wirkung der Chorda-Lingualisreizung und ihre Beeinflussung durch Atropin. *Arch. Exptl. Pathol. Pharmakol.*, **170**, 560

170. Beznák, A. (1932). Die autacoide Aktivitat des venosen Blutes von sezernierenden Submaxillardrusen. *Arch. Ges. Physiol.*, **229**, 719

171. Gibbs, O. S. and Szeloczey, J. (1932). Die humorale Uebertragung der Chorda tympani-Reizung. *Arch. Exptl. Pathol. Pharmakol.*, **168**, 64

172. Henderson, V. E. and Roepke, M. H. (1933). On the mechanism of salivary secretion. *J. Pharmacol. Exp. Therap.*, **47**, 193

173. Henderson, V. E. and Roepke, M. H. (1933). Ueber den lokalen hormonalen Mechanismus der Parasympathikusreizung. *Arch. Exp. Pathol. Pharmakol.*, **172**, 314

174. Emmelin, N. and Muren, A. (1950). Acetylcholine release at parasympathetic synapses. *Acta Physiol. Scand.*, **20**, 13

175. Emmelin, N. (1960). Is there a leakage of acetylcholine from postganglionic parasympathetic nerve endings? *Nature (London)*, **185**, 297

176. Assarson, N. and Emmelin, N. (1964). On the mechanism of the 'degeneration secretion' of saliva. *J. Physiol. (London)*, **170**, 17P

177. Emmelin, N. (1965). Action of transmitters on the responsiveness of effector cells. *Experientia*, **21**, 57

178. Emmelin, N. and Stromblad, B. C. R. (1958). A 'paroxysmal' secretion of saliva following parasympathetic denervation of the parotid gland. *J. Physiol. (London)*, **143**, 506

179. Emmelin, N. and Trendelenburg, U. (1972). Degeneration activity after parasympathetic or sympathetic denervation. *Ergebnisse der Physiologie*. Vol. 66, 147 (Berlin: Springer-Verlag)

180. Dean, P. M. and Matthews, E. K. (1972). Pancreatic acinar cells: measurement of membrane potential and miniature depolarization potentials. *J. Physiol. (London)*, **225**, 1

181. Fritz, M. E. (1971). Membrane potentials in parotid glands of cats with degeneration secretion. *Amer. J. Physiol.*, **220**, 1025

182. Nordenfelt, I. (1965). *Acetylcholine Synthesis in Salivary Glands*. (Thesis), 1 (Lund: Hakan Olsson)

183. Nordenfelt, I. (1967). Metabolism of transmitter substances in salivary glands. *Secretory Mechanisms of Salivary Glands*, 142 (L. H. Schneyer and C. A. Schneyer, editors) (New York: Academic Press)

184. Stromblad, B. C. R. (1957). Supersensitivity caused by denervation and by cholinesterase inhibitors. *Acta Physiol. Scand.*, **41**, 118

185. Leaders, F. E. and Pan, P. J. (1967). Local cholinergic–adrenergic interaction in the dog salivary gland preparation. *Arch. Intern. Pharmacodyn.*, **165**, 71

186. Hilton, S. M. and Lewis, G. P. (1955). The cause of the vasodilatation accompanying activity in the submandibular salivary gland. *J. Physiol. (London)*, **128**, 235

187. Emmelin, N. and Engstrom, J. (1960). On the existence of specific secretory sympathetic fibres for the cat's submaxillary gland. *J. Physiol. (London)*, **153**, 1

188. Ohlin, P. (1965). *Secretory Responses of Innervated and Denervated Submaxillary Glands of Rats.* (Thesis). *Acta Univ. Lund.* Sect. II, No. 7, 1

189. Norberg, K.-A. and Olson, L. (1965). Adrenergic innervation of the salivary glands in the rat. *Z. Zellforsch.*, **68**, 183

190. Ehinger, B., Garrett, J. R. and Ohlin, P. (1967). Adrenergic nerves in the major salivary glands of the rabbit. *Experientia*, **23**, 924

191. Freitag, P. and Engel, M. B. (1970). Autonomic innervation in rabbit salivary glands. *Anat. Rec.*, **167**, 87

192. Garrett, J. R. and Holmberg, J. (1972). Effects of surgical denervations on the autonomic nerves in parotid glands of dogs. *Z. Zellforsch.*, **131**, 451

193. Young, J. A. and Martin, C. J. (1971). The effect of sympatho- and parasympathomimetic drugs on the electrolyte concentration of primary and final saliva of the rat submaxillary gland. *Pflügers Arch.*, **327**, 285

194. Dische, Z., Kahn, N., Rothschild, C., Danilchenko, A., Licking, J. and Wang, S. C. (1970). Glycoproteins of submaxillary saliva of the cat: Differences in composition produced by sympathetic and parasympathetic nerve stimulation. *J. Neurochem.*, **17**, 649

195. Kahn, N., Mandel, I., Licking, J., Wasserman, A. and Morea, D. (1969). Comparison of the effects of parasympathetic and sympathetic nervous stimulation on cat submaxillary gland saliva. *Proc. Soc. Exp. Biol. Med.*, **130**, 314

196. Euler, U. S. v. and Purkhold, A. (1951). Effect of sympathetic denervation on the noradrenaline and adrenaline content of the spleen, kidney and salivary glands in the sheep. *Arch. Physiol. Scand.*, **24**, 212

197. Euler, U. S. v. and Ryd, G. (1963). Effect of sympathetic denervation and adrenalectomy on the catecholamine content of the rat submaxillary gland. *Acta Physiol. Scand.*, **59**, 62

198. Stromblad, B. C. R. (1960). Adrenaline–noradrenaline content of the submaxillary gland of the cat. *Experientia*, **16**, 417

199. Cattell, M., Wolff, H. G. and Clark, D. (1934). The liberation of adrenergic and cholinergic substances in the submaxillary gland. *Amer. J. Physiol.*, **109**, 375

200. Emmelin, N. and Muren, A. (1951). Sensitization of the submaxillary gland to chemical stimuli. *Acta Physiol. Scand.*, **24**, 103

201. Stromblad, B. C. R. (1960). Effect of denervation of cocaine on the action of sympathomimetic amines. *Brit. J. Pharmacol. Chemotherap.*, **15**, 328

202. Koppanyi, T. and Maling, H. M. (1972). The effects of pretreatment with reserpine, α-methyl-*p*-tyrosine, or prostaglandin E₁ on adrenergic salivation. *Proc. Soc. Exp. Biol. Med.*, **140**, 787

203. Emmelin, N. and Engstrom, J. (1960). Parotid pain during treatment with bretylium. *Lancet*, **II**, 263

204. Emmelin, N. and Engstrom, J. (1961). Supersensitivity of salivary glands following treatment with bretylium or guanethidine. *Brit. J. Pharmacol. Chemotherap.*, **16**, 315

205. Emmelin, N. and Holmberg, J. (1965). Neuroglandular effects of bretylium and guanethidine studied on salivary glands of cats. *J. Oral Therap. Pharmacol.*, **2**, 24

206. Dale, H. H. (1906). On some physiological actions of ergot. *J. Physiol. (London)*, **34**, 163

207. Emmelin, N. (1955). Sympatholytic agents used to separate secretory and vascular effects of sympathetic stimulation in the submaxillary gland. *Acta Physiol. Scand.*, **34**, 29

208. Thulin, A. (1972). On the β-adrenergic receptors in salivary glands of rats and dogs. *Experientia*, **28**, 420

209. Ekstrom, J. (1969). 4-(2-hydroxy-3-isopropylaminopropoxy) acetanilide as a β-receptor blocking agent. *Experientia*, **25**, 372

210. Cowley, L. H. and Shackleford, J. M. (1970). An ultrastructural study of the submandibular glands of the squirrel monkey, Saimiri sciureus. *J. Morphol.*, **132**, 117

211. Martin, C. J. and Young, J. A. (1971). A microperfusion investigation of the effects of a sympathomimetic and a parasympatho-mimetic drug on water and electrolyte fluxes in the main duct of the rat submaxillary gland. *Pflügers Arch.*, **327**, 303

212. Schneyer, L. H., Thavornthon, T. and Schneyer, C. A. (1971). Isoproterenol-stimulated sodium absorption from perfused submaxillary excretory duct of rat. *Fed. Proc. (Fed. Amer. Soc. Exp. Biol.*, **30**, 606

213. Mangos, J. A. and McSherry, N. R. (1969). Micropuncture study of sodium and potassium excretion in rat parotid saliva: role of aldosterone. *Proc. Soc. Exp. Biol. Med.*, **132**, 797

214. Martinez, J. R. and Martinez, A. M. (1972). Effects of ADH and dibutyryl cyclic-AMP on submaxillary secretion in the dog. *Europ. J. Pharmacol.*, **18**, 375

215. Harrop, T. J. and MacKay, B. (1968). Electron microscopic observations on myoepithelial cells and secretory nerves in rat salivary glands. *J. Can. Dental Assoc.*, **34**, 480

216. Emmelin, N., Garrett, J. R. and Ohlin, P. (1969). Motor nerves of salivary myoepithelial cells in dogs. *J. Physiol. (London)*, **200**, 539

217. Emmelin, N. and Holmberg, J. (1967). The presence of Beta-receptors in the submaxillary gland of the dog. *Brit. J. Pharmacol. Chemotherap.*, **30**, 371

218. Emmelin, N., Ohlin, P. and Thulin, A. (1969). The pharmacology of salivary myoepithelial cells in dogs. *Brit. J. Pharmacol. Chemotherap.*, **37**, 666

219. Emmelin, N. and Gjorstrup, P. (1972). On the function of salivary myoepithelial cells. *J. Physiol. (London)*, **225**, 25P

220. Emmelin, N. and Gjorstrup, P. (1973). On the function of myoepithelial cells in salivary glands. *J. Physiol. (London)*, in press

221. Norberg, K.-A. and Hamberger, B. (1964). The sympathetic adrenergic neuron. Some characteristics revealed by histochemical studies on the intraneuronal distribution of the transmitter. *Acta Physiol. Scand., Suppl.* **238**, 1

222. Bernard, C. (1858). De l'influence de deux ordres de nerfs qui determinent les variations de couleur de sang veineux dans les organes glandulaires. *Compt. Rend.*, **47**, 245

223. Schachter, M. (1970). Vasodilatation in the submaxillary gland of the cat, rabbit, and sheep. *Handbuch der Experimentellen Pharmakologie*, Vol. 25, 400 (E. G. Erdos, editor) (Berlin: Springer-Verlag)

224. Karpinsky, E., Barton, S. and Schachter, M. (1971). Vasodilator nerve fibres to the submaxillary gland of the cat. *Nature (London)*, **232**, 122

225. Hilton, S. M. and Lewis, G. P. (1957). Functional vasodilatation in the submandibular salivary gland. *Brit. Med. Bull.*, **13**, 189

226. Hilton, S. M. (1960). *Polypeptides which affect Smooth Muscles and Blood Vessels*, 258 (M. Schachter, editor) (Oxford: Pergamon Press)

227. Gautvik, K. (1970). *Studies on Vasodilator Mechanisms in the Submandibular Salivary Gland in Cats.* (Thesis). (Oslo: Universitetsforlaget)

228. Mellander, S. (1971). Systemic circulation: Local control. *Ann. Rev. Physiol.*, **32**, 313

229. Lundvall, J. (1972). Tissue hyperosmolality as a mediator of vasodilatation and transcapillary fluid flux in exercising skeletal muscle. *Acta Physiol. Scand. Suppl.*, **379**, 1

230. Kjellmer, I. (1965). Studies on exercise hyperemia. *Acta Physiol. Scand. Suppl.*, **244**, 1

231. Darke, A. C. and Smaje, L. H. (1972). Dependence of functional vasodilatation in the cat submaxillary gland upon stimulation frequency. *J. Physiol. (London)*, **226**, 191

7
Gastric Secretion

S. J. KONTUREK
Medical Academy Krakow, Poland

7.1 INTRODUCTION

The stomach secretes small ions, water and macromolecules into the gastric lumen, and gastrin into the circulation. Gastric secretion is controlled by the autonomic nervous system, hormones, the functional capacity of the gastric mucosa and the gastric circulation. Secretion can be divided into basal and postprandial periods, which, in turn, can be subdivided into phases according to the site origin of the secretory stimulus: cephalic, gastric, and intestinal. The stimulation of acid secretion during the cephalic and gastric phases has the same dual mechanism, namely, direct cholinergic activation of oxyntic glands and cholinergic release of gastrin. The vagus and gastrin are strikingly interdependent in stimulating secretion. The acid concentration of gastric juice is determined by the rate of secretion, by the buffering effect of food and by diffusion of acid into the mucosa. The gastric mucosa resists rapid diffusion of acid back from the juice. Damage to the mucosa hastens this back-diffusion of acid with development of erosive lesions.

7.2 ANATOMICAL CONSIDERATIONS

7.2.1 Structural basis of gastric secretion

The surface area of gastric mucosa in man is *ca.* 800 cm^2. It may be divided into three different zones, each lined by specific types of glands: cardiac, oxyntic and pyloric glands.

The cardiac gland area is a small ring *ca.* 0.5–4.0 cm wide around the gastroesophageal junction. It consists of tubular, highly-branched, and coiled glands containing mucous cells and few or no peptic or oxyntic cells. Cardiac glands secrete mucosubstances and small amounts of electrolytes.

The oxyntic gland area, occupying the fundus and body of the stomach, comprises 75–80% of the total gastric mucosal area. A surface epithelium of columnar cells covers this area. The mucosa contains numerous invaginations or gastric pits penetrating *ca.* one-quarter of its thickness. Approximately 100 pits occupy 1 mm^2, with 3–7 oxyntic glands emptying into each of them. Oxyntic glands, numbering *ca.* 35 million, are straight or slightly-coiled tubules composed of four types of secretory cells: mucous neck cells, oxyntic (parietal) cells, peptic (chief) cells and argentaffin cells.

The neck of each oxyntic gland is lined with mucous cells which are precursors of surface epithelium, parietal and peptic cells. Oxyntic cells, interspersed with mucous neck cells in the midportion of glands, produce acid and intrinsic factor. Peptic cells, encountered chiefly at the base of the glands, secrete pepsinogens. Mucus is produced by the mucous cells of the entire stomach. Argentaffin cells, heterogenous cells found in the mucosa of the entire alimentary canal, are able to reduce silver ion. The chromaffin and argentaffin substances stored in the cytoplasmatic granules are probably the specific products of endocrine function[1]. These cells have no contact with the glandular lumen, suggesting an unknown endocrine activity.

The oxyntic gland area is separated from the pyloric gland area by a transitional zone containing both gland types.

The pyloric gland area constitutes 15–20% of the total gastric mucosal area. It is lined by simple branched tubular glands composed of cells resembling the mucous cells in the neck and base of the oxyntic glands. In the middle third of the thickness of the mucosa, gastrin-producing cells (G-cells) can be localised by immunofluorescence[2]. Pyloric glands contain few or no oxyntic cells and secrete a juice of alkaline mucus and some electrolytes, such as calcium phosphate, bicarbonates, and chlorides of sodium and potassium.

Electron microscopy reveals specialised structures in oxyntic, peptic and mucous cells[3,4]. Oxyntic cells show an extensive tubular network of canaliculi, which start at the base of the cell and, after a tortuous course, open into the apical cell surface. The luminal surfaces of oxyntic cells contain numerous long microvilli, the membranes of which are a continuation of the lining of the canaliculi. Oxyntic cells contain a remarkably large number of mitochondria at the base of the cells. These organelles are important in providing the energy needed for oxyntic cells to produce high concentrations of hydrochloric acid.

The peptic cells contain numerous zymogen granules in the cytoplasm close to the apical portion of cells, which immunofluorescence has shown to be pepsinogen I granules[5]. Similar granules containing pepsinogen II can be localised in cells of the pyloric glands.

Mucous neck cells and surface epithelial cells are characterised by varying amounts of secretory granules, containing different mucosubstances in the apical portion of the cells.

7.2.2 Growth and renewal of gastric mucosa

The surface epithelium of the gastric mucosa is constantly renewed and replaced by desquamation of old cells and migration of new cells from mitotic foci at the bottom of the gastric pits and at the glandular necks[6,7]. The newly-formed cells differentiate into oxyntic and peptic cells. The turnover time of mucous cells is *ca.* 2–6 days.

When the gastric mucosa is injured, the repair process starts from the margin of the damage[6]. If only the surface layer is removed, epithelial cells quickly cover the area. Depending on the extent of damage, cells can be replaced within a few hours to a few days. If the gastric glands are extensively destroyed, as in a peptic ulcer, the lesion requires weeks to heal. After the defect fills with granulation tissue, the surface epithelial cells are renewed rapidly and migrate over the defect. Subsequently, the epithelium invaginates, forming the pits which are slowly transformed into glands in which specialised cells finally develop.

7.2.3 Nerve and blood supply of the stomach

The parasympathetic innervation of the stomach[8] consists of branches of the anterior and posterior vagal trunks, which are formed from the oesophageal plexus. The anterior trunk contains elements of the right and left vagus, as does the posterior trunk. Branches of the anterior trunk reach the ventral surface, while those of the posterior trunk are distributed to the dorsal surface of the stomach. Extragastric branches of vagal nerves innervate the liver, gall bladder, pancreas and intestines.

The preganglionic efferent fibres of the vagus nerves supplying the stomach synapse with the ganglia of the myenteric plexus of Auerbach and the submucosal plexus of Meissner, forming a dense network in the muscle and submucosa, respectively. The cells of the plexuses exhibit morphologic characteristics suggesting that they are not all of the same type. They probably constitute secondary parasympathetic ganglion cells, associative or inter-nuncial cells and sensory cells. The post-ganglionic fibres of the intrinsic plexuses innervate the secretory cells and participate in the local intramural reflexes.

The sympathetic innervation of the stomach derives from the 6th to 10th spinal nerves, which terminate mainly in the celiac ganglia from whence the postganglionic fibres reach the stomach. Synapses of pre- and post-ganglionic sympathetic fibres occur beyond the celiac ganglion on gastric arterial walls. Most of these fibres accompany the gastric arteries and mix with vagal fibres in the gastric wall.

The autonomic nervous system of the stomach also includes afferent fibres which are the pathways for visceral pain sensation and the vagovagal reflexes which influence gastric secretion. Pain fibres are absent from the vagus, and pain sensations arising from the stomach are conveyed by way of splanchnic afferent nerves to the spinal cord via thoracic dorsal nerve roots.

Blood is supplied to the stomach by the three branches of the celiac artery: left gastric, splenic, and hepatic arteries. Branches of these arteries form an extensive submucosal network of anastomoses[9]. The mucosal arteries, arising as branches of the submucosal plexus, penetrate to the mucosa and divide, forming a capillary network around the gastric glands. A small area of the lesser curvature does not show the submucosal plexus and mucosal arteries originate directly from the arterial chain along the lesser curvature.

7.2.4 The gastric mucosal barrier

The phrase 'gastric mucosal barrier' is a physiological concept referring to the ability of the mucosa to prevent rapid penetration by hydrogen ions from the gastric lumen into the interstitial space and the rapid diffusion of sodium ions in the opposite direction. Davenport[10,11] has called attention to its potential importance in gastric disease. The barrier has no proven anatomic correlate, although it is tempting to visualise surface epithelial cells and the tight junctions between adjacent cells as a physical barrier.

Normally, the lipoprotein layer that forms the plasma membrane is relatively impermeable to ions, whereas it is permeable to un-ionised and fat-soluble substances which can easily diffuse across the layer; many damaging agents are either un-ionised or fat-soluble substances (Figure 7.1).

Numerous agents can damage the mucosa: hydrochloric acid in high concentration (*ca.* 250 mN), aliphatic acids (such as acetic, propionic and butyric acids), natural detergents (such as bile salts and lysolecithin), ethanol in concentrations above 10%, and salicylic and acetylsalicylic acids in acid solutions. A common damaging agent is aspirin, which dissociates poorly at an acid pH (pK_a=3.5), but being lipid-soluble, readily penetrates the apical cell membrane of gastric cells, enters the cells, and becomes un-ionised, thereby causing toxic effects[10].

When the mucosa is damaged, acid diffuses into the mucosa and releases histamine from injured cells[12]. Histamine stimulates acid secretion and causes vasodilation and heightened permeability of capillary walls to proteins[13]. The mucosa becomes oedematous, and interstitial fluid filters across the mucosa into the gastric lumen. The net damaging effect is that sodium, potassium and proteins leak into the lumen and hydrogen ions enter the

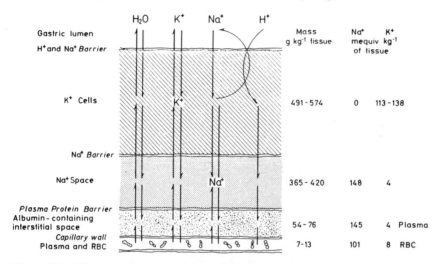

Figure 7.1 Electrolyte anatomy of the oxyntic gland area of canine gastric mucosa. The mucosa is divided into spaces or volumes of distribution determined physiologically. Volumes and concentrations appear on the right. The thickness of the arrows denotes the relative ease with which the components can cross the barriers. In normal circumstances, but especially when the mucosa is damaged, electrolytes may move from plasma across the mucosa between cells as well as through them. (From Davenport[11], courtesy of Year Book Medical Publishers.)

mucosa. Acid in the mucosa stimulates intramural reflexes, resulting in increased acid and pepsin secretion[14]. It also may destroy the mucosal capillaries, producing interstitial haemorrhage and even overt bleeding[15]. Topical damage is usually reversible, but with strong and repeated insults the mucosa may develop bleeding erosions[16].

7.3 METHODS OF STUDYING GASTRIC SECRETION

7.3.1 Preparations

The ideal preparation for studying gastric secretion would be the *in situ* stomach of a conscious subject whose gastric juice is uncontaminated by other secretions and food. In the intact stomach, however, certain phenomena cannot be studied, particularly the importance of specific mechanisms which determine the pattern of secretion. Various preparations have been used which can be divided into *in vivo* and *in vitro* categories. *In vivo* methods can be further subdivided into those involving conscious and anaesthetised animals. This chapter will describe only the preparations using conscious animals (Figure 7.2).

In the standard test of human gastric secretory function, an indwelling gastric tube is introduced through the nose or mouth into the stomach, with the tip placed in the most dependent part of the organ under fluoroscopic

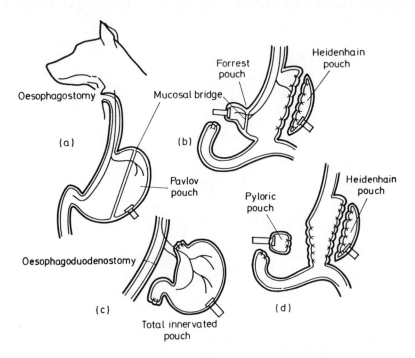

Figure 7.2 Types of gastric pouches: (a) innervated fundic pouch (Pavlov pouch) in the dog with oesophageal fistula; (b) vagally denervated fundic pouch (Heidenhain pouch) and innervated antral pouch (Forrest pouch); (c) innervated pouch of the entire stomach; (d) vagally-denervated fundic pouch (Heidenhain pouch) and vagally-denervated pyloric pouch. (From Magee[141], by courtesy of Charles C. Thomas, Publisher.)

control. Gastric content is aspirated continuously, and the specimens are analysed for volume, pH, HCl, pepsin and electrolyte content. The major limitation of this technique is incompleteness of collection due to the escape of gastric juice into the duodenum and the contamination of gastric juice with biliary, pancreatic and intestinal juices. Non-absorbable dyes or isotopes infused through a separate tube into the stomach during the collection of gastric juice may allow a fairly accurate estimation of the amount of juice recovered. Continuous aspiration permits about 90% recovery of gastric content when gastric secretory rate is high, but recovery is far less under basal conditions. The reflux of intestinal content into the stomach can be prevented by using a gastroduodenal tube with a rubber cuff mounted over the tube midway between the gastric and duodenal orifices. At the beginning of each study, the cuff is inflated distal to the pyloric sphincter to prevent reflux of duodenal content into the stomach. Gastric secretion is collected during basal conditions and in response to various secretory stimuli[17].

The first observation on gastric secretion was made by Beaumont[18,19] in 1833 on Alexis St. Martin, who had sustained a post-traumatic gastric fistula. Since that time, gastric fistulas have been extensively employed in laboratory animals. The technique includes the introduction of a metal or plastic cannula into the body of the stomach, close to the antrum, to allow optimal drainage and diversion of gastric acid away from the antral and duodenal mucosa, thereby preventing the triggering of acid-sensitive gastric inhibitory mechanisms located in the antrum and duodenum[20]. Gastric fistulas permit the study of intact stomachs with fully preserved innervation. They are useless, however, in secretory studies of response to food. For this purpose, portions of the stomach can be isolated from the main stomach as gastric pouches. In general, pouches of the fundic gland area are of three types: vagally innervated, vagally denervated but with sympathetic fibres still intact, and completely denervated or transplanted pouches. In addition, pouches of the entire stomach and of the antral gland area, both vagally innervated or denervated, are used for special purposes[20].

Vagal denervation is accomplished by transecting the wall of the stomach, whereas innervation is preserved by constructing a mucosal septum, leaving the remaining seromucosal layers of the wall intact. The vagally-innervated pouch invented by Pavlov[21] is constructed from the midportion of the greater curvature of the stomach and is assumed to represent the secretory patterns of the main stomach. Stimulation by sham feeding causes both the pouch and the main stomach to secrete in parallel.

The vagally-denervated pouch, described by Heidenhain[22], is constructed from the same region of the stomach as a Pavlov pouch. Although all vagal branches passing across the anterior and posterior walls of the stomach are severed, the Heidenhain pouch may receive vagal input from branches entering the celiac ganglia which accompany sympathetic nerves along the blood vessels to the pouch. Heidenhain pouches may respond minimally to insulin hypoglycaemia, but this could be due to vagal release of gastrin rather than direct vagal stimulation of oxyntic glands in the pouch. Surgical transformation of a Pavlov pouch into a Heidenhain pouch (by dividing the septum between the pouch and the rest of the stomach) markedly diminishes both acid response to a meat meal and pepsin secretion[23].

Farrell and Ivy[24] prepared a completely denervated pouch by transplanting a Heidenhain pouch into the mammary gland region of the abdominal wall, with complete separation of the pouch from its original neurovascular pedicle. This form of autotransplantation was used to prove the existence of a humoral stimulus for the gastric secretory response to food.

A pouch of the entire stomach with oesophagoduodenal anastomosis was made by Ivy and his co-workers[25] to study the intestinal phase of gastric secretion. Feeding a dog with such a pouch resulted in the stimulation of gastric secretion. The possibility cannot be excluded that a pouch of the entire stomach may retain some vagal innervation. These animals are difficult to keep in good health because of severe diarrhoea, probably resulting from vagotomy and subsequent exocrine pancreatic insufficiency. Pouches of the entire stomach, with intact vagal innervation, have also been constructed, but the high ensuing secretory rate in these preparations makes it hard to keep the animals alive.

Studies on the release of gastrin require the separation of the antral gland area from the fundic region to prevent acidification of antral mucosa and inhibition of gastrin release. For this purpose, a pouch is fashioned from the antral region. It may retain full vagal innervation when separated from the remaining stomach by a double-walled mucosal septum[26]. Vagally-denervated antral pouches are created by transection of all layers of the wall and division of blood vessels and nerves at the lesser curvature[27,28]. The formation of a totally denervated antral pouch requires autotransplantation to the abdominal wall and division of all blood vessels and nerves to the pouch, which now receives its blood supply from the newly-formed vessels of the abdominal wall.

In antral pouch preparations, the fundic–antral border must be defined precisely. For this purpose, pH measurements by an intragastric pH glass electrode are used[29]. This procedure has limited value because the pH differences between these two regions may not be great, but, by combining pH measurement with excision of a band at the pH transition, one can get 'pure' antral pouches.

The cephalic phase of gastric secretion is initiated by stimuli emanating from the brain. In dogs, this phase can be activated by sham feeding with an oesophageal fistula preparation[30]. Cervical oesophagostomy can be performed by a double-barrelled cutaneous oesophagostomy or by the cannulation of the exteriorised oesophagus[20]. For the latter purpose[31], the oesophagus is mobilised through the left side of the neck and covered by a skin flap in the first stage of the operation. In the second stage, a cannula is passed into the oesophagus through the mouth and inserted into the oeso-phageal opening. During experiments, the cannula is opened and the distal oesophagus is ligated so that the swallowed food does not reach the stomach. Between experiments, the swallowed food passes into the stomach.

Studies on the influence of the small intestine on gastric secretion are usually performed in animals provided with isolated intestinal loops. A Thiry loop has the proximal end of the intestinal segment closed to form a blind pouch, and the distal end is exteriorised as a mucous fistula. A Thiry–Vella loop is open to the abdominal wall at both ends. Meyer et al.[32] prepared dogs with intestinal loops for the study of the release of gut hormones. Cuffs were placed around the pylorus and at different levels of the small intestine. This permitted isolation of intact small bowel segments for per-fusion by inflating balloons within the lumen under the cuffs. The proximal part of the duodenum containing the duodenal bulb can be isolated without denervation by the formation of a double mucosal septum at the pylorus. The duodenum is transected just above the entrance of the common bile duct and either brought directly to the skin to form a cutaneous fistula or anastomosed to an isolated segment of ileum and then brought to the skin as a mucous fistula.

7.3.2 Measurements of gastric secretion

Gastric secretion can be studied under basal conditions and in response to a variety of stimuli such as gastrin or gastrin analogues, histamine or its analogue betazole (Histalog), insulin, 2-deoxy-D-glucose and others.

Basal gastric secretion refers to interdigestive or fasting secretion and is usually collected as four sequential 15-min aspirates. Secretion is also measured overnight (for 12 h), but it is uncomfortable for the patient and has little diagnostic advantage over a 1-h morning collection. Basal secretion is conventionally referred to as 'basal acid output' (BAO) and is expressed in milliequivalents per hour (mequiv h^{-1}). Average basal acid secretion is greater in males than in females and the normal BAO value is *ca.* 2 mequiv h^{-1}, the range being from 0 to 5 mequiv h^{-1} [33].

Secretory stimuli are given in various ways and usually in doses producing maximal (highest observed) acid secretory rates. For maximal acid secretion, the following subcutaneous doses are used in patients: histamine diphosphate 40 μg kg^{-1}, betazole 1500 μg kg^{-1}, and pentagastrin 6 μg kg^{-1}. Confusion has arisen over the terminology used to express the stimulated gastric acid secretion. The highest observed acid secretion is best tested by measurement of 'peak acid output' (PAO) during the hour after administration of the secretory stimulus using the two consecutive highest periods of acid output. If 10 min collections are used, this peak 20 min output is multiplied by three. If 15 min collections are used, the peak 30 min output is multiplied by two to express the results for convenience as mequiv h^{-1}. PAO is distinguished from 'maximum acid output' (MAO) which, according to Baron[33], refers to the total acid output during the first hour after injection of the secretory stimulus. Makhlouf *et al.*[34], on the other hand, use the term 'calculated maximum response' (CMAO), which is calculated from dose-response data using graded doses of any gastric secretagogue. It refers to the maximal response of the stomach attainable at an infinite dose of single stimulus. In normal human subjects, PAO and MAO depend on the age, sex and population studied. The average normal value[35] is *ca.* 20 mequiv h^{-1} for adults, and the range is 5–40 mequiv h^{-1}. In patients with duodenal ulcers, the dose of gastric stimulus, e.g. pentagastrin, required for a half-maximal response (D_{50}) is significantly lower and CMAO is significantly greater than in normal human subjects, suggesting either an increased sensitivity of parietal cells to secretagogues or an increased parietal cell mass.

The insulin test[36], used to determine the completeness of vagotomy, includes intravenous administration of 0.2 unit kg^{-1} soluble insulin. Gastric secretion is collected for 2–3 h and venous blood is obtained for blood glucose concentrations. Criteria suggestive of an incomplete vagotomy[37] include:

(a) an increase in the volume of gastric secretion after insulin,

(b) BAO greater than 2 mequiv h^{-1};

(c) an increase in acid concentration of 20 mequiv l^{-1} over the highest preinsulin level or an increase greater than 10 mequiv l^{-1} if basal gastric juice is achlorhydric; and

(d) an increase in acid output exceeding 2 mequiv h^{-1} in any postinsulin hour.

The principal controversy over the insulin test concerns the quantity of secreted acid which indicates incomplete vagotomy. To avoid further confusion, Grossman[38] has recently suggested reporting the results of the insulin test in absolute units of secretion rather than as a positive or negative test. This way might allow better prognostic interpretation of the test.

7.4 COMPOSITION OF GASTRIC JUICE

Gastric juice represents a mixture of secretions from oxyntic, peptic and mucous cells. The composition of this juice may also be contaminated with saliva, duodenal secretion or food. In addition, some gastric ions diffuse back from the lumen into plasma.

Gastric juice is a complex solution of two primary components:

(a) an acidic component containing hydrochloric acid and water produced by parietal cells; and

(b) an alkaline component containing pepsinogen, produced by peptic cells and electrolytes such as chloride, sodium and potassium, which originate in several types of cells.

The variation in the composition of gastric secretion has not been explained satisfactorily, although several hypotheses have been advanced. Since Pavlov[21], the most popular concept has been the two-component hypothesis developed by Hollander[39] and, more recently, by Makhlouf et al.[40]. Parietal cells are postulated to secrete hydrogen ions at a constant concentration of ca. 170 mequiv l^{-1}, the variation in acid concentration in the juice depending on the rate of non-parietal cell secretion of the alkaline component. Both components mix in the lumen; when the secretory rate of the acidic component increases, the proportion of alkaline material decreases. Non-parietal secretion is probably of extracellular origin and contains much sodium; sodium concentration declines in gastric juice as that of hydrogen ion rises. It was found, however, that the concentration of acid in gastric juice usually decreases linearly as the concentration of sodium increases over only a limited range. When the results are examined over the range of 0–170 mM, the relation is curvilinear.

According to Roseman[41], the chloride concentration in gastric secretion does not change with the acidity of the juice. Oxyntic gland cells separate a solution of sodium chloride of constant concentration from plasma and convert a variable proportion to hydrochloric acid. However, the range of acid concentration in Roseman's experiments collected from a gastric fistula was only 90–149 mM. Cooke and Grossman[42], using Heidenhain pouch secretion, found that chloride concentration may increase somewhat at acid concentrations above 150 mM.

The Teorell hypothesis[43,44] explains the curvilinear relation between the concentration of chloride and acid by assuming that the primary acidic secretion is isotonic with plasma and consists of hydrochloric acid and a fairly constant concentration of potassium chloride. During the course of secretion, some of the hydrogen ions are exchanged across the mucosa for sodium ions. At low secretory rates, the back diffusion of hydrogen ions from the lumen to plasma exceeds the movement of chloride in the opposite direction. With increasing acidity, the acid and chloride concentrations rise together, to *ca.* 160 and 170 mM, respectively. The Teorell hypothesis predicts a sudden rise in chloride concentration when the acid concentration is in the range of 110–150 mM. The extent to which the primary acidic component is modified depends on the time the acid remains in contact with the mucosa and on the ionic permeability of the mucosa.

Neither of these hypotheses appear to be completely correct. As mentioned above, the two-component hypothesis predicts linearity, whereas the back-diffusion theory predicts a curvilinear relation between the hydrogen ion concentration and the sodium concentration in gastric juice. The available data fit both linear and curvilinear models equally well. The problem cannot be settled by present methods. Probably a mixture of concepts would better explain the available data on the composition of gastric juice[45].

7.5 SECRETION OF INORGANIC SUBSTANCES

7.5.1 Gastric hydrochloric acid

Hydrochloric acid is secreted into the gastric lumen by the parietal cells. The striking characteristic of these cells is their elaborate system of membranes, classified as vesicles, tubules and cisterns. The intracellular canaliculi lined with microvilli communicate with the apical surface of the plasma membrane and are implicated in acid secretory activity[46]. Evidence exists that acid appears in the canaliculi in a concentration reaching about 160 mN[47].

The mechanism of hydrogen ion secretion against an enormous concentration gradient requires energy which is generated in oxyntic cells mainly by aerobic metabolism and to a lesser degree by glycolysis. According to the 'ATPase' theory[48], the energy available from the ATP hydrolysis is transferred to a protein carrier which moves protons against an electrochemical gradient. The gastric mucosa contains two kinds of ATPases: one activated by anions (chloride or bicarbonate) and the other activated by potassium and inhibited by ouabain. Since the mucosa also secretes anions, the anion-activated ATPase is probably an integral part of the secretory mechanism.

The 'redox' theory of acid secretion postulates the existence of an extra-mitochondrial oxidation–reduction reaction[49]. With the oxidation of substrate by dehydrogenase on one side of the membrane, protons are released to the other side without participation of ATP.

Data concerning the biochemical pathways involved in acid secretion are fragmentary and derive from studies of *in vitro* mucosa. Certainly they are too unreliable to confirm either an ATP-dependent or a redox-dependent process.

Intracellular control of acid secretion is poorly understood, but evidence suggests the involvement of cyclic 3'5'-AMP (cAMP) in gastric acid secretion[50]. Exogenous cAMP stimulates acid secretion by isolated frog gastric mucosa and secretion stops after cAMP is exhausted. Caffeine and theophylline inhibit the activity of phosphodiesterase, an enzyme which catabolises cAMP, raises the tissue content of cAMP, and stimulates acid secretion.

However, canine experiments also suggest that the gastric adenyl cyclase–cAMP system is not involved in the control mechanism of acid secretion[51].

Parietal cells consume oxygen in proportion to acid output. The ratio of hydrogen ions produced to oxygen molecules consumed by the gastric mucosa is less than two. During hydrogen ion secretion into the gastric lumen, equal numbers of bicarbonate ions are released into the blood. Parietal cells contain a high concentration of the enzyme carbonic anhydrase, which catalyses the hydration of carbon dioxide derived from metabolism or from the blood. The carbonic acid provides hydrogen ions to neutralise the hydroxyl ions left behind in the acid-secreting oxyntic cells. This reaction produces bicarbonate ions which are discharged into the venous blood. The amount of bicarbonate released into the blood during secretion is directly proportional to the amount of acid secreted. The excess bicarbonate in the blood during acid secretion is known as the alkaline tide and can be used to indirectly estimate gastric acid secretion during a meal[52].

Hydrogen ion concentration in gastric juice is a function of the rate of secretion. As secretion accelerates, hydrogen ion concentration rises and sodium concentration falls. Potassium and chloride concentrations remain within a fairly narrow range. The maximal concentration of hydrogen ions found in man is *ca.* 150 mN; in the dog, it is *ca.* 160 mN. The relationship between the concentration of hydrogen ions and the rate of secretion is not invariable, however. Gastric juice high in acid can sometimes be obtained at low secretory rates, e.g. during prolonged histamine stimulation. Theoretically, the maximal acidity which could be achieved by the stomach corresponds to pure parietal secretion and is almost isotonic with a solution of pure hydrochloric acid mixed with small amounts of potassium (166 mN Cl^-, 149 mN H^+, and 17 mN K^+). The variation in the composition of gastric juice depends upon the parietal and non-parietal secretions. The latter secretion has a composition similar to that of extracellular fluid (137 mN Na^+, 6 mN K^+, 117 mN Cl^-, and 25 mN HCO_3^-).

7.5.2   Sodium, potassium and chloride

Sodium ion concentration in gastric juice varies inversely with the rate of secretion and with the hydrogen ion concentration. Under basal conditions, the sodium concentration reaches its highest level, while during maximal stimulation it falls to its lowest value (*ca.* 10 mequiv l^{-1}). During a stable secretory period induced by histamine or gastrin, sodium content in gastric juice remains constant.

Sodium in gastric juice is derived from non-parietal components of both fundic and pyloric glands and from transmucosal diffusion[45]. The main source of sodium is non-parietal secretion, the composition of which is identical with that of interstitial fluid. Interestingly, the sodium content rises transiently just after the stimulation of gastric secretion with histamine or gastrin, or after added cholinergic stimulation. This can be explained by a transient increase in capillary filtration under these conditions. The subsequent fall of sodium content to a steady state may indicate local circulatory adjustment. The diffusion of sodium across the mucosa contributes only slightly to the sodium concentration in gastric juice. However, after damage of the gastric mucosa with topical aspirin, sodium diffuses into the juice in larger amounts[11].

Potassium concentration in gastric juice is higher than that in plasma, varying in man from 8 to 20 mN. It rises after stimulation with various agents, but thereafter parallels hydrogen ion secretion. In a steady secretory rate, the potassium concentration is related to secretory rate and acid output, whereas in an unstable secretory state, the concentration of potassium bears no relationship to these variables of gastric secretion. Potassium in gastric juice comes partly from the intracellular potassium of parietal cells and partly from other gastric mucosal cells[53].

The chloride concentration in gastric juice (170 mN) is higher than that in plasma (108 mN). The mucosal surface of the oxyntic gland area is electrically negative to the serosal surface. The potential difference (p.d.) is *ca.* 60 mV in unstimulated mucosa and is significantly lower after secretory stimulation[54]. Chloride is secreted against an electrochemical gradient by an active process. This chloride pump probably resides in oxyntic cells, where it is located in the parietal cell, and is loosely coupled with the proton pump by an unknown mechanism[55]. The potential difference (p.d.) across the mucosa of the pyloric gland area is small (10 mV) compared with that of the oxyntic gland area[56]. The p.d. across the duodenal mucosa is opposite in direction, i.e., with a positive mucosal surface and a negative serosal surface. When the probe passes the pyloric sphincter, the potential reverses abruptly; this phenomenon may be used to locate a pyloric sphincter[57].

7.5.3 Water flow through gastric mucosa

Secretion of gastric juice requires a large movement of water through the mucosa[58]. The main force pulling water from the cell toward the gastric lumen is an osmotic gradient created by actively transported hydrogen and chloride ions; these are the major components creating the osmotic pressure of gastric juice. The osmotic pressure of unstimulated secretion in man may vary considerably (170–276 mosmal), depending upon the acidity and rate of gastric secretion. When the acidity and rate of secretion are low, the osmotic pressure falls; as the acidity and rate of secretion rise, the osmotic pressure also increases. Although the osmolarity of gastric juice is in equilibrium with the osmolarity of the blood plasma flowing through the capillaries that envelop the gastric glands, the osmotic pressure of gastric juice is not always isotonic with plasma. Osmolarity of gastric secretion also depends upon the water permeability of the membranes lining the surfaces of gastric mucosal cells. The channels of water movement have not been determined, although a transcellular route through pores of the cell membrane[59] and passage through tight junctions between the cells have been proposed[60].

Water moves across the gastric mucosa in both directions. The flux rate from the gastric lumen to blood can be estimated from the disappearance of water labelled with deuterium oxide placed in the stomach. The rate of water absorption from the stomach is affected only slightly by the tonicity of the gastric content, probably due to a diffusion barrier preventing large net movement of water when hyper- or hypo-tonic solutions are applied to the gastric mucosa[61]. In the unstimulated stomach, large fluxes of water occur in each direction, but no net water movement takes place. During the stimulation of gastric secretion, despite large movements of water from the mucosa in the lumen, flux of water from the lumen to the blood remains high[62].

7.6 SECRETION OF ORGANIC SUBSTANCES

7.6.1 Pepsinogens and pepsins

Gastric secretion is a mixture of water, electrolytes and macromolecules which include enzymes, mucosubstances, blood-group substances and other biologically-active materials (e.g., vitamin B_{12} binders, gastrone and gastric intrinsic factor).

Among the gastric enzymes, the most important in the digestive process are the proteases[63]. The gastric mucosa secretes inactive zymogens called pepsinogens. They are synthesised and stored as granules in the peptic cells, in non-granular form in mucous neck cells of oxyntic glands, in some cells of pyloric glands and in Brunner's glands. The granules containing pepsinogens accumulate in the unstimulated cells and induce a negative feed-back mechanism to slow new synthesis. In the unstimulated state, only small amounts of pepsinogens are secreted into the gastric lumen and this is compensated by new synthesis. After secretory stimulation, the granules are discharged into the glandular lumen, producing an initial rise in pepsin concentration in gastric juice. As secretory stimulation continues, peptic cells become depleted of granules. The depletion of all zymogen granules in peptic cells depends upon the strength and duration of the stimulus and requires an average of 6–18 h. During prolonged stimulation, pepsinogen secretion is sustained, despite lack of further formation of enzymic zymogen granules. The granules begin to reappear from 6 h after cessation of stimulation.

In the presence of acid, pepsinogens with a mol. wt. of 42 500 are converted to pepsins with a mol. wt. of *ca.* 35 000. The conversion process to pepsin begins below pH 5 and then proceeds autocatalytically, cleaving several basic peptides from the zymogen molecules. The pH for optimal activity of pepsins varies from 1.8 to 3.5, depending upon the pepsin species and the substrate. Pepsins are irreversibly inactivated at neutral or alkaline pH.

Pepsinogens and pepsins are a heterogenous group of enzymatic proteins which can be subdivided by chemical and immunological methods. Using agar-gel electrophoresis for the separation, Samloff[64,65] found eight proteolytic fractions in gastric juice, seven of which were inactivated by alkali and considered as pepsinogens (pepsinogens 1–7). One fraction was alkali-stable and was termed the 'slow-moving protease'.

All pepsinogens can be subdivided into two immunologically-unrelated groups: group I (pepsinogens 1–5) and group II (pepsinogens 6 and 7). Group I pepsinogens are found only in the oxyntic gland area where they are formed in peptic cells and mucous neck cells. Group II pepsinogens come from the oxyntic gland area as well as from the pyloric gland area and Brunner glands. The slow-moving protease was found also in jejunal mucosa and probably represents tissue cathepsins. Groups I and II pepsino-gens, immunologically distinct, can be localised in cells by an immunofluores-cence method[66]. One group can also be distinguished from another by using appropriate substrates; e.g., group II pepsins do not split synthetic substrate N-acetyl-L-phenylalanyl-L-di-iodotyrosine, which is hydrolysed by group I pepsins[64].

Basal secretion of pepsin is continuous but relatively small. The strongest stimuli for pepsin secretion include: feeding and cholinergic stimulation induced by insulin hypoglycaemia, sham feeding, the administration of stable choline esters or local cholinergic stimulation evoked by gastric distention[67]. In man, histamine stimulation causes an initial peak pepsin output, representing a 'wash-out' phenomenon. With prolonged histamine infusion, pepsin secretion continues to rise, indicating that histamine is a definite stimulus of pepsin secretion[68]. Gastrin and related peptides, such as pentagastrin and tetragastrin, also stimulate pepsin secretion in man[69]. Maximal pepsin output to histamine, gastrin and related peptides can be achieved at the dose level which is submaximal for acid secretion. A supra-maximal dose of histamine inhibits, while that of gastrin does not affect pepsin secretion in man. Intestinal hormones, such as secretin, cholecystokinin and its analogue, caerulein, inhibit gastrin-stimulated acid secretion in man and dog and stimulate pepsin secretion when acting alone[70,71]. More especially, secretin, given exogenously or released endogenously by duodenal acidifica-tion, strongly stimulates pepsin secretion. Cholecystokinin can inhibit pepsin secretion when acting with gastrin. Other hormonal peptides either inhibit pepsin secretion (e.g. gastric inhibitory peptide) or leave pepsin secretion unchanged (glucagon and calcitonin)[72]. Prostaglandins (PGA_1, PGE_1, and PGE_2) inhibit pepsin response to food and to histamine[73].

Cholinergic blockage by atropine results in strong inhibition of pepsin secretion elicited by all modes of stimulation. Vagotomy decreases basal pepsin secretion and abolishes that evoked by vagal stimulation but not by food in man and in dog[75]. Pepsin dose response curves to gastrin, pentagastrin and histamine are all shifted to the right and therefore larger doses of these stimuli are needed to achieve the prevagotomy level of pepsin secretion[75].

Damage of the gastric mucosa by topical application of highly-concen-trated hydrochloric acid, acetic acid or ethanol elicits an increase in pepsin output, indicating that back-diffusion of hydrogen ion stimulates pepsin secretion[76]. Since atropine given parenterally prevents this increase of pepsin secretion, it has been suggested that a local cholinergic reflex is involved in this stimulation. Acid at physiological concentrations also stimulates pepsin secretion. This may be the most important regulatory mechanism of pepsin secretion[76].

7.6.2 Gastric mucus secretion

The gastric mucosa, like other epithelial tissues of the gastrointestinal tract, is coated by a continuous film of mucin called gastric mucus. This film is a three-dimensional gel, synthesised and secreted by columnar epithelial cells and mucous neck cells in the oxyntic gland area and by the cells of the pyloric gland area. The major stimulants of mucus secretion are local mucosal irritation and cholinergic stimulation[77]. Feeding, gastrin and histamine do not affect mucus secretion[78].

Gastric mucus consists of various macromolecules such as glycoproteins, proteins and mucopolysaccharides which are built in a stable structure maintained by electrostatic forces supplied by the charged sulphate and carboxyl end-groups and hydrogen bonding[79]. This spatial organisation is unaffected by pepsin but it is highly mobile and sensitive to increasing ionic strength and decreasing pH. These environmental changes can destroy the mucus structure because they reduce the hydrogen bonds, suppress the electrostatic forces and free the individual macromolecules. Once detached from the main gel, the macromolecules are shifted from the gel form dissolved in gastric juice to the deposit precipitated by acid as 'visible' mucus.

The principal constituents of gastric mucus are glycoproteins sharing a common structure, namely a protein core surrounded by multiple carbohydrate side chains. The carbohydrate compounds constitute *ca.* 85% of glycoprotein content and include sialic acid, hexose (galactose and mannose) and acetylhexosamine (acetyloglucosamine and acetylogalactosamine) fucose. The relative concentrations of these carbohydrates and their spatial arrangements are responsible for the physical characteristics of glycoproteins[79].

Glycoproteins may be acidic or neutral according to the presence or absence of acidic sialic acid or sulphated residues. The major glycoprotein of the mucus gel can be separated from other smaller compounds by ultrafiltration followed by chromatography in urea solutions. It contains galactose, fucose and *N*-acetyloglucosamine, and *N*-acetylogalactosamine and *N*-acetyloneuraminic acid, which all form a prosthetic carbohydrate with a protein compound composed mainly of such amino acids as serine, threonine, proline and alanine[79].

Although neutral glycoproteins form the bulk of the mucosubstances, sulphated glycoproteins have also been isolated from the gastric juice of man and dog. Histoautoradiographic studies performed after injection of radiosulphate showed that the isotope was quickly incorporated into gastric mucus and detected in the gastric mucosa of species secreting sulphated glycoproteins. In man, however, the sulphated glycoproteins have been shown to be a contaminant of gastric juice originating in upper digestive secretion, mainly in saliva[80].

Mucopolysaccharides extracted from gastric juice are a mixture of chondroitin sulphates composed mainly of hexosamine, uronic acid and sulphate. They are present in large amounts in dogs but in only negligible amounts in man.

Mucoproteins containing polysaccharides as prosthetic groups linked to small protein moieties are responsible for the viscosity of gastric mucus. They form important organic compounds, such as blood-group substances, intrinsic factor and gastrone[81]. About 78% of normal individuals secrete blood-group substances A, B and H into gastric juice; they are called 'secretors'. The individuals of blood group O do not secrete substances A and B, but some of them secrete substance H which appears to be present to a lesser degree in people belonging to other blood groups. ABH non-secretors are more susceptible to gastric and duodenal ulcers than secretors.

Group A subjects have a higher predilection for tumours arising in areas of production of blood-group substances, e.g. in the stomach[82].

Gastrone[82] is an endogenous depressant of gastric secretion, consisting of at least two materials. One is a mucus-like substance with a mol. wt. of *ca.* 100 000; it is less active and is resistant to peptic digestion. The other is a glycoprotein, with a mol. wt. between 10 000 and 40 000; it is a potent inhibitor easily degraded by pepsin. The first compound is responsible for the inhibitory activity of acid gastric juice and the second for that of anacid gastric juice. The physiological role of gastrone has not been established.

Some polysaccharides present in mucus, particularly sulphated muco-substances, inhibit pepsin activity due to their interaction with protein substrate, which is not hydrolysable by pepsin. Their physiological role is doubtful because they are present in human gastric juice in small concentration and are ineffective in the pH range of normal gastric juice.

Gastric juice contains small amounts of serum proteins. The passage into gastric juice of excessive amounts of serum protein, mainly albumin, has been observed in Menetrier's disease, in acute gastritis, in gastric cancer, and after damage of the gastric mucosal barrier.

7.6.3   Intrinsic factor secretion

Intrinsic factor (IF), a mucoprotein with a mol. wt. of *ca.* 55 000, is secreted by the gastric mucosa. It is necessary for the absorption of vitamin B_{12} from the ileum. IF binds vitamin B_{12} in a non-dialysable complex and passes it on to specific receptors of the ileal mucosa promoting its absorption. Besides IF, which is a specific or primary binder of B_{12}, gastric juice possesses non-specific or secondary B_{12} binders, which can be separated by using auto-antibodies to IF obtained from the serum of pernicious anaemia patients. These antibodies block only the specific B_{12} binder (IF), without affecting non-specific binders. IF can be measured *in vitro* by radio immunoassay and *in vivo* by following the absorption of radio isotopically-labelled vitamin B_{12}[82,83].

The cellular origin of IF in gastric mucosa can be traced by autoradio-graphy using radioactive-labelled B_{12}. The origin of IF differs by species; in man it is produced by parietal cells[83]. IF is stored in the gastric mucosa and released spontaneously in small amounts into the juice. After stimulation of gastric secretion, IF secretion abruptly rises, followed by a prolonged plateau of secretion slightly above the basal level. Gastric stimulation with agents such as histamine, gastrin, gastrin-related peptides, insulin or cholinergic stimulants elicits an elevation in IF output, markedly exceeding the amounts of IF required for normal absorption of vitamin B_{12}. The capacity of the gastric mucosa to secrete IF usually correlates closely with its ability to secrete acid[84]. In patients with pernicious anaemia, the B_{12}-binding capacity of gastric juice is markedly reduced due to the deficiency of IF. Patients with atrophic gastritis and achlorhydria, with or without pernicious anaemia, have increased circulating antibodies to parietal cells in their serum. About half of the patients with pernicious anaemia also have intrinsic factor antibodies which circulate in the blood and may inhibit the production of IF.

7.7 CONTROL OF GASTRIC SECRETION

Gastric secretion depends upon several interrelated mechanisms: the autonomic nervous system, hormones, the parietal cell mass and the mucosal circulation. The major physiological stimulant of gastric secretion is the ingestion of a meal which elicits neurohormonal stimulation of acid and pepsin secretion.

7.7.1 Stimulants of gastric secretion

Substances in the body which stimulate gastric acid secretion are acetylcholine, gastrin, cholecystokinin and histamine. Acetylcholine is released in the gastric wall by the stimulation of pre- and post-ganglionic vagal fibres; it transmits the excitation from postganglionic nerve endings to oxyntic or pyloric glands. Cholinergic impulses reach gastric glandular cells via the vagus nerves or intramural reflexes; released acetylcholine directly stimulates oxyntic glands to produce acid and pepsin or causes gastrin cells in the pyloric glands to elaborate gastrin.

Gastrin is a peptide hormone released mainly by cholinergic reflexes from the specialised endocrine cells of the pyloric gland area (G-cells). Long vagovagal reflexes initiated by sham feeding or insulin hypoglycaemia cause a large release of gastrin. Also, short intramural reflexes, occurring in response to local chemical or mechanical stimuli and acting in the antrum, may cause the release of gastrin in amounts sufficient to provoke a maximal rate of acid secretion. A detailed description of the chemical characteristics and assay of gastrin appears in the first chapter of this volume.

The spectrum of physiological effects of gastrin covers all major gastrointestinal activities, including secretion, motility and absorption. In the stomach, gastrin is a strong stimulant of acid secretion and a moderate stimulant of pepsin and intrinsic factor secretion. Gastrin and acetylcholine are strongly interdependent as stimulants of gastric secretion. They potentiate one another in stimulating parietal glands.

Histamine is a potent gastric secretagogue producing peak rates of acid secretion comparable to those evoked by gastrin or pentagastrin in man and in laboratory animals. Although the concept that histamine is the final common local stimulator of parietal cells has received much attention in the past, results from more recent experiments seem to indicate that acid secretion is not causally related to histamine release or metabolism. The evidence that endogenous histamine plays no important role in gastric secretion has been summarised in the opening chapter of this volume. Recent studies on methyl derivatives of histamine[145], possible products of histamine methylation in gastric mucosa, which are more potent gastric secretagogues than histamine, and the discovery of histamine H_2-receptor antagonists[146] tip the balance of the opinion towards the idea of histamine mediation in gastric secretion.

Other stimulants of gastric secretion include calcium, alcohol and caffeine. Acute elevation of serum calcium induced by intravenous calcium infusion elicits an increase in gastric-acid secretion and the serum gastrin level in man[85] and in some laboratory animals (monkeys, cats, and ferrets). The stimulatory effect of calcium on gastric-acid secretion is probably due to the increase of gastrin release and to the potentiation of the action of available gastrin on oxyntic cells. Interestingly, calcium infusion evokes a greater increase in serum gastrin in patients with gastrin-producing tumours (Zollinger–Ellison syndrome) than in normal subjects and may be useful as a test in differentiating patients with this disorder from hypersecretors without the excess gastrin production.

Ethanol is a stimulant of gastric secretion, both after oral intake and intravenous administration. It probably acts by releasing gastrin[86]. When applied topically in high concentrations, ethanol damages the gastric mucosa[11].

Caffeine stimulates gastric acid secretion when given alone and potentiates the gastric response to other stimuli, such as gastrin or histamine. Its stimulatory effect is also probably due to gastrin release[87].

7.7.2 Relation between maximal response and parietal cell mass

Card and Marks[88] established a correlation between the highest observed acid response to histamine and the number of parietal cells in the gastric mucosa of man and dog. The relationship was nearly linear, and the slope was such that a maximal rate of acid secretion of 20 mequiv h^{-1} with histamine stimulation corresponded to a total parietal cell population of one billion cells. The estimate of parietal cell number or mass based on the highest secretory response is correct only for normal conditions. Under certain instances, such as after vagotomy[89] or antrectomy[90], the highest acid response declines markedly; in dog[91] but not in man[92], it can be at least partly restored to the preoperative level by the administration of a stable choline ester or gastrin (Figure 7.3).

7.7.3 Blood flow and gastric secretion

Gastric mucosal blood flow estimated by the aminopyrine clearance technique[93,94] revealed that increased blood flow *per se* cannot initiate or augment gastric secretion. On the other hand, blood flow plays an important permissive role in the sense that adequate flow is required for acid secretion. Various stimuli of gastric secretion, such as gastrin, histamine and vagal stimulation, augment mucosal blood flow by two major mechanisms:
    (a) the direct action of secretory stimuli on vascular smooth muscle, and
    (b) the release of local vasodilator substances by increased metabolism.

The inhibition of gastric secretion induced by vasodilators, such as isoproterenol[93], secretin[93], glucagon[95], or prostaglandins[96], lowers mucosal blood flow. In these cases, however, the ratio of mucosal blood flow to secretory rate does not decline. This suggests that the primary action of the secretory inhibitor is not via reduced blood flow. When secretion is inhibited by a vasoconstrictor, such as vasopressin[93] or norepinephrine[96], the ratio of mucosal blood flow to secretion does decline, suggesting that the mechanism of inhibition does operate via reduced blood flow.

7.7.4 Stimulation of gastric secretion. Phases of gastric secretion

Gastric secretion is customarily divided into basal (spontaneous, un-stimulated, interprandial) and postprandial (stimulated, digestive) periods. The postprandial period corresponds to the fed state and can be further subdivided into cephalic, gastric and intestinal phases, according to the organ from which the neurohumoral stimulus originates. The division into phases is artificial, because in the natural course of secretion all phases begin

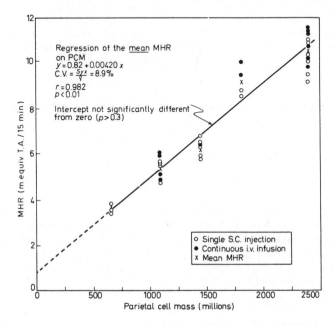

Figure 7.3 Relationship between highest histamine response and parietal cell mass. (From Marks et al.[142], by courtesy of *Amer. J. Physiol.*)

almost simultaneously and overlap in time. In addition, the mechanisms by which natural secretory stimuli evoke secretion during cephalic and gastric phases is basically similar, namely, direct cholinergic action on the parietal cells and cholinergic release of gastrin from the pyloric glands. For these reasons, it is meaningless to attribute to each of these phases a certain fraction in the total secretory response during feeding.

7.7.4.1 Basal secretion

Basal secretion of acid in humans is usually tested after an overnight fast. It varies considerably from person to person and in one person from time to time. A circadian rhythm[97] of acid secretion exhibits the lowest output in the morning between 5 and 11 a.m. and the highest output at night between 2 p.m. and 1 a.m. The factors responsible for basal secretion probably depend upon constant gastrin release, tonic vagal stimulation, and the release of intestinal inhibitors. The abolition of basal secretion requires removal of both sources of stimulation, namely, the vagus nerves and the antrum. Vagotomy reduces basal acid secretion but does increase fasting serum gastrin in man[98]. Antrectomy lowers the fasting gastrin level in the serum and acid output in the gastric juice[98].

7.7.4.2 Cephalic phase

The cephalic phase refers to the stimulation of gastric secretion by factors acting in the region of the head. The stimuli for the cephalic phase include the thought, expectation, sight, taste, smell, chewing and swallowing of palatable food. Factors evoking conditioned reflexes established by pairing of unconditioned and indifferent stimuli, such as light or sound, can also be effective. The cephalic phase is mediated entirely by the vagus. The importance of vagal nerves was recognised by the classical demonstration in Pavlov's laboratory[30] that intact vagi were required for the cephalic phase induced by sham feeding. Besides sham feeding, the cephalic stimulation of gastric secretion can be elicited by insulin hypoglycaemia or 2-deoxy-D-glucose (2-DG) glucocytopenia[99].

The precise area in the central nervous system which controls vagal impulses remains unidentified[100]. The stimuli are transmitted from the cortex and subcortical area (mainly from the limbic system) to the anterior hypothalamus and next to the medullary vagal centres. These impulses then proceed via vagal nerves either directly to oxyntic glands where they stimulate acid and pepsin secretion or to pyloric glands where they release gastrin. The gastric secretory response to sham feeding appears after a latent period of 5–7 min and continues as a copious acidic secretion for as long as 3 h after the food has been eaten and forgotten.

Cephalic stimulation elicited by insulin hypoglycaemia or sham feeding results in secretion of acid from a vagally-innervated pouch. It also raises the level of immunoreactive circulating gastrin (Figure 7.4)[101]. Denervation of the antral region or injection of atropine completely abolishes the plasma gastrin response to cephalic stimulation, indicating the importance of vagal gastrin release[102]. The secretory response of the vagally innervated stomach to insulin hypoglycaemia is not abolished by antrectomy. Therefore, the response is not due to an elevation of circulating gastrin but depends upon direct vagal stimulation of oxyntic glands. In the dog[91] but not in man[92], the response of a vagally-innervated stomach to sham feeding is greatly reduced by antrectomy and can be restored to preantrectomy level by infusion of exogenous gastrin in a subthreshold dosage. This indicates that vagal influences in the cephalic phase can be subdivided into the stimulation by vagally-released gastrin, vagal activation of the oxyntic glands and gastrin sensitisation of the oxyntic glands to the action of vagal cholinergic impulses (Figure 7.5)[91].

The response to sham feeding was also demonstrated in man with an oesophageal fistula and a gastric fistula, or with intubation of the oesophagus by a gastrostomy tube used to drain the stomach postoperatively after surgery for duodenal ulcer[92]. When the patient ate, the food passed from the oesophagus to the exterior through the oesophageal fistula or gastrostomy tube. The peak sham feeding response was *ca.* 50% of the maximal response to exogenous gastrin. Antrectomy in man was shown to markedly diminish

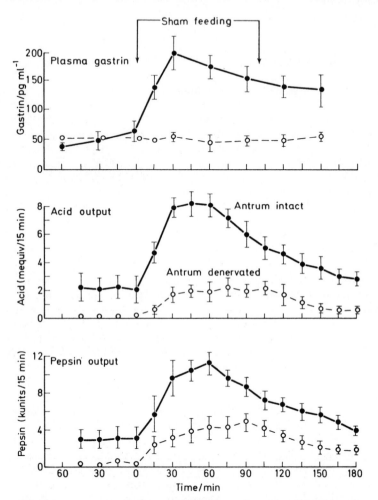

Figure 7.4 Plasma gastrin, and acid and pepsin output from the main stomach during sham feeding for 100 min. (From Tepperman *et al.*[143], by courtesy of *Gastroenterol.* and Williams and Wilkins Co.)

the response of sham feeding, but unlike the response in the dog, subthreshold doses of exogenous gastrin did not potentiate this response[92].

Vagal release of gastrin was demonstrated by Uvnäs[103] who showed that antrectomy in cats abolished or markedly reduced the acid response to electrical stimulation of vagal nerves. These findings were doubted for years until Dragstedt *et al.*[104] recognised that acid bathing the antral mucosa inhibited release of gastrin. Vagally-mediated gastrin release can be prevented almost completely by irrigation of the antral mucosa with acid, although the secretory response of a Pavlov pouch to cephalic stimulation in dogs with an

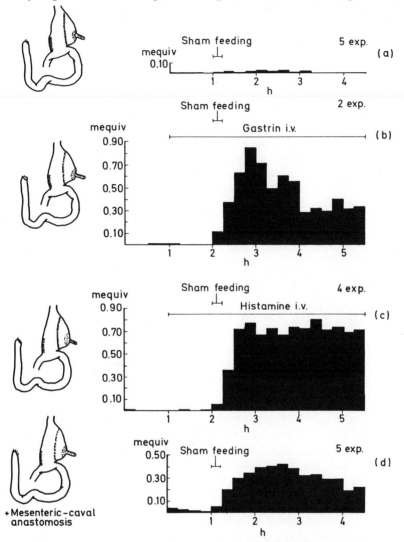

Figure 7.5 Mean acid responses to sham feeding in a canine Pavlov pouch after resection of gastrin-producing regions: (a) sham feeding alone; (b) sham feeding and concomitant injection of gastrin in *ca.* $\frac{1}{5}$ of the threshold dose; (c) sham feeding and concomitant injection of histamine just below the threshold dose; (d) sham feeding after anastomosis of the superior mesenteric vein to the inferior vena cava. (From Olbe[91], by courtesy of Munksgaard.)

acidified antrum is only partially reduced. The incomplete effect in the innervated pouch is due to direct vagal stimulation of oxyntic glands which is unaltered by antral acidification[105].

7.7.4.3 Gastric phase

Pavlov was aware that the cephalic phase of vagal reflex excitation could not account for the entire gastric secretory response to food. With Edkin's[106] discovery of gastrin, the gastric phase as the hormonal component of the gastric response to food was established. In the last decade, rapid progress in gastrointestinal endocrinology has led to the isolation, chemical characterisation and synthesis of gastrin, and has established an interdependence between the vagus and the antrum in their stimulation of acid and pepsin secretion from the fundus.

The gastric phase of gastric secretion can be defined as that fraction of the secretory response occurring when a stimulus acts in the region of the stomach. It begins with copious secretory volume containing high concentrations of acid and pepsin. This phase may continue 3–4 h after the intake of food.

Four components of the gastric phase have been documented:

(a) mechanical stimulation of the innervated fundic gland area, producing long vagovagal reflexes that activate the oxyntic glands, as shown by a markedly increased acid and pepsin response in the Pavlov pouch to distention;

(b) mechanical stimulation of the denervated fundic gland area, causing local reflex activation of oxyntic glands, as evidenced by slightly increased acid response in the Heidenhain pouch to distention;

(c) mechanical stimulation of pyloric gland area, resulting in local reflex stimulation of gastrin cells to produce gastrin; and

(d) chemical stimulation of the pyloric gland area, producing local reflex gastrin release from gastrin cells[107].

In the last two situations, the stimulation of gastrin release was demonstrated by an increase of both circulating gastrin and acid secretion from the totally denervated or transplanted fundic pouch.

The mechanisms involved in gastrin release from the antral gland area in the gastric phase have been intensively studied since Edkin's work, but Grossman et al.[108] offered the first conclusive proof in 1948 that an antral hormone is liberated from the pyloric gland region of the stomach. They used distention to stimulate an antral pouch and found heightened acid secretion from the transplanted fundic pouch. Concurrent stimulation with a subthreshold dose of stable choline ester (urecholine) potentiated acid secretion due to the increased sensitivity of gastrin cells to local stimulation and greater responsiveness of oxyntic glands to gastrin[108].

The same mechanisms have been proposed[107] for both the cephalic and gastric phases of gastric secretion. In this view, the gastric phase is mediated entirely by cholinergic reflexes, which may be initiated by mechanical or chemical stimulation of receptors of the oxyntic or pyloric gland areas. Impulses then travel by way of long vagal reflexes or through the local intramural nerve plexuses to reach the neuro-effector junction in the vicinity of either pyloric or oxyntic glands. Acetylcholine is proposed as the final chemostimulator which might stimulate acid and pepsin secretion or cause gastrin release (Figure 7.6)[107].

This simplified picture of the cholinergic mediation of gastrin release has been challenged by the finding that atropine given systemically does not inhibit the release of immunoassayable gastrin in response to feeding in man and in the dog[109] (Figure 7.7). Perhaps neural release of gastrin is resistant to atropine, or an alternative mechanism may be involved in this release such as direct stimulation of gastrin cells by food.

Although atropine fails to depress gastrin release in response to feeding, gastrin release in the gastric phase is still thought to be mediated mainly by reflexes[110]. Since vagal denervation apparently interferes very little with gastrin release by agents acting locally in the pyloric region, this release appears to be mediated mainly by intramural reflexes. Neural pathways involved in gastrin release from gastrin cells can be blocked by local anaesthetics (xylocaine), which, however, do not affect stimulation with acetylcholine applied topically to the pyloric mucosa. This indicates that acetylcholine acts directly on gastrin cells to release gastrin. The ganglionic blocking agent, hexamethonium, blocks the action of local mechanical and chemical stimuli

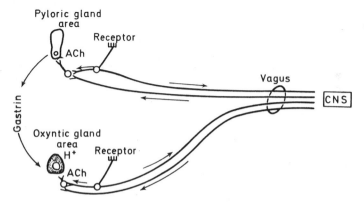

Figure 7.6 Diagram of the postulated intramural and vagal innervation involved in the release of gastrin from pyloric gland area and in the stimulation of oxyntic glands in the pyloric gland area. (From Grossman[144], by courtesy of *Physiologist*.)

but, as expected, does not alter the effect of acetylcholine[111]. Atropine, applied topically to the pyloric mucosa, blocks all known stimulants releasing gastrin, including acetylcholine[112]. However, this conclusion may be premature since it is unknown whether atropine applied topically to the pyloric mucosa can be absorbed into the circulation and block gastrin action at the level of the parietal cells. The action of topically applied atropine should, therefore, be reinvestigated, using gastrin radioimmunoassay.

All local stimuli releasing gastrin, including acetylcholine, are pH-dependent, and the irrigation of the pyloric mucosa with an acid solution at a pH below 2 causes an inhibition of gastrin release by all known mechanisms. Apparently, then, acid acts on the same site as atropine, namely, on the gastrin-producing cells. The pH threshold for inhibition of gastrin release varies, depending upon the type of release; it is about pH 3 for amino acids and *ca.* pH 1.5 for alcohols, distension and vagal stimulation[113].

The factors responsible for gastrin release after food intake remain undefined. Ingested proteins seem to be the most active gastrin releasers; proteins buffer gastric acid, cause distention and chemically stimulate.

Many early studies on gastrin release used crude extracts of liver and meat. Recently, numerous pure chemical substances have been recognised as potent stimulants of gastrin release. Most active releasers include small molecular

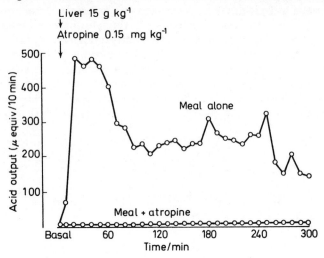

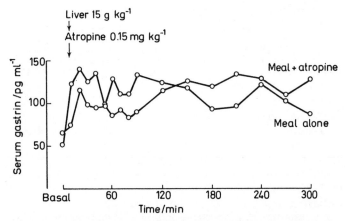

Figure 7.7 Effect of subcutaneous administration of atropine 0.15 mg kg^{-1} on the Pavlov pouch acid response to 15 g kg^{-1} beef liver meal (upper graph) and on the serum gastrin response to a meal (lower graph). (From Cesendes *et al.*[102], by courtesy of *Gastroenterol.* and Williams and Wilkins Co.)

amino acids, such as glycine, alanine and serine (in both L- and D-isomeric forms), ethanol and propanol, acetic and proprionic acids, and bile salts. The structure–function relationship[110] of gastrin releasers reveals that the most effective compounds are small molecules containing two or three carbon atoms with a terminal alcohol or carboxyl group. It is noteworthy that the gastrin-releasing potency of acetylcholine applied topically markedly exceeds that of all other chemical and mechanical stimuli. With acetylcholine irrigation, the antral mucosa can release enough gastrin to elicit acid secretion from the oxyntic glands equal to the maximal response during stimulation with exogenous gastrin. Under natural conditions, however, relatively little gastrin is released, but its action on the oxyntic glands is potentiated greatly by direct cholinergic stimulation; this results in high rates of gastric secretion during feeding[110].

7.7.4.4 Intestinal phase

Intestinal stimulation of gastric secretion begins when food enters the duodenum. This phase has not been as well documented as the cephalic or gastric phases because the intestinal mucosa also contains inhibitory substances which can suppress gastric secretion stimulated in all phases. The intestinal phase is thought to involve one or more hormones released from the intestinal mucosa by distension, acetylcholine, or digestive products.

The intestinal phase of gastric secretion was recognised long ago by Pavlov[21], but definitive proof of its existence was provided by Ivy et al.[114]. They used dogs with a vagotomised pouch of the entire stomach and an oesophagoduodenal anastomosis. Feeding the dogs caused increased gastric secretion starting 1 h later—unless the food was predigested, in which case secretion started earlier. Sircus[115], using dogs with a Heidenhain pouch and a Thiry–Vella loop of the distal duodenum and proximal jejunum, found that irrigation of the loop with intestinal chyme, obtained from another animal digesting a meat meal (or acid solution or distention of the loop) provoked acid secretion from the pouch. This observation was taken as evidence of the hormonal nature of the intestinal phase, and the term 'intestinal gastrin' was applied to this hormone. Whether the chemical structure and the mechanism of release of intestinal gastrin are the same as those of the antral hormone remains uncertain, however (Figure 7.8).

When the immunochemical method was used to detect gastrin in the extracts from intestinal mucosa[116], the upper duodenal mucosa of man was found to contain concentrations of gastrin almost as high as the antral mucosa, whereas gastrin concentrations in distal duodenum and jejunum dropped sharply. This is consistent with the recent observation that the plasma gastrin response to food passing from the stomach to the duodenum in peptic ulcer patients is essentially unaltered by antrectomy[117]. Food is also capable of releasing significant amounts of gastrin from extragastric sources in patients with total gastrectomy. Yalow and Berson[116] reported that a large proportion of circulating gastrin has the characteristics of 'big' gastrin, a molecule larger than heptadecapeptide gastrin ('little' gastrin). The ratio of big to little gastrin is higher in duodenal than in antral mocosa. The plasma concentration of big gastrin increases in response to food, suggesting that the upper gut might contribute considerably to this postprandial gastrin increase.

Whether intestinal gastrin is the only hormone responsible for the intestinal stimulation of gastric secretion remains unclear. Species differences have been found in the content of immunoreactive gastrin in the upper duodenum;

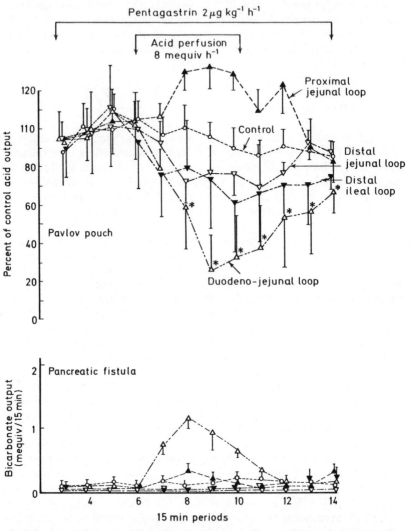

Figure 7.8 Effect of acidification at various levels of the small intestine on pentagastrin-induced gastric acid secretion from Pavlov pouch and on pancreatic bicarbonate secretion. (From Konturek et al.[130], by courtesy of *Amer. J. Physiol.*)

laboratory animals, such as hogs or dogs, have much less gastrin in the upper duodenum than man. Studies on dogs, however, indicate that in addition to intestinal gastrin, another hormone is released from the intestinal mucosa. This inference has been supported by the findings that acid secretion from the Heidenhain pouch increases when acid is instilled into the jejunum, despite the absence of a concomitant increase in the serum gastrin level[118,119]. Apparently the Heidenhain pouch response to feeding is much higher than the maximal response to exogenous gastrin, suggesting that another potent intestinal stimulatory hormone may operate in the intestinal phase of gastric secretion in dogs. Since cholecystokinin exhibits the full range of physiological activity of gastrin and is released from the intestinal mucosa by the digestive products of protein and fat, this hormone might be responsible for a part of the intestinal stimulation of gastric secretion.

Control of the intestinal phase also involves a cholinergic component. This inference is supported by evidence that a subthreshold dosage of stable choline ester (bethanechol) markedly enhances the gastric secretory response to food in the gut, whereas atropine and topical anaesthetics (in the gut) abolish the response[120].

7.7.5 Inhibition of gastric secretion

Secretory outputs of various gastric components in response to a meal depend on the interplay of many stimulatory and inhibitory factors. Several inhibitory mechanisms have been demonstrated by which acid and pepsin secretion may be depressed.

Inhibition of gastric secretion is usually classified as central, antral, and intestinal in origin. This division is artificial to the extent that various inhibitory and stimulatory processes are normally interrelated.

7.7.5.1 Gastric inhibition of central origin

Cephalic stimulation of gastric secretion elicited by feeding is based on the sensation of appetite. The inhibition of appetite by emotional or environmental influences depresses or abolishes the vagal reflex excitation in the cephalic phase. This has been demonstrated by introduction of food directly into the stomach of conscious dogs with the Pavlov pouch without the dog being aware of the food. The exclusion of the cephalic phase prolongs the whole process of digestion[121].

The same area of the hypothalamus concerned with the control of food intake has also been found to influence gastric secretion[100]. Stimulation with an electrode in the ventromedial nucleus of the hypothalamus of conscious rats, dogs or monkeys inhibits secretion during feeding. Higher levels of the visceral nervous system in primates are probably involved in the inhibition of acid secretion that accompanies stressful stimuli, probably through the release of catecholamines.

7.7.5.2 Antral gastric inhibitory mechanisms

Acidification of the antral mucosa suppresses tonic release of gastrin as well as gastrin released by various chemical and mechanical stimuli or by vagal stimulation[122]. In all these instances, gastric secretion is inhibited. Antral acidification represents a negative feed-back because gastrin is a stimulant of gastric acid secretion. When acid enters the antral region and contacts the pyloric glandular mucosa, it slows and eventually stops further gastrin release. Apparently gastrin release by vagal stimulation, distention and alcohol has a lower threshold for inhibition (pH 1.5) than other releasers, such as amino acids or acetylcholine (pH 3.0) (Figure 7.9)[123].

It is generally held that the inhibition of gastric secretion triggered by acid bathing the antral mucosa is probably due to the decreased release of gastrin. However, it has also been postulated in the past that a special inhibitory

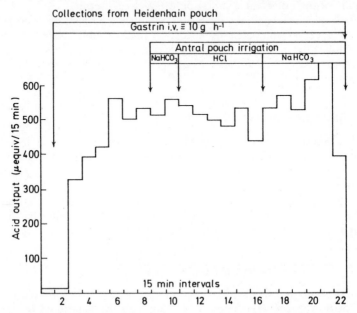

Figure 7.9 Heindenhain pouch acid response to gastrin during antral pouch irrigation with 0.1 N bicarbonate or 0.1 N HCl. The irrigation of the pyloric gland area affected the secretion of acid from the denervated fundic pouch in response to gastrin. (From Gillespie and Grossman[123], by courtesy of *Amer. J. Physiol.*)

factor is released from the antral mucosa[124]. The term 'antral chalone' has been applied to this hormone to indicate its capacity to inhibit all forms of gastric acid stimulation. No convincing evidence is available, however, that an antral chalone exists and plays any physiological role. One possible candidate for the role of antral chalone is a substance extracted from the mucus of antral and whole stomach juice, called gastrone[82]. The physiological significance of gastrone is unknown and its relationships to other inhibitory substances in saliva (sialogastrone) and urine (urogastrone) have not been established.

7.7.5.3 Duodenal gastric inhibitory mechanisms

The existence of duodenal mechanisms inhibiting gastric acid secretion has been recognised for more than 50 years. The introduction of acids, fat and hypertonic solutions into the duodenum of man and dog is known to inhibit acid secretion. Since the inhibition was demonstrated in dogs with vagally denervated and transplanted fundic pouches, inhibitory mechanisms were thought to operate through the humoral pathways. The term 'entero-gastrone'[125] has been applied to a hormone released by acid, fat and hypertonic solutions in the intestine.

In 1904, Sokolov[126] first demonstrated that duodenal acidification inhibits the gastric secretory response to a meal. Since then, a number of studies in man and in laboratory animals revealed that acid in the duodenum inhibits basal and gastrin or food-induced acid secretion. The strongest inhibitory mechanism is confined to the upper part of the duodenum, particularly the duodenal bulb, which is claimed to release a special inhibitory hormone named bulbogastrone[127]. The pH-sensitive inhibitory mechanism located in the duodenal bulb was found to be effective after transplantation of the bulb, suggesting that a hormonal factor is involved in the mediation of bulbar inhibition.

Acidification of the duodenum releases secretin which, in addition to stimulation of pancreatic bicarbonate and fluid secretion, also causes inhibition of gastric acid secretion. Studies have shown that the duodenal pH required to inhibit gastric secretion (pH 4.5) correlates well with the pH required to stimulate pancreatic secretion[128]. Secretin is recognised as one of the enterogastrones released by acid in the intestine, having a possible physiological role in the feed-back inhibition of gastric secretion. The inhibitory effect of secretin varies among different species; e.g. in man[128] this inhibition shows competitive kinetics, whereas in the dog it is non-competitive[129]. Some doubt exists, however, about the significance of secretin release for the inhibition of gastric secretion in response to food, because under normal conditions the only part of the duodenum in which the pH drops below the threshold for secretin release is the duodenal bulb. Evidence suggests that the duodenal bulb, which plays a critical role in gastric secretory inhibition, releases only small amounts of secretin, and that bulbar inhibition of the stomach cannot be attributed solely to release of secretin from the duodenal mucosa (Figure 7.10)[130,131].

Other secretin-related peptides have been isolated from intestinal mucosal extracts, such as gastric inhibitory peptide (GIP)[132], enteric glucagon and vasoactive inhibitory polypeptide (VIP) with glucagon-like and secretin-like activity[133]. GIP was found to strongly inhibit both acid and pepsin secretion induced by histamine, pentagastrin and insulin[132]. The ability of GIP to inhibit histamine-stimulated acid secretion satisfies one of the criteria for the claim that this peptide could be the enterogastrone released by fat introduced into the duodenum. The elucidation of the physiological role of GIP in the gastric-inhibitory mechanism requires the demonstration that it is released from the duodenum by a physiological mechanism and that it can be identified in the blood.

Pancreatic and enteric glucagons were shown to inhibit gastric and pancreatic secretion in response to various stimuli, such as gastrin, histamine and food[134]. Since glucagon is effective in relatively small doses, equivalent to those released endogenously by certain amino acids during digestion and absorption of protein in the lumen of the small bowel, this hormone may play a role in the inhibition of gastric secretion under physiological conditions. VIP also inhibits gastric secretion, but its importance is unknown[133].

The inhibition of gastric secretion by a fat meal or by duodenal instillation of fat has been well documented[135-137]. Since the products of lipid digestion, namely fatty acids dispersed as soap micelles or monolein bile-stabilised micelles, stimulate the release of both cholecystokinin and secretin[138] from the intestinal mucosa, possible combinations of these two hormones released by a fatty meal potentiate one another in inhibiting gastric secretion. Also,

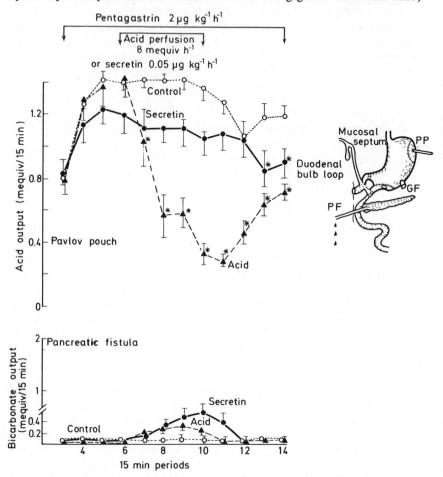

Figure 7.10 Effect of acidification of the duodenal bulb on the Pavlov pouch acid response to pentagastrin and on pancreatic bicarbonate secretion. Exogenous secretin given in a dose producing equal rates of bicarbonate secretion does not affect the Pavlov pouch response to pentagastrin. (From Konturek *et al.*[130], by courtesy of *Amer. J. Physiol.*)

other releasers of cholecystokinin, such as the products of protein digestion (mainly L-isomers of essential amino acids) might inhibit gastrin-induced gastric secretion. In man and in the dog[139], cholecystokinin is a partial agonist of gastric secretion[140].

Inhibition of gastric secretion by hyperosmotic solutions in the duodenum probably operates through the activation of osmoreceptors and the release of one or more inhibitory hormones[118]. The inhibitory enterogastric reflex might also be responsible for this inhibition[131].

References

1. Rubin, W. (1972). Endocrine cells in the normal human stomach. *Gastroenterology*, **63**, 784
2. McGuigan, J. E. and Greider, M. H. (1971). Correlative immunochemical and light microscopic studies of the gastrin cell of the antral mucosa. *Gastroenterology*, **60**, 223
3. Ito, S. (1967). Anatomical structure of the gastric mucosa. *Handbook of Physiology Alimentary Canal*, Vol. 2, Sec. 6, 705 (C. F. Code, editor) (Washington, D.C.: American Physiological Society)
4. Toner, P. G., Carr, K. E. and Wynburn, G. M. (1971). *The Digestive System. An ultrastructural Atlas and Review*, 37. (New York: Appleton-Century-Croft)
5. Samloff, I. M. (1971). Cellular localization of group I pepsinogens in human gastric mucosa by immunofluorescence. *Gastroenterology*, **60**, 185
6. Myhre, E. (1968). Regeneration of gastric mucosa. *The Physiology of Gastric Secretion*, 75 (L. S. Semb and J. Myren, editors) (Baltimore: The Williams and Wilkins Co.)
7. Crean, G. P., Marshall, M. W. and Rumsey, R. D. E. (1969). Parietal cell hyperplasia induced by the administration of pentagastrin (ICI 50,123) to rats. *Gastroenterology*, **57**, 147
8. Burge, H. (1968). The anatomy of the abdominal vagus with special reference to bilateral selective nerve section. *The Physiology of Gastric Secretion*, 27 (L. S. Semb and J. Myren, editors) (Baltimore: The Williams and Wilkins Co.)
9. Michels, N. A. (1955). *Blood supply and anatomy of the upper abdominal organs.* (Philadelphia: J. B. Lippincott)
10. Davenport, H. W. (1967). Salicylate damage to the gastric mucosal barrier. *New. Engl. J. Med.*, **276**, 1307
11. Davenport, H. W. (1971). *Physiology of the Digestive Tract*, 93 (Chicago: Year Book Medical Publishers)
12. Johnson, L. R. (1968). The source of histamine released during damage to the gastric mucosa by acetic acid. *Gastroenterology*, **54**, 8
13. Davenport, H. W. (1966). Fluid produced by the gastric mucosa during damage by acetic and salicylic acids. *Gastroenterology*, **50**, 487
14. Johnson, L. R. (1971). Pepsin output from the damaged canine Heidenhain pouch. *Amer. J. Dig. Dis.*, **16**, 403
15. Davenport, H. W. (1964). Gastric mucosal injury by fatty and salicylic acids. *Gastroenterology*, **46**, 245
16. Ivey, K. J. (1971). Gastric mucosal barrier. *Gastroenterology*, **61**, 247
17. Brooks, A. M. and M. I. Grossman. (1970). Effect of secretin and cholecystokinin on pentagastrin stimulated gastric secretion in man. *Gastroenterology*, **59**, 114
18. Beaumont, W. (1959). *Experiments and Observations on the Gastric Juice and the Physiology of Digestion.* (New York: Dover Publications, Inc.)
19. Beaumont, W. (1847). *The Physiology of Digestion.* (Burlington, Vt.: Chaunsey Goodrich)
20. Emas, S., Swan, K. G. and Jacobson, E. D. (1967). Methods of studying gastric secretion. *Handbook of Physiology Alimentary Canal*, Vol. 2, Sec. 6, 743 (C. F. Code, editor) (Washington, D.C.: American Physiological Society)
21. Pavlov, I. P. (1910). *The Work of the Digestion Glands.* 7 (W. H. Thompson, editor) (London: Griffin)
22. Heidenhain, R. (1879). Über die Absonderung der Fundusdrüsen des Magens. *Arch. Ges. Physiol.*, **19**, 148
23. Andersson, S. and Grossman, M. I. (1965). Effect of vagal denervation of pouches on gastric secretion in dogs with intact or resected antrums. *Gastroenterology*, **48**, 449
24. Farrel, J. I. and Ivy, A. C. (1926). Studies on the motility of the transplanted gastric pouch. *Amer. J. Physiol.*, **76**, 227

25. Ivy, A. C., Lim, R. K. S. and McCarty, J. E. (1925). Contributions to the physiology of gastric secretion. II. The intestinal phase of gastric secretion. *Quart. J. Exp. Physiol.*, **15**, 55

26. Zeljony, G. P. and Savich, V. V. (1911–1912). Concerning the mechanism of gastric secretion. *Proc. Soc. Russ. Physicians St. Petersburg*

27. Klemensiewicz, R. (1875). Über den Succus pyloricus. *Sitzberg, Kaiserlichen Akad. Wiss.*, **71**, 249

28. Heidenhain, R. (1878). Über die Pepsinbildung in den Pylorusdrüsen. *Arch. Ges. Physiol.*, **18**, 169

29. Moe, R. E. and Klopper, P. J. (1966). Demonstration of the functional anatomy of the canine gastric antrum. *Amer. J. Surg.*, **111**, 80

30. Pavlov, I. P. and Schumowa-Simanowskaja, E. O. (1895). Beitrage zur Physiologie der Absonderungen. *Arch. Anat. Physiol.*, Anat. Abt. 53

31. Olbe, L. (1959). Esophageal cannula dog, a simple mode of preparation for sham-feeding experiments. *Gastroenterology*, **37**, 460

32. Meyer, J. H., Way, L. W. and Grossman, M. I. (1970). Pancreatic bicarbonate response to various acids in the duodenum of dog. *Amer. J. Physiol.*, **219**, 964

33. Baron, J. H. (1970). The clinical use of gastric function test. *Scand. J. Gastroent.*, *Suppl.*, **6**, 9

34. Makhlouf, G. M., McManus, J. P. A. and Card, W. I. (1966). A quantitative statement of the two-component hypothesis of gastric secretion. *Gastroenterology*, **51**, 455

35. Isenberg, J. I., Best, W. and Grossman, M. I. (1972). The effect of graded doses of pentagastrin in gastric acid secretion in duodenal ulcer and non-duodenal ulcer subjects. *Clin. Res.*, **20**, 222

36. Hollander, F. (1946). Insulin test for the presence of intact nerve fibres after vagal operations for peptic ulcers. *Gastroenterology*, **7**, 607

37. Gillespie, G., Elder, J. B., Smith, I. S., *et al.* (1972). Analysis of basal acid secretion and its relation to the insulin response in normal and duodenal ulcer subjects. *Gastroenterology*, **62**, 903

38. Grossman, M. I. (1972). Personal communication

39. Hollander, F. (1952). Gastric secretion of electrolytes. *Fed. Proc. (Fed. Amer. Soc. Exp. Biol.)*, **11**, 706

40. Makhlouf, G. M., McManus, J. P. A. and Card, W. I. (1966). A quantitative statement of the two-component hypothesis of gastric secretion. *Gastroenterology*, **51**, 149

41. Roseman, R. (1907). Contribution to the physiology of digestion. The properties and composition of the dog's gastric juice obtained by sham feeding. *Arch. Ges. Physiol.*, **118**, 467

42. Cooke, A. R. and Grossman, M. I. (1965). Electrolytes in gastric juice after adrenalectomy and glucocorticoid administration. *Physiologist*, **8**, 139

43. Teorell, R. (1939). On the permeability of the stomach mucosa for acids and some other substances. *J. Gen. Physiol.*, **23**, 263

44. Teorell, R. (1947). Electrolyte diffusion in relation to the acidity regulation of the gastric juice. *Gastroenterology*, **9**, 425

45. Hunt, J. N. and Wan, B. (1967). Electrolytes of mammalian gastric juice. *Handbook of Physiology, Alimentary Canal*, Vol. 2, Sec. 6, 781 (C. F. Code, editor) (Washington, D.C.: American Physiological Society)

46. Sedar, A. W. and Friedman, M. H. F. (1961). Correlation of the fine structure of the gastric parietal cell (dog) with functional activity of the stomach. *J. Biophys. Biochem. Cytol.*, **11**, 349

47. Villegas, L. and Sananes, L. (1971). Fluxes and cellular resistences in frog gastric mucosa. *Gastric Secretion*, 131 (G. Sachs, E. Heinz and K. J. Ullrich, editors) (New York and London: Academic Press)

48. Kasbekar, D. K. and Durbin, R. P. (1965). An adenosine triphosphatase from frog gastric mucosa. *Biochim. Biophys. Acta*, **105**, 472

49. Hersey, S. J., High, W. L. and Jobis, F. F. (1971). Optical measurements of intracellular reactions in gastric mucosa. *Gastric Secretion*, 239 (G. Sachs, E. Heinz and K. J. Ullrich, editors) (New York and London: Academic Press)

50. Harris, J. B., Nigon, K. and Alonso, D. (1969). Adenosine-3',5'-monophosphate: intracellular mediator for methylxantine stimulation of gastric secretion. *Gastroenterology*, **57**, 377
51. Mao, C. C., Shanbour, L. L., Hodgins, D. S. and Jacobson, E. D. (1972). Cyclic adenosine-3',5'-monophosphate (cyclic AMP) and secretion of the canine stomach. *Gastroenterology*, **63**, 427
52. Rune, S. J. (1966). Comparison of the rates of gastric secretion in man after ingestion of food and after maximal stimulation with histamine. *Gut*, **7**, 344
53. Davenport, H. W. (1965). Potassium fluxes across the resting and stimulated gastric mucosa: Injury by salicylic and acetic acids. *Gastroenterology*, **49**, 238
54. Durbin, R. P. (1968). Electrical potential difference of the gastric mucosa. *Handbook of Physiology Alimentary Canal*. Vol. 2, Sec. 6, 879 (C. F. Code, editor) (Washington, D.C.: American Physiological Society)
55. Forte, J. G. (1970). Hydrochloric acid secretion by gastric mucosa. *Membrane and ion transport*. Vol. 3, 111 (E. E. Bittar, editor) (London: Willey–Interscience)
56. Geall, M. G., Phillips, S. F. and Summerskill, W. H. J. (1970). Profile of gastric potential difference in man. *Gastroenterology*, **58**, 437
57. Andersson, S. and Grossman, M. I. (1965). Profile of pH, pressure, and potential difference at gastroduodenal junction in man. *Gastroenterology*, **49**, 364
58. Moody, F. G. (1971). Water flow through gastric secretory mucosa. *Gastric Secretion*, 432 (G. Sachs, E. Heinz and K. J. Ullrich, editors) (New York and London: Academic Press)
59. Obrink, K. J. and Waller, M. (1965). The transmucosal migration of water and hydrogen ions in the stomach. *Acta Physiol. Scand.*, **63**, 175
60. Diamond, J. M. (1971). Standing-gradient model of fluid transport in epithelia. *Fed. Proc. (Fed. Amer. Soc. Exp. Biol.)*, **30**, 6
61. Altamirano, M. (1969). Action of concentrated solutions of nonelectrolytes on the gastric mucosa. *Amer. J. Physiol.*, **216**, 33
62. Code, C. F., Higgins, J. A., Moll, J. C., Orvis, A. L. and Scholer, J. F. (1963). The influence of acid on the gastric absorption of water, sodium and potassium. *J. Physiol.*, **166**, 110
63. Hirschowitz, B. I. (1967). Secretion of pepsinogen. *Handbook of Physiology, Alimentary Canal*, Vol. 2, Sec. 6, 889 (C. F. Code, editor) (Washington, D.C.: American Physiological Society)
64. Samloff, I. M. (1971). Pepsinogens, pepsins, and pepsin inhibitors. *Gastroenterology*, **60**, 586
65. Samloff, I. M. and Townes, P. L. (1970). Electrophoretic heterogenity and relationship of pepsinogens in human urine, serum and gastric mucosa. *Gastroenterology*, **57**, 659
66. Samloff, I. M. (1971). Cellular localization of group I pepsinogens in human gastric mucosa by immunofluorescence. *Gastroenterology*, **61**, 185
67. Cooke, A. R. (1969). Acid and pepsin secretion in response to endogenous and exogenous cholinergic stimulation and pentapeptide. *Aust. J. Exp. Biol. Med. Sci.*, **47**, 197
68. Konturek, S. J., Szybinski, Z. and Horzela T. (1967). Effect of medical vagotomy on acid and pepsin responses to histamine and pentagastrin in man. *Scand. J. Gastroent.*, **2**, 311
69. Jepson, K., Duthie, H. L. and Fawcett, A. N. (1968). Acid and pepsin response to gastrin I, pentagastrin, tetragastrin, histamine and pentagastrin snuff. *Lancet*, **2**, 139
70. Brooks, A. M., Isenberg, J. and Grossman, M. I. (1969). The effect of secretin, glucagon, and duodenal acidification on pepsin secretion in man. *Gastroenterology*, **57**, 159
71. Stening, G. F. and Grossman, M. I. (1969). Gastrin-related peptides as stimulants of pancreatic and gastric secretion. *Amer. J. Physiol.*, **217**, 262
72. Cohen, N., Mazure, P., Dreiling, P. A. and Janowitz, H. D. (1960). Effect of glucagon on histamine-stimulated gastric secretion in man. *Gastroenterology*, **39**, 48
73. Robert, A., Nezamis, J. E. and Phillips, J. P. (1967). Inhibition of gastric secretion by prostaglandins. *Amer. J. Dig. Dis.*, **12**, 1073

74. Cardis, D. T. and Smith, G. (1968). Gastric secretion and anticholinergic drugs. *Brit. J. Surg.*, **55**, 185
75. Emas, S. and Grossman, M. I. (1967). Effect of truncal vagotomy on acid and pepsin responses to histamine and gastrin in dogs. *Amer. J. Physiol.*, **212**, 1007
76. Johnson, L. R. (1972). Regulation of pepsin secretion by topical acid in stomach. *Gastroenterology*, **62**, 766
77. Gerard, A. (1968). Glycoproteins in canine gastric mucosa. *Arch. Biol. (Liege)*, **79**, 1
78. DeGraef, J., Gerard, A., Lev, R. and Glass, O. B. J. (1968). Secretion of acid and neutral mucosubstances in the dog stomach. *The Physiology of Gastric Secretion*, 124 (L. S. Semb and J. Myren, editors) (Baltimore: The Williams and Wilkins Co.)
79. Schrager, J. (1969). The composition and some structural features of the principal gastric glycoprotein. *Digestion*, **2**, 73
80. Lambert, R., Andre, C. and Bernard, A. (1971). Origin of the sulfated glycoprotein in human gastric secretions. *Digestion*, **4**, 234
81. Glass, G. B. J., Mori, H. and Pamer, T. (1969). Measurement of sulfated glycoproteins in human gastric juice under fasting conditions and following stimulation with histamine, pentagastrin and insulin. *Digestion*, **2**, 124
82. Glass, G. B. J. (1968). Proteins in gastric secretion. *The Physiology of Gastric Secretion*, 456 (L. S. Semb and J. Myren, editors) (Baltimore: The Williams and Wilkins Co.)
83. Twoney, J. J., Laughter, A. H. and Jordan, P. H. (1971). Studies into human IF secretion. *Amer. J. Dig. Dis.*, **16**, 1075
84. Jeffries, G. H. (1967). Gastric secretion of intrinsic factor. *Handbook of Physiology Alimentary Canal*, Vol. 2, Sec. 6, 919 (C. F. Code, editor) (Washington, D.C.: American Physiological Society)
85. Reeder, D. D., 'Jackson, B. and Ban, J. *et al.* (1970). Influence of hypercalcemia on gastric secretion and serum gastrin concentration in man. *Ann. Surg.*, **172**, 540
86. Elwin, C. and Uvnäs, B. (1966). Distribution and local release of gastrin. *Gastrin*, 69 (M. I. Grossman, editor) (Berkeley and Los Angeles: University of California Press)
87. Cohen, M. M., Debas, H. T., Holubitsky, I. B. and Harrison, R. C. (1971). Caffeine and pentagastrin stimulation of human gastric secretion. *Gastroenterology*, **61**, 440
88. Card, W. I. and Marks, I. N. (1960). The relationship between the acid output of the stomach following 'maximal' histamine stimulation and parietal cell mass. *Clin. Sci.*, **19**, 147
89. Konturek, S. J., Wysocki, A. and Oleksy, J. (1968). Effect of medical and surgical vagotomy on gastric response to graded doses of pentagastrin and histamine. *Gastroenterology*, **54**, 392
90. Broome, A. and Olbe, L. (1968). Studies on the mechanism of the antrectomy-induced supression of the maximal acid response to histamine in duodenal ulcer patients. *Scand. J. Gastroent.*, **4**, 281
91. Olbe, L. (1966). Vagal release of gastrin. *Gastrin*, 83 (M. I. Grossman, editor) (Berkeley and Los Angeles: University of California Press)
92. Knutson, U. and Olbe, L. (1971). Significance of antrum in gastric acid response to sham feeding in duodenal ulcer patients. *Gastrointestinal Hormones and Other Subjects*, 25 (E. H. Thaysen, editor) (Copenhagen: Munksgaard)
93. Jacobson, E. D., Linford, R. H. and Grossman, M. I. (1966). Gastric secretion in relation to mucosal blood flow studied by a clearance technic. *J. Clin. Invest.*, **45**, 1
94. Jacobson, E. D. (1968). Clearances of the gastric mucosa. *Gastroenterology*, **54**, 434
95. Lin, T. M. and Warrick, M. W. (1971). Effect of glucagon on pentagastrin-induced gastric acid secretion and mucosal blood flow. *Gastroenterology*, **61**, 328
96. Jacobson, E. D. (1970). Comparison of prostaglandin E_1 norepinephrine and the gastric mucosal circulation. *Proc. Soc. Exp. Biol. Med.*, **133**, 516
97. Moore, J. G. and Englert, E. (1972). Circadian rhythm of gastric acid secretion in man. *Nature (London)*, **226**, 1261

98. McGuigan, J. E. and Trudeau, W. L. (1972). Serum gastrin levels before and after vagotomy and pyloroplasty or vagotomy and antrectomy. *New Engl. J. Med.*, **286,** 184

99. Hirschowitz, B. I. and Sachs, G. (1965). Vagal gastric secretory stimulation by 2-deoxy-D-glucose. *Amer. J. Physiol.*, **209,** 452

100. Brooks, F. P. (1967). Central neural control of acid secretion. *Handbook of Physiology Alimentary Canal*, Vol. 2, Sec. 6, 805 (C. F. Code, editor) (Washington, D.C.: American Physiological Association)

101. Nilsson, G., Simon, J. and Yalow, R. S. (1972). Plasma gastrin and gastric acid response to sham feeding and feeding in dogs. *Gastroenterology*, **63,** 51

102. Csendes, A., Walsh, J. H. and Grossman, M. I. (1972). Effects of atropine and antral acidification on gastrin release and acid secretion in response to insulin and feeding in dogs. *Gastroenterology*, **63,** 257

103. Uvnäs, B. (1942). The part played by the pyloric region in the cephalic phase of gastric secretion. *Acta Physiol. Scand., Suppl.*, **4,** 13

104. Dragstedt, L. R., Woodward, E. R. Oberhelman, J. A. Jr., *et al.* (1951). Effect of transplantation of antrum of stomach on gastric secretion in experimental animals. *Amer. J. Physiol.*, **165,** 386

105. Olbe, L. (1966). Vagal release of gastrin. *Gastrin*, 83 (M. I. Grossman, editor) (Berkeley and Los Angeles: University of California Press)

106. Edkins, J. S. (1906). The chemical mechanism of gastric secretion. *J. Physiol. (London)*, **34,** 183

107. Grossman, M. I. (1968). The gastric phase of gastric secretion. *The Physiology of Gastric Secretion*, 249 (L. S. Semb and J. Myren, editors) (Baltimore: The Williams and Wilkins Co.)

108. Grossman, M. I., Robertson, C. R. and Ivy, A. C. (1948). The proof of a hormonal mechanism for gastric secretion, the hormonal transmission of the distension stimulus. *Amer. J. Physiol.*, **153,** 1

109. Nilsson, G., Simon, J., Yallow, R. S. and Berson, S. A. (1972). Plasma gastrin and gastric acid responses to sham feeding and feeding in dogs. *Gastroenterology*, **63,** 51

110. Grossman, M. I. (1970). Gastrin and its activities. *Nature (London)*, **228,** 1147

111. Schofield, B. (1966). Inhibition by acid of gastrin release. *Gastrin*, 171 (M. I. Grossman, editor) (Berkeley and Los Angeles: University of California Press)

112. Schofield, B., Redford, M., Grabham, A. H. and Nuaimi, K. (1967). Neural factors in the control of gastrin release. *Gastric Secretion, Mechanisms and Control*, 91 (T. K. Schnitka, J. A. L. Gilbert and R. C. Harrison, editors) (London: Pergamon Press)

113. Anderson, S. and Elwin, C. F. (1968). Influence of acidity on release of gastrin by chemical agents. *The Physiology of Gastric Secretion*, 296 (L. S. Semb and J. Myren, editors) (Baltimore: The Williams and Wilkins Co.)

114. Ivy, A. C., Lim, R. K. S. and McCarthy, J. E. (1925). Contributions to the physiology of gastric secretion. II. The intestinal phase of gastric secretion. *Quart. J. Exp. Physiol.*, **15,** 55

115. Sircus, W. (1953). The intestinal phase of gastric secretion. *Quart. J. Exp. Physiol.*, **38,** 91

116. Yalow, R. S. and Berson, S. A. (1971). Further studies on the nature of immuno-reactive gastrin in human plasma. *Gastroenterology*, **43,** 457

117. Stern, D. H. and Walsh, J. H. (1972). Release of duodenal gastrin in man. *Clin. Res.*, **20,** 223

118. Konturek, S. J. and Grossman, M. I. (1965). Effect of perfusion of intestinal loops with acid, fat or dextrose on gastric secretion. *Gastroenterology*, **49,** 481

119. Emas, S. and Grossman, M. I. (1969). Response of Heidenhain pouch to histamine, gastrin and feeding before and after truncal vagotomy in dogs. *Scand. J. Gastroent.*, **4,** 497

120. Webster, D. R. and Armour, J. C. (1932). Effect of pyloric obstruction on gastric secretion. *Trans. R. Soc. Can.*, **26,** 109

121. Pavlov, I. P. (1910). *The Work of the Digestive Glands*, 99 (W. H. Thompson, editor) (London: Griffin)

122. Andersson, S. and Olbe, L. (1964). Inhibition of gastric acid response to sham feeding in Pavlov pouch dogs by acidification of antrum. *Acta Physiol. Scand.*, **61**, 55

123. Gillespie, I. E. and Grossman, M. I. (1962). Effect of acid in pyloric pouch on response of fundic pouch to injected gastrin. *Amer. J. Physiol.*, **203**, 557

124. Thompson, J. C. (1966). The question of an antral chalone. *Gastrin*, 193 (M. I. Grossman, editor) (Berkeley and Los Angeles: University of California Press)

125. Kaulbersz, J. and Konturek, S. J. (1962). Comparison of enterogastrone derived from various sections of the small intestine. *Gastroenterology*, **43**, 457

126. Sokolov, A. P. (1904). *Thesis*, St. Petersburg

127. Uvnäs, B. (1971). Role of the duodenum in inhibition of gastric secretion. *Scand. J. Gastroent.*, **6**, 113

128. Berstad, A. and Petersen, H. (1970). Dose response relationship of the effect of secretin on acid and pepsin secretion in man. *Scand. J. Gastroent.*, **5**, 647

129. Johnson, L. R. and Grossman, M. I. (1969). Characteristics of inhibition of gastric secretion by secretin. *Amer. J. Physiol.*, **217**, 1401

130. Konturek, S. J., Tasler, J. and Obtulowicz, W. (1971). Duodenal mechanisms for inhibiton of gastric secretion in dogs. *Amer. J. Physiol.*, **220**, 1091

131. Konturek, S. J. and Johnson, L. R. (1971). Evidence for an enterogastric reflex for the inhibition of gastric acid secretion. *Gastroenterology*, **61**, 667

132. Pederson, R. A. and Brown, J. C. (1972). Inhibition of histamine-, pentagastrin- and insulin-stimulated canine gastric secretion by pure 'gastric inhibitory polypeptide'. *Gastroenterology*, **62**, 393

133. Said, S. I. and Mutt, V. (1972). Isolation from porcine intestinal wall of a vasoactive octacosapeptide related to secretin and to glucagon. *Europ. J. Biochem.*, **28**, 199

134. Ginsberg, W. B., Levine, R. A. and Washington, A. (1972). Effect of glucagon on histamine- and pentagastrin-stimulated canine gastric acid secretion and mucosal blood flow. *Gastroenterology*, **63**, 45

135. Feng, T. P., Hou, H. C. and Lim, R. K. S. (1929). On the mechanism of the inhibition of gastric secretion by fat. *Chin. J. Physiol.*, **3**, 371

136. Debas, H. T., Bedi, B. S. and Gillespie, G. *et al.* (1969). Mechanism by which fat in the upper small intestine inhibits gastric secretion. *Gastroenterology*, **56**, 483

137. Swan, K. G., Konturek, S. J., Jacobson, E. D. and Grossman, M. I. (1966). Inhibition of gastric secretion and motility by fat in the intestine. *Proc. Soc. Exp. Biol. Med.*, **121**, 840

138. Meyer, J. H. and Grossman, M. I. (1972). Release of secretin and cholecystokinin. *Gastrointestinal Hormones*, 43 (L. Demling, editor) (Stuttgart: Georg Thieme Verlag)

139. Konturek, S. J., Tasler, J. and Obtulowicz, W. (1972). Role of gastric vagal innervation in the action of cholecystokinin on gastric secretion. *Gastrointestinal Hormones*, 69 (L. Demling, editor) (Stuttgart: Georg Thieme Verlag)

140. Grossman, M. I. (1970). Gastrin, cholecystokinin and secretin act on one receptor. *Lancet*, **1**, 1088

141. Magee, D. F. (1962). *Gastrointestinal Physiology*, 92 (Springfield: Charles C. Thomas Publisher)

142. Marks, I. N., Komarov, S. A. and Shay, H. (1960). Maximal acid secretory response to histamine and its relation to parietal cell mass in the dog. *Amer. J. Physiol.*, **199**, 579

143. Tepperman, B. L., Walsh, J. H. and Preshaw, R. M. Effect of antral denervation on gastrin release by sham feeding and insulin hypoglycemia in dogs. *Gastroenterology* (in the press)

144. Grossman, M. I. (1963). Integration of neural and hormonal control of gastric secretions. *Physiologist*, **6**, 349

145. Black, J. W., Duncan, W. A. M. and Durant, C. J. (1972). Definition and antagonism of histamine H_2-receptors. *Nature*, **236**, 385

146. Code, C. F., Maslinski, S. M., Massini, F. and Navert, H. (1972). Methyl histamines and gastric secretion. *J. Physiol.* (*London*) **38**, 557

8
Pancreatic Exocrine Secretion

R. M. PRESHAW
University of Toronto

8.1 INTRODUCTION

The pancreas secretes digestive enzymes, water and electrolytes into the duodenum, usually in response to ingestion of food. This organ also elaborates and secretes hormones that regulate metabolism (an endocrine function of the pancreatic islets which will not be further considered in this chapter).

Several comprehensive reviews have recently appeared concerning various aspects of the exocrine function of the pancreas[1-9]. This review deals primarily with experimental work which sheds new light on earlier concepts of pancreatic function.

8.2 MORPHOLOGY

The pancreas is a typical exocrine gland, with most of its cells arrayed in acini. Acinar cells are characterised by the presence of zymogen granules, an extensive intracellular membrane network and numerous mitochondria[10]. A lumen can be recognised in the centre of most acini; the acinar cells frequently have microvilli derived from their luminal membrane, but the luminal surface may appear smooth[11]. More often, sections show centro-acinar cells apparently separating certain of the zymogen-containing cells from the lumen. Centro-acinar cells are paler-staining and have few formed elements in their cytoplasm, apart from mitochondria[10]. These cells are believed to be the initial components of the glandular duct system (Figure 8.1).

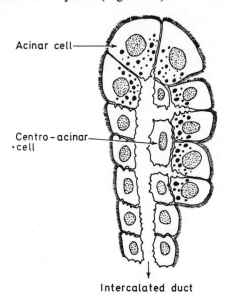

Acinar cell

Centro-acinar cell

Intercalated duct

Figure 8.1 Diagram of the pancreatic acinus (From Ekholm and Edlund[11], by courtesy of *J. Ultrastruct. Res.* and Academic Press.)

Duct lumens which apparently lack acinar cells in their wall are designated intercalary ducts. The centro-acinar cells forming the structure of the ducts are separated from other tissues by a definite space, and thus have a continuous basement membrane. Ekholm and Edlund[11] distinguished two types of cell in the small ducts: one identical to the centro-acinar cell, and the other appearing more dense and containing vacuoles, often in large numbers. Like the acinar cells, duct cells are separated from each other by small intercellular spaces, with junctional complexes in the region of the apical surface. Duct cells also have microvilli, of varying shape and size, which bulge into the lumen.

Large intralobular ducts are ensheathed by connective tissue, derived partly from septa between lobules of the gland. These ducts are lined by columnar epithelial cells, with occasional interspersed goblet cells. In the main duct itself, small mucus glands may be identified near its duodenal termination[12].

Considerable doubt surrounds the exact mechanism of formation of pancreatic juice (see Section 8.3). Histologic studies have precisely delineated the role of the acinar cell in the synthesis and secretion of enzyme protein but have done little to elucidate the problem of water and solute transport in the gland. The microscopic appearance of the various cells forming the duct system permits no conclusions about permeability factors or the localisation of any more complex transport processes in any particular area.

8.3 FORMATION OF PANCREATIC JUICE

8.3.1 Water

Mammalian pancreatic juice, collected from a catheter inserted in the main duct where it enters the duodenum, is iso-osmotic with plasma and contains HCO_3^- in a concentration possibly four or five times the concentration of this anion in blood[1]. As indicated elsewhere in this text, the formation of specialised secretions by epithelial tissues is thought to depend upon a primary solute transport process, with water accompanying solute movement in accordance with osmotic gradients. Diamond[13] has pointed out that virtually all fluid-transporting epithelial structures are characterised by long, narrow, dead-end channels. Solute transported into these channels would be expected to diffuse down its concentration gradient toward the open end, while water would enter the lumen across the channel walls to further reduce osmolality. Given anatomic restrictions on the size of the channel, and of course the presence of one blind end, water and solute would flow from the open end, even with adverse hydraulic pressure gradients.

In man, the main pancreatic duct is over 10 cm long, and the luminal radius at its widest point is approximately 2–6 mm. At their origin, the intercalated ducts have a radius of 0.1–2.0 μm, since they may appear to be filled by a solitary zymogen granule—which has a mean diameter of 4–6 μm[11]. According to Diamond and his associates, water-solute coupling by means of a standing osmotic gradient will occur if solute transport processes are located appropriately to long, narrow channels closed at one end[13-15]. A mathematical analysis of this model system[16] was restricted to channels with an internal radius less than 1 μm (so that the time needed for radial diffusion equilibrium could be disregarded) and with a length less than 200 μm. Channels of this size are present in epithelia in which water transport has been studied most intensively (gall bladder, small intestine, etc.). Given values for solute diffusion coefficients, transport rates, and osmotic water permeability (in the range observed in epithelial tissues), Diamond and Brossert calculated that this mechanism could easily provide flows at the required velocity, the secreted fluid being either hypertonic or isotonic with respect to the bathing solution available.

If such a standing osmotic gradient exists in the secreting pancreas, it could reside in the duct system or in the potential intercellular spaces between secreting cells. In the latter case, little or no osmotic gradient would be detected in the duct system proper. The existence of a standing gradient in the duct system is perhaps more plausible, since the anatomic requirements are already present. As with the lateral intercellular spaces in the gall bladder mucosa and elsewhere, there is little reason to believe that the solution present in the smaller pancreatic ducts is well stirred. While the main pancreatic duct of the cat contains smooth muscle elements and contracts spontaneously and rhythmically[17], this may not be true of smaller ducts and the extent of stirring produced by these contractions is unknown. In the pancreatic duct system, any advantage derived from the increased length of the channels relative to those in gall bladder epithelium could be offset by the increased radius, which would require a longer time to achieve radial diffusion equilibrium. Diamond and Brossert[16] calculated that an isotonic solution could be produced in blind-ended channels less than 200 μm long if solute transport were restricted to 10–100 μm lengths near the blind end. There seems little reason why solute transport in the pancreas must extend over much greater lengths of the ducts.

Diamond and Brossert concluded that determination of the presence of standing osmotic gradients in secreting epithelia would depend on (1) direct measurement of solute concentrations in the region of active transport, or (2) localisation of the solute transport process toward the blind end of the channel. Few attempts have been made to measure solute concentration in samples obtained from various parts of the pancreatic duct system. Only one report has appeared of a hypertonic fluid in smaller pancreatic ducts; in the *in vitro* rabbit pancreas, Swanson and Solomon[18] obtained duct samples by micropuncture during spontaneous secretion and after secretin stimulation. During spontaneous secretion, samples were isotonic with the bathing solution, but during secretin stimulation samples from ducts with radii approximately 25 μm exhibited values of 320–340 mOsm kg^{-1} H$_2$O (bathing solution 300 mOsm kg^{-1}). This suggests that water flow in the pancreas is coupled to solute transport by means of a standing osmotic gradient in the smaller ducts. The failure to demonstrate such a gradient during spontaneous secretion means that either the duct responsible for solute transport lengthens during stimulation or simply that the transport process is located somewhere more proximal in the duct system. Therefore, this argument also fails to identify the site of solute transport in the gland.

8.3.2 Electrolytes

Schultz (Chapter 3, Electrophysiology) has indicated how analysis of transport processes is restricted to studying what happens in the boundary phases of a system. Structural investigations of the membranes involved, in terms of specific diffusion pathways or intramembrane interactions, remain rudimentary. For many years, speculation about the formation of pancreatic juice was restricted to derivations from measurements of the differences between the ionic content of blood and that of pancreatic juice issuing from a catheter in the main pancreatic duct. Only recently have measurements been made of electrochemical gradients across the smaller ducts. Perhaps now the minimum transport processes required to form pancreatic juice can be defined.

As with measurements of duct fluid osmolality, few attempts have been made to determine the potential difference across duct or acinar cells. Reber, Wolf and Lee[19] recorded a potential difference (PD) of -2 to -6 mV (lumen negative) across the rabbit pancreatic duct both *in vivo* and *in vitro*. Secretin caused an increase in lumen negativity. Schulz, Yamagata and Weske[20] found similar PDs in rabbit pancreatic ducts after correction for a diffusion potential between pancreatic juice and the salt bridge used. These were little altered by secretin. In anaesthetised cats, Way and Diamond[21] recorded a mean resting PD of $+2.0 \pm 0.3$ mV (lumen positive) after correction for junction potentials. Intravenous injection of an effective dose of secretin raised the luminal PD to a maximum of -4.9 ± 0.2 mV within 1 min, a total change of about 7 mV. In these studies, the pancreatic duct was also perfused with exogenous solutions at rates high enough to render negligible changes in concentration produced by addition of secretin-stimulated juice. Here, secretin administration was associated with a PD shift of 2.7 mV in the same direction as that observed previously. Swanson[22] found that the PD in the duct system of the *in vitro* rabbit pancreas was in the range -7 to -8 mV.

If one accepts the argument (Section 8.3.1) that solute transport takes place in smaller rather than in larger ducts, the PD at the site of solute transport in the secreting cat or rabbit pancreas is probably a few mV negative from lumen to bathing solution. The resistance of the solution between larger and smaller ducts is presumably small. Application of the Nernst equation for concentrations of Na^+, K^+, Cl^-, and HCO_3^- in pancreatic juice and plasma (or bathing solution) indicates that, at least in the cat and rabbit, the observed concentrations of Na^+, K^+, and Cl^- in pancreatic juice are below electrochemical equilibrium, and HCO_3^- is above. If one disregards any higher concentrations possibly existing in local-standing osmotic gradients, at least the presence of HCO_3^- in pancreatic juice must be associated with an active process. The presence of the other ions in pancreatic juice could be attributed entirely to electrochemical gradients, or other processes which might include specific transport mechanisms.

The conclusion that Na^+ and K^+ may be present in pancreatic juice simply due to electrochemical gradients has been challenged by investigators using several approaches. Using the *in vitro* preparation of rabbit pancreas, Rothman and Brooks[23] showed that removing Na^+ from the bathing solution or replacing Na^+ with Li^+ stopped secretion within 30 min. In a similar preparation, reduction of bath Na^+ from 143 to 54 mM inhibited secretion by 92%[24]. In the juice of the isolated, perfused cat pancreas, Na^+ concentration was kept constant at approximately 160 mM while perfusate Na^+ was progressively reduced to 70 mM[25]. Reduction of perfusate Na^+ below 70 mM caused a sharp fall in secretory rate. Ridderstap and Bonting[26, 27] have described the presence of a Na^+-K^+-activated ATPase in canine and rabbit pancreas homogenates. This enzyme system was inhibited by ouabain and other cardiac glycosides, which similarly inhibited pancreatic flow rate in both the intact dog and the isolated rabbit pancreas. Ridderstap and Bonting concluded that the secretory cells of the pancreas possess a Na^+ pump which actively extrudes Na^+ from the cell, and that this is apparently the primary rate-limiting step in exocrine pancreatic secretion, as previously found for the secretion of aqueous humour and for the formation of cerebrospinal fluid[27]. Way and Diamond[21] suggested it was hardly surprising that pancreatic cells have a Na^+-K^+-activated ATPase, which might be used to regulate cell volume and intracellular ionic concentrations. Conceivably, its inhibition might interfere with several cellular functions, including transport processes. This objection cannot be applied to the observation that juice Na^+ is maintained constant at 160 mM in the perfused cat pancreas when perfusate Na^+ concentration is reduced to 70 mM[25]. Assuming that the PD in the smaller ducts or acini did not become markedly electronegative in the last experiment (PD was not recorded in these studies), this perhaps best affirms the presence of a transport process for Na^+ in the formation of pancreatic juice.

8.3.3 Bicarbonate

Unlike the case of Na^+, the involvement of an active process in forming a HCO_3^--rich pancreatic juice seems indisputable. Its exact nature remains unclear, but several hypotheses have been forwarded.

Carbonic anhydrase is present in pancreatic cells in fairly low concentrations[28], and inhibitors of carbonic anhydrase reduce pancreatic flow rate and bicarbonate output in man[29], cat[30], and dog[31]. The activity present in the pancreas has been measured in homogenates of the whole gland. Maren[32] pointed out that local concentrations in the acinar cells or elsewhere might be considerably higher. A report that carbonic anhydrase can be localised to duct cells histochemically[33] has been rejected on the basis that the method used was not specific for this enzyme[34].

Rawls et al.[35] calculated that the amount of carbonic anyhdrase present in pancreatic tissue (0.34 µmol kg^{-1}) could catalyse the reaction

$$CO_2 + H_2O \rightarrow H_2CO_3 \rightarrow HCO_3^- + H^+$$

so that a 25-g canine pancreas would produce 10 000 µmol HCO_3^- min^{-1}. This theoretical rate greatly exceeds the observed rate of HCO_3^- output in pancreatic juice. In the dog, pancreatic HCO_3^- output can attain rates of nearly 150 µmol min^{-1} (assuming a 25-g pancreas)[1]. One difficulty with this theory is that potent inhibitors of carbonic anhydrase, such as acetazolamide, are apparently incapable of completely inhibiting pancreatic flow rate and bicarbonate output. However, Rawls et al. calculated that even during >99% inhibition of the enzyme, the uncatalysed hydration of CO_2 would proceed fast enough to explain the residual HCO_3^- output. In this scheme, CO_2 could be derived from either pancreatic metabolism or from external sources. CO_2 can penetrate membrane structures more easily than HCO_3^-. It is reasonable to suggest that hydration of CO_2 catalysed by carbonic anhydrase occurs in the pancreatic cell near the luminal membrane. Simon et al.[36] described the presence in pancreatic homogenates of an ATPase which is stimulated severalfold by HCO_3^-. They suggested that this may be responsible for Cl^-–HCO_3^- exchange across the luminal membrane (Figure 8.2).

The theory that carbonic anhydrase plays a primary role in pancreatic bicarbonate secretion has been criticised. Claims have been made that acetazolamide can inhibit sodium[37] and chloride[38] transport, and it remains possible that the inhibitory action of this agent on pancreatic secretion is not mediated solely by its specific effect on carbonic anhydrase.

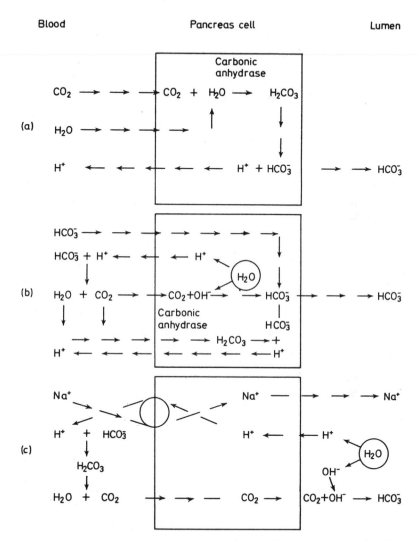

Figure 8.2 Possible models for pancreatic HCO_3^- transport. (A) model based on carbonic anhydrase; (B) model based on HCO_3^- transport mechanism; (C) model based on Na^+-H^+ exchange

In the anaesthetised dog, labelled bicarbonate introduced into the blood appears promptly in pancreatic juice[39]. Case et al.[40] demonstrated that sodium ^{14}C-bicarbonate in the perfusate of the cat pancreas, isolated in vivo, reaches a half-maximal value in pancreatic juice within 3 min. The same authors noted that flow rate in this preparation is directly proportional to perfusate bicarbonate concentration. When bicarbonate is omitted, flow almost stops. These observations have generated the hypothesis that juice bicarbonate is derived mainly from plasma bicarbonate (Figure 8.2B). Basically this reduces the function of the pancreatic secretory cell to a transport system for bicarbonate. According to this theory, the presence of carbonic anhydrase in pancreatic tissue is an embarrassment, and Case et al.[40] postulated an additional mechanism to explain its presence. They adopted an old suggestion of Davies[41] that perhaps the primary event in the pancreatic cell is the splitting of water into hydrogen and hydroxyl ions. H^+ would move out of the cell into plasma (perhaps by a specific transport process) where it would react with HCO_3^- to form CO_2. This CO_2 would re-enter the cell to combine with OH^- (under the influence of carbonic anhydrase) and form HCO_3^-, which would then presumably enter the specific HCO_3^- transport process and pass into the duct (Figure 8.2B). Comparison with Figure 8.2A shows that this latter cycle does not really differ much from the straightforward carbonic anhydrase hypothesis outlined above.

To this reviewer, it appears that too much emphasis has been placed on the rapid transfer of labelled HCO_3^- from one phase (perfusate) to another (juice). As Case et al.[40] recognised, labelled HCO_3^- introduced into their perfusate solution undergoes the following reaction:

$$[^{14}C]HCO_3^- + H^+ \rightarrow [^{14}C]H_2CO_3 \rightarrow [^{14}C]CO_2 + H_2O$$

The initial reaction of HCO_3^- with H^+ is rapid and the dehydration of H_2CO_3 becomes rate-limiting[42]. Calculated from the velocity constant for this first-order reaction at 37 °C in the absence of a catalyst, the half-time is 9 ms[43]. In the presence of blood, red cell carbonic anhydrase would further accelerate the reaction. The conclusion seems unavoidable that the appearance of labelled HCO_3^- in pancreatic juice in these two separate types of experiments could have resulted from either of the mechanisms outlined in Figure 8.2A and 8.2B.

Theories dependent upon a transport process for HCO_3^- do not adequately explain the finding that various weak acids can successfully substitute for HCO_3^- in pancreatic secretion. In the isolated, perfused cat pancreas, Schulz and her colleagues[44, 45] demonstrated that the low flow rate produced by omitting HCO_3^- from the perfusing fluid could be increased up to fivefold by substituting sulphamerazine or glycodiazine. In the rabbit pancreas, isolated in vitro, acetate, formate, propionate, or butyrate can partially substitute for HCO_3^-[46]. In both preparations, the weak acid anion was found in pancreatic juice in concentrations up to three times greater than those present in the perfusate or bathing solution.

Conceivably these weak acids are transported by a mechanism which normally handles only HCO_3^-. H_2CO_3 is also a weak acid, of course, and the recorded restoration of pancreatic flow rates in the cat pancreas by substitution with sulphamerazine or glycodiazine is unimpressive. For example, the mean flow rate in the presence of HCO_3^- is 28 µl min^{-1}, during substitution with phosphate is 2.5 μl min^{-1}, and during substitution with sulphamerazine it is 7.6 μl min^{-1}[144]. On the other hand, substitution of acetate for bicarbonate in the bathing solution of the isolated rabbit pancreas is said to produce flow rates up to 90% of normal[46].

A more attractive hypothesis, offering a simpler explanation for the findings with weak acids, involves replacement of a mechanism for transport of HCO_3^- into the duct lumen with active transport of H^+, but in the opposite direction. In this scheme, OH^- remaining in the duct would be available to combine with CO_2 to form HCO_3^-, and buffering of OH^- could be accomplished by other weak acids. The ability of the weak acid to restore pancreatic flow rate in the HCO_3^--free state would depend on its ability to reach the site of hydroxyl ion formation. Schulz et al.[44] have provided evidence that nonionic diffusion of the lipid-soluble weak acid is critical to this process.

At this stage, one can only echo the contention of Schulz[45] that resolution of these theories depends upon knowledge of boundary phases of the pancreatic secretory cell unavailable at present. This requires measurement of the electrochemical gradients for both H^+ and HCO_3^- across both the serosal and luminal membranes of the secreting cell. Using bromothymol blue, Schulz estimates that the interior of the secretory cell has a pH 'far lower than 7', and has measured a PD of -50 mV relative to interstitial fluid. This argues against a passive transport process at the luminal cell membrane, suggesting instead an active mechanism.

On the other hand, Swanson and Solomon[24] used measurements of the distribution of 5,5-dimethyl-2,4-oxazolodinediane (DMO) to calculate that the mean intracellular pH in whole rabbit pancreas was 7.25 when the bathing solution was held at 7.4. They also obtained a PD value of about -40 mV across the cell membrane (exact cell not specified). Although this calculation may not accurately measure the pH in the cell responsible for secretion of solute, these workers were encouraged to find that the distribution of H^+ between cell and bathing solution was far from an equilibrium. Combining this information with experiments confirming the inhibitory action of ouabain and low concentrations of sodium on pancreatic flow rate, they have suggested that a Na^+–H^+ exchange mechanism exists at the serosal membrane linked indirectly to metabolism through the Na^+–K^+ pump. The normal Na^+ gradient from blood to the interior of the cell is sufficient to move H^+ out of the cell on a one-to-one basis against a pH difference. Na^+ entering the cell would be handled by the usual Na^+–K^+ pump and might be transported into the duct lumen. One model based on this Na^+–H^+ exchange mechanism is depicted in Figure 8.2C.

8.3.4 Site of solute transport

Definition of the transport site demands precise definition of the electrochemical gradients at all points in the system. A start has been made to gather this critical information. The micropuncture technique has been used to obtain samples from various levels in the pancreatic duct system, permitting some estimate of the changes occurring in the secreted fluid during passage through the duct system to the duodenum.

Reber and Wolf[47] obtained samples from ducts with an average radius of 50–100 μm in the unstimulated pancreas of the anaesthetised rabbit. HCO_3^- and Cl^- concentrations were the same as those from samples taken from a catheter in the main duct. Using an identical preparation, Schulz et al.[20] found a decline in Cl^- concentration from smaller to larger ducts in one series of experiments, and, in another series, a rise in Cl^- concentration from samples assumed to be from acini compared with main duct samples. In both series, secretion was stimulated by secretin. Schulz et al. also injected a plasma sample into an 'interlobar' duct (size unstated), using a technique adapted from renal tubule micropuncture in which the sample is kept in situ by means of a split oil drop. In the unstimulated gland, chloride concentration changed little after 3–6 min in the duct, and volume (measured with inulin in the sample) was also unchanged. However, during secretin stimulation, both Cl^- and inulin concentrations fell, indicating addition of fluid to the sample. Since the fall in inulin concentration ratio was greater than the fall in Cl^-, secretin must have caused secretion of a Cl^--containing fluid into these ducts.

Mangos and his colleagues[48, 49] have described micropuncture studies in the pancreas of both rat and rabbit. In both species, micropuncture samples termed 'acinar fluid' were obtained at widely varying flow rates under the influence of secretin, but the concentrations of Na^+, K^+ and Cl^- appeared reasonably constant (Table 8.1). The surprising feature is the low Cl^- concentration in acinar samples from the rabbit compared with those from the rat. Cl^- concentrations in samples from 'interlobular' ducts in both species resemble those found in main duct collections. In the rat, Cl^- appears to be lost between acinus and the intermediate-sized duct.

Table 8.1   Mean ($\pm$ SD) ionic concentrations in acinar fluid of rat and rabbit pancreas

(From Mangos et al.[48], by courtesy of Amer. J. Physiol.)

	Ionic concentrations (mequiv l^{-1})	
Ion	Rat	Rabbit
Na^+	149 $\pm$ 4	157 $\pm$ 3
K^+	6.7 $\pm$ 1	3.1 $\pm$ 1
Cl^-	114 $\pm$ 4	43 $\pm$ 3

Concentrations did not alter significantly at varying flow rates.

Mangos et al.[48] found that Cl^- and HCO_3^- concentrations in final pancreatic juice vary in the rat and rabbit in different directions with changes in flow rate (Figure 8.3). Previous studies, mainly in the cat and dog, had led workers to believe that the mammalian pancreas secretes a HCO_3^--poor fluid at low flow rates, which changes to a HCO_3^--rich fluid at high flow rates (Cl^- changing reciprocally with HCO_3^-). That the rabbit behaves in 'classical' fashion is small compensation, for this discovery means that the primary solute transported in the rat, at least, is unlikely to include HCO_3^-. Whether the rat, rabbit, cat, or dog pancreas represents the typical mammalian pancreas is also

an open question. Wormsley[50] has measured human duodenal contents during
secretin stimulation and has also found a decline in HCO_3^- concentration at
high recovery rates. It seems premature to assume that the human pancreas
functions more like that of the rat than that of the rabbit, cat, or dog, since
changes in the ionic composition of fluid recovered from the human duodenum during secretin stimulation are not necessarily due to changes in pancreatic juice ionic composition. Clearly, this matter needs further investigation
in man.

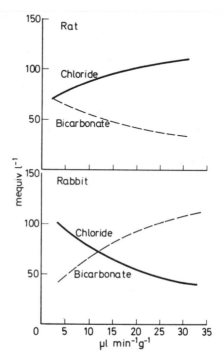

Figure 8.3 Relationship between concentrations of HCO_3^- and Cl^- in pancreatic juice and flow rate in the rat and
rabbit. (From Mangos *et al.*[48], by courtesy of *Amer. J. Physiol.*)

In other studies using the split oil drop technique, Mangos *et al.*[49] injected
pancreatic fluid into 'interlobular' ducts of the rat pancreas. When stimulated
with secretin, Cl^- concentration fell in these samples, but no change in inulin
concentration ratio occurred. These findings indicate that Cl^- moves out of
the rat pancreatic ducts under the influence of secretin. Presumably, Cl^- is
replaced by HCO_3^- entering the duct. Thus, these findings agree with conclusions derived from studies on main duct and acinar fluid composition in this
species by the same authors. Mangos *et al.* suggested a one-to-one exchange
of Cl^- for HCO_3^- in the secretin-stimulated rat ducts. Despite the absence of
PD measurements, they proposed that this Cl^- movement must be ascribed
to active transport.

These findings superficially resemble those reported earlier for split oil drop
microperfusion in the rabbit pancreas by Schulz *et al.*[20]. However, the inverse
relationship between Cl^- and HCO_3^- at varying flow rates in rabbit pancreatic
juice (Figure 8.3) and the ionic composition of acinar fluid (Table 8.1) indicate

transductal fluxes of anions in directions opposite those found in the rat. Thus, Cl^- must enter the lumen in exchange for HCO_3^-. This precisely opposes the conclusion of Schulz that Cl^- moves out of the rabbit duct lumen during secretin stimulation.

As previously considered, pancreatic juice may contain solute at concentrations greatly different from those in interstitial fluid and blood. Movement of solute according to these electrochemical gradients occurs across regions of the duct which play no specific role in solute transport. The only question is whether these fluxes are great enough to significantly change the final product entering the intestine. Several attempts have been made to investigate ionic distribution across the main pancreatic duct by perfusing solutions of known composition along isolated segments. In the rabbit, Reber et al.[19] found that, at low flow rates, a simulated pancreatic juice lost HCO_3^- and gained Cl^-. At higher flow rates (not specified) the concentration changed little. In the cat pancreas, Case et al.[30] found similar loss of HCO_3^- and a gain of Cl^- from a simulated pancreatic juice perfused through the main duct. However, little apparent net flux occurred at rates greater than 40 µl min^{-1}. In the same preparation, secretin stimulated flow rates up to 200 µl min^{-1}. The conclusion seems reasonable that, in cats, movement of ions across the walls of the main duct is insignificant when secretion has been stimulated. Way and Diamond[21] examined the permeability of the main feline pancreatic duct to the four major ions in pancreatic juice by a similar perfusion technique, but using a higher flow rate (330 µl min^{-1}). By using solutions of widely different composition, they were able to calculate that the permeability ratios for the common ions across the main duct wall resemble the ratios of their free-solution mobilities in similar dilute solutions, indicating that the main duct plays no specialised role in discriminating between these ions.

8.3.5 Enzyme secretion

The pancreatic acinar cell synthesises large quantities of digestive enzymes and enzyme precursors (zymogens). These are stored in specialised granules before discharge into the duct lumen on ingestion of food. The following stages have been defined by Palade, Siekevitz, and Caro[51]:

(1) Incorporation of amino acids into secretory protein on ribosomes attached to the membrane of the rough-surfaced endoplasmic reticulum.
(2) Transport of the newly synthesised protein into the cisternae of the rough-surfaced endoplasmic reticulum.
(3) Intracellular transfer of the protein to the Golgi region where it is packaged into the zymogen granule.
(4) Migration of zymogen granules to the luminal surface of the cell where passage of granular content occurs into the ducts.

The details of these processes have been explored by investigators at Rockefeller University[52-61].

In the guinea-pig, the entire process of synthesis, concentrative packaging, storage and release takes about 1–2 h. In 1967, Jamieson and Palade remarked that the general secretory cycle in the acinar cell was fairly well understood, but that the forces, molecular events and control mechanisms at each step awaited elucidation[57]. These authors have since demonstrated that intracellular transport of secretory proteins can be dissociated from protein synthesis; i.e. almost total inhibition of protein synthes is by cyclohexamide has relatively little effect on intracellular movement of pulse-labelled protein[58]. With protein synthesis inhibited by cyclohexamide, intracellular transport of secretory protein is unaltered by inhibitors of glycolysis, but is sensitive to respiratory inhibitors (cyanide) and inhibitors of oxidative phosphorylation (dinitrophenol)[59]. Evidence was found that endogenous fatty acids are the primary oxidisable substrate in acinar tissue.

The mature zymogen granule isolated from acinar cells contains highly concentrated protein[62]. Studies on isolated granules have revealed surprising stability in water, sucrose, or urea solutions, while enzyme content is easily extracted above pH 7, or by various electrolyte solutions[63, 64]. This indicates either that the zymogen granule membrane is remarkably impermeable to water, which seems unlikely, or that proteins exist in the granule in the form of an osmotically inactive aggregate[60].

Discharge of the stored protein into the duct lumen depends upon respiratory energy sources[65, 66], but is not greatly altered by blocking protein synthesis[60]. This energy-dependent process is activated by the specific secretagogues of the pancreas (acetylcholine and cholecystokinin). Secretagogues, however, have little or no effect on intracellular transport of the secretory proteins. Morphologic studies of granule secretion[52] clearly indicate fusion of granule membrane with apical cell membrane and movement of protein into the duct lumen by exocytosis. The step which requires coupling to a source of energy remains uncertain. Because secretion continues for at least 90 min in the presence of inhibitors of protein synthesis[60], the cell must reuse intracellular membranes during the secretory process. Otherwise it would be difficult to see how the membrane of the secretory granule could continue to be formed, with synthesis of membrane protein at a standstill. According to the morphologic studies, the membrane of granules probably fuse with and contribute to the membrane of the acinar cell surface during the discharge process. Presumably this excess membrane is reintroduced into the intracellular secretory cycle. An actual increase in apical surface area has been observed in secreting parotid acinar cells[67], which return to relatively normal size about 2 h after stimulation has been stopped.

The formation of zymogen granules was originally interpreted as a storage mechanism prominent in the absence of specific stimulation, since the numbers of visible granules rose with starvation and granules were discharged after refeeding. This view was supported by recovery from postmicrosomal supernates of the major portion of the amylase measured in pancreatic cell homogenates[68]. Moreover, secretion of enzyme protein continued unabated from cells apparently depleted of zymogen granules[69]. Jamieson and Palade take the opposite view—that intracellular transport of secretory protein occurs primarily within membrane-bound compartments[61]. They explained the earlier findings as perhaps due to rupture of small, membrane-bound vesicles during homogenisation and to the presence of much smaller granules in the secreting cell, which would not appear prominent on light microscopy.

The control of enzyme synthesis in the acinar cell might be strictly secondary to excitation of granular discharge. Control might also be directly mediated by the same agents responsible for the onset of secretion. The current evidence is conflicting. Most *in vitro* studies, in which secretagogues have induced discharge of secretory protein, have failed to reveal effects of the same agents on enzyme synthesis[61, 65, 70-72]. In contrast, feeding or administration of the same stimulants to the whole animal has been found to enhance pancreatic protein synthesis[73-75]. Some workers have failed to confirm this effect; they proposed that the rate of protein synthesis in the pancreas is constant[76]. Morisset and Webster demonstrated dissociation of the effects of cholecystokinin and a choline ester on protein synthesis in the rat pancreas, depending on whether they studied the pancreas in the intact animal or used an *in vitro* preparation of the pancreas from the same species[77]. Thus, stimulants of enzyme secretion probably do enhance synthesis in the intact animal (one positive finding generally being worth at least two negative findings). But they make it even more difficult to determine whether this effect is direct or secondary to some other part of the secretory cycle.

8.4 STIMULUS–SECRETION COUPLING

When a specific first or extracellular messenger interacts with its receptor site on a cell surface, a membrane-bound enzyme is activated (adenylate cyclase) which increases the intracellular concentration of adenosine 3′,5′-cyclic monophosphate (cAMP)[78]. In order to implicate cAMP as a second messenger in the function of a given tissue, Sutherland and his colleagues proposed a number of criteria which must be met: (1) increase in intracellular cAMP in response to the first messenger (hormone or stimulant); (2) ability of exogenous cAMP (or analogues) to mimic the action of the first messenger; (3) ability of methylxanthines to mimic or potentiate the first messenger (these agents inhibit hydrolysis of cAMP); and (4) presence in the tissue of dependent protein kinase. We shall summarise here the evidence implicating cAMP as the second messenger in the exocrine pancreas.

   (1) In the anaesthetised cat, secretin, cholecystokinin, and acetylcholine increase cAMP concentrations in samples of pancreatic tissue[79].
   (2) Kulka and Sternlicht[80] found that cAMP and several analogues would increase the rate of protein secretion by the *in vitro* mouse pancreas. Similar results were obtained in the rabbit[81, 82] and rat[77, 83]. On the negative side, using the perfused cat pancreas, Case and Scratcherd[84] could demonstrate no effect of dibutyryl cAMP on enzyme secretion, but found augmentation of water and electrolyte output.
   (3) Theophylline produced a small increase in protein or enzyme output from the isolated rabbit pancreas[81, 82] and from the perfused cat pancreas[84], and enhanced protein output in response to cholecystokinin in the cat[84, 85] and rabbit[82] and to dibutyryl cAMP in the rat[83].

The evidence implicating cAMP in stimulus–secretion coupling in the exocrine pancreas is persuasive. Most of the work has mainly concerned enzyme secretion, with much less attention given to water and electrolyte secretion. (Secretin has been found to increase adenylate cyclase activity in isolated fat cell membranes[86, 87].)

  The relationship between the second messenger function of both cAMP and calcium has been emphasised by Rasmussen[88]. In pancreatic tissue preloaded with $^{45}Ca^{2+}$, cholecystokinin and acetylcholine increased both enzyme secretion and Ca^{2+} outflux[89]. Hokin has demonstrated that Ca^{2+} is an essential component of the medium for enzyme extrusion in isolated pancreas slices[90]. This has been confirmed in another *in vitro* system[91]. These results support the concept that perhaps Ca^{2+} is another second messenger in the acinar cell. However, Rasmussen *et al.*[91] quote data on the effect of choline esters on cAMP accumulation in pancreatic tissue at varying external Ca^{2+} levels which suggest that Ca^{2+} is the key second messenger, and that cAMP should be relegated to a lesser role.

8.5 REGULATION OF EXOCRINE PANCREATIC FUNCTION

8.5.1 Basal rate of secretion

Pancreatic secretion is generally assumed to proceed slowly during starvation. The exact rate of this basal secretion in any species, from mouse to man, is unknown. It is also uncertain how this basal secretion depends upon intrinsic processes within the gland or upon resting levels of function of excitatory systems of the gland. Uncertainty about the exact rate of resting secretion is not due to absence of measurements, but to interference with the organism that is necessary to measure secretory rate. For example, the pancreatic response to a meal may be assessed in dogs by diverting all pancreatic juice to the exterior using a cannula placed in the main duct. If pancreatic juice, as it is produced, is measured and immediately replaced into the duodenum, the total amount secreted in response to the meal is much less than in experiments where the secreted juice is not returned to the intestine[93]. As B. F. Skinner has written: 'When privacy is invaded with scientific instruments, the form of stimulation is changed; the scales read by the scientists are not the private events themselves'[94].

Experiments with isolated glands or preparations of pancreatic tissues or cells indicate that the ratio between resting levels of secretory activity and stimulated levels may be unremarkable. For example, the resting rate of flow of pancreatic juice in the isolated rabbit pancreas *in vitro* is about 300 µl h^{-1} (compared with approximately 50 µl h^{-1} in the anaesthetised rabbit); it increases about 30% with secretin stimulation[95]. Fragments of rat pancreas *in vitro* release amylase into the medium at a steady rate which may be doubled by introduction of stimulants like cholecystokinin or a choline ester[77]. Few would argue that these basal levels of secretory activity in such preparations indicate the resting levels of secretion in the intact animal. The rates of activity of *in vitro* preparations are much more likely to represent not only intrinsic cellular processes but also the absence of normal regulatory influences, e.g. features normally maintaining the integrity of membranes and therefore reducing normal rates of enzyme leakage from the cell.

8.5.2 Neural regulation

The neural transmitters, acetylcholine and norepinephrine, influence pancreatic secretory rates. Davies *et al.* discovered the effect of acetylcholine on isolated pancreatic tissues in 1949[96]. Confirmatory experiments have been summarised by Hokin[2]. In recent years, acetylcholine or its more stable analogues have been reported to: (1) increase the rate of efflux of labelled protein from isolated cells derived from guinea-pig pancreas[72]; (2) accelerate the rate of zymogen granule discharge from guinea-pig pancreatic slices[62]; (3) increase the movement of amylase into the medium from fragments of rat pancreas[77, 83, 91]; (4) increase the output of enzymes by the isolated, perfused cat pancreas[79] (but have little effect on rate of secretion in the same preparation); and (5) increase the enzyme output from the *in vitro* rabbit pancreas[82, 97].

In the intact animal, local or systemic acetylcholine or its analogues are known to release the hormone gastrin, which has an excitatory action on pancreatic secretion (see Chapter 1, Gastrointestinal Hormones). This makes it somewhat uncertain just where acetylcholine or its analogues are acting when administered *in vivo*, but presumably the main effect is directly on pancreatic tissue. An added complication is the possibility that gastrin itself may potentiate the effect of acetylcholine on certain tissues.

Injected into the dorsal lymph sac, acetylcholine increases pancreatic secretory rate and decreases granule count in the pancreas of starved specimens of *Rana esculenta*[98]. Methacholine increases the enzyme output of the pancreas in the anaesthetised cat[99]. And when acetylcholine is injected into the celiac artery of the anaesthetised pig, there is a short-lasting spurt of pancreatic juice containing an increased amount of amylase[100]. (This response persists after resection of the stomach and entire intestine, ruling out a contribution from gastrin and other gastrointestinal hormones.)

In the mouse pancreas, acinar cell membrane potentials were found to be approximately -40 mV[101], agreeing with previous reports[45, 44]. Spontaneous miniature depolarisation potentials are frequent and their amplitude is enhanced by addition of physostigmine. Addition of acetyl-B-methylcholine causes a depolarisation of approximately 15 mV.

Clearly, acetylcholine in the intact animal is released in the pancreas by postganglionic parasympathetic fibres, which are easily demonstrated in the rat, cat and rabbit[102]. The lengthy physiological history of parasympathetic stimulation and the pancreas was well summarised in 1967 by the late Dr J. Earl Thomas[3].

The effects of vagal stimulation vary widely from species to species. Electrical vagal stimulation increases flow rate and enzyme output in the rabbit[97], but the action on flow rate is unremarkable (as in the dog)[3]. In the anaesthetised pig, vagal stimulation produces an astonishing increase in pancreatic flow rate, as well as an increase in enzyme output[100]. This effect persists unchanged after extirpation of the stomach and intestine and after administration of enough atropine to abolish the increase in enzyme output. No definite conclusion can be reached about the nature of this atropine-resistant vagal effect on water and electrolyte secretion[103]. This species variation in pancreatic response to vagal stimulation occurs in other reported studies. For example, English cats undergo no increase in pancreatic flow rate on vagal stimulation[104], but cats from the south of Sweden may secrete over 1 ml of juice in 10 min during vagal excitation[105].

In the conscious state, a vagal reflex is initiated by the sight, smell and taste of food. In the experimental animals, this reflex can be studied by shamfeeding, in which ingested food is diverted to the exterior by an oesophageal fistula. Pancreatic flow rate and protein output reflexly increases in the dog under circumstances suggesting that the pancreatic effect cannot be attributed to secondary stimulation by passage of gastric contents into the intestine[106]. In a tortuous argument, it was suggested that the action of shamfeeding on the pancreas was mediated mainly by gastrin released by vagal action on the gastric antrum. Supportive evidence was published by Orahood et al.[107], who performed experiments wherein the pancreatic response to vagal stimulation was compared before and after the vagal supply to both pancreas and stomach was cut. In man, the sight and taste of an appetising French meal was shown to increase pancreatic flow rate and bicarbonate and enzyme output[108]. In subjects unable to secrete any gastric acid, however, a similar procedure caused a rise in enzyme output from the pancreas, while the increase in bicarbonate output was insignificant[109].

It has always seemed surprising that this vagal reflex appears so prominent in the dog, an animal which habitually gulps food when given half a chance. Perhaps in this species, as in others, the most important system activating the parasympathetic outflow to the exocrine pancreas is related to the vagovagal reflex discovered in 1959 by Harper et al[110]. These authors found that stimulation of the central cut end of one vagus nerve would augment pancreatic secretion, as long as the other vagus was intact. It was quickly suggested that distention of the stomach was a means of activating a vagovagal reflex to the pancreas[111]. Others have confirmed the finding that gastric distention acts mainly on pancreatic enzyme secretion[112].

Splanchnic nerve stimulation or norepinephrine inhibits pancreatic secretion. (The relationship between the vasomotor effects of sympathetic stimulation and secretion has been summarised by Thomas[3] and by Grayson in Chapter 4 of this volume.) Recent evidence allows dissociation of the effect on blood flow and the secretory processes. Barlow et al.[113] found that a-adrenergic agents inhibit pancreatic secretion produced by secretin infusion under conditions where blood flow to the pancreas does not fall. Hubel[114] demonstrated that norepinephrine reduces the secretory rate of the isolated in vitro rabbit pancreas (which, of course, lacks vascular perfusate). As Hubel observed, the finding that these drugs directly inhibit the secretory cell does not mean that splanchnic stimulation also acts through a direct effect of a neurotransmitter on the pancreatic cell. The sympathetic nerves could act indirectly through vasomotor changes or by a combination of both vasomotor and direct effects.

8.5.3 Hormonal regulation

In the first chapter of this volume, Johnson summarised the chemical nature, mechanism of release and effects on the pancreas of the three prime gut hormones: gastrin, secretin and cholecystokinin. (In this section, as elsewhere in this volume, 'cholecystokinin' is used in preference to 'pancreozymin' or 'cholecystokinin–pancreozymin'; but note that nomenclature in physiology, as in geography, often ignores priorities in discovery.) A complex relationship exists between the parasympathetic nervous system and the release and effects of these hormones and there is evidence of interaction between these three substances in their various effects. One should therefore consider the evidence that these hormones act directly on the pancreatic secretory cell.

Davies *et al.* found that cholecystokinin would accelerate movement of zymogen granules from the cells of the isolated cat pancreas[96]. Further studies on this effect were summarised by Hokin and Hokin[65]. More recently, similar findings were reported from studies of isolated fragments of mouse[80] or rat pancreas[77, 91]. Caerulein, a decapeptide isolated from amphibian skin with a structure allied to cholecystokinin, induced discharge of labelled protein from isolated acinar cells[72], and a pentapeptide derived from the gastrin molecule increased extrusion of amylase from the *in vitro* mouse pancreas[80]. No reports have appeared of an action of secretin on isolated pancreatic fragments or slices, but this hormone has only a weak effect on enzyme secretion *in vivo*[115], and changes in water and electrolyte flux in isolated cells or tissues have not been studied. In the isolated rabbit pancreas, secretin augments flow rate slightly, as already noted[23].

Does the interaction of secretin and the pancreas indicate the presence of a purposeful feed-back system aimed at maintaining a constant duodenal pH? The relationships illustrated in Figure 8.4 are well established, at least in the dog. Secretin release from the duodenum depends upon luminal acidification.

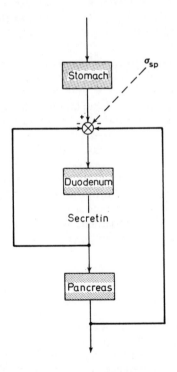

Figure 8.4 Relationship between stomach and pancreas and duodenal lumen pH; σ_{sp} is a supposed luminal pH set-point (see text)

Secretin augments pancreatic HCO_3^- output, which would reduce the degree of luminal acidification. Secretin also inhibits gastric acid output and gastric emptying (see Chapter 1). Although gastric emptying has been claimed to be accelerated by the introduction of alkaline solutions into the duodenum[116], no good evidence is available that introduction of bicarbonate into the duodenum inhibits the resting rate of pancreatic secretion or the pancreatic response to exogenous secretin. Apparently the system illustrated in Figure 8.4 can deal effectively only with changes in duodenal pH due to increasing H^+ concentration—the natural event. Introduction of strongly alkaline fluids into the duodenum does not commonly occur, but presumably would not be handled efficiently. While this tends to undermine the idea that the system has a set-point to which it approximates (σ_{sp} in Figure 4.8), this still could be an example of feed-back control. The pattern and purpose defines a feed-back system, and not the pattern alone[117]. If the purpose of the pancreas is to maintain a near-neutral duodenal pH, then this system is an example of feed-back control. On the other hand, in the absence of feeding, little acid may be produced by the gastric glands (see Chapter 7), and subsequent acidification of the duodenal lumen may be nonexistent, resulting in a minimal release of secretin. This indicates that the secretin–pancreas system is not an example of feedback in the same sense as, for example, the autoregulation of flow through small vessels by oxygen lack.

8.5.4 Interaction

Johnson has pointed out in Chapter 1 that an interaction occurs between the gastrointestinal hormones, and between these hormones and the parasympathetic outflow in controlling alimentary gland secretion. For a discussion of problems of defining potentiation between gut hormones, the interested reader is referred elsewhere[118-120].

Harper recently concluded that, during digestion, secretin probably does not potentiate the effect of cholecystokinin on enzyme output by the pancreas. Perhaps the only interaction is between cholecystokinin, gastrin and vagal impulses and the action of secretin on water and electrolyte output[9]. In anaesthetised cats the potentiating effect of cholecystokinin, gastrin extracts and vagal excitation on secretin-induced pancreatic flow was ascribed to an increase in blood flow to the gland[104]. This interaction was confirmed in canine experiments by Henriksen and Worning[121], who noted no indication of interaction in stimulating protein output. In man, a combination of a low dose of secretin with a high dose of cholecystokinin was found to produce rates of pancreatic bicarbonate output equalling those following a high dose of secretin[122]. No interaction between these two agents could be demonstrated on the output of amylase. In a further study, a high dose of secretin decreased the human pancreatic enzyme response to cholecystokinin[123]. In conscious cats, cholecystokinin administered alone caused little or no stimulation of pancreatic flow rate, but had a marked effect when combined with a low dose of secretin[124, 125]. Potentiation between exogenous secretin and cholecystokinin in accelerating flow and bicarbonate output in dogs is mimicked by the infusion of phenylalanine into the duodenum when secretin is given intravenously[126]. (Amino acids are potent releasing agents for cholecystokinin.) As in the other studies quoted, no definite evidence was found for interaction between cholecystokinin and secretin acting on pancreatic enzyme output.

Interaction between the parasympathetic nervous system and gastrointestinal hormones may also be studied through the effects of anticholinergic drugs or surgical denervation on pancreatic responses to the hormones. In a review of the effects of vagotomy on pancreatic function in 1967, the results were assessed as 'variable'[5]. This opinion still appears valid. Vagotomy has recently been reported to have no effect on secretin-stimulated pancreatic flow rate in the dog[127], to sensitise the canine pancreas to exogenous secretin[128], and to reduce secretion and bicarbonate output in response to exogenous secretin in man[129]. In three studies[127, 129, 130], vagotomy was said to have little or no effect on the rate of enzyme output in response to cholecystokinin. Several workers had previously found atropine to depress pancreatic responses (for summary, see Preshaw[3]), but Henriksen reported no effect of atropine on secretin-stimulated pancreatic secretion in conscious dogs and a significant increase in flow rate in response to cholecystokinin[127]. In contrast, Konturek et al.[131] showed that atropine causes a consistent reduction in secretin-stimulated flow rate and bicarbonate output in conscious dogs.

The potentiation between various modes of exciting the pancreas and the action of secretin on flow rate and bicarbonate output explains an annoying contradiction. As recognised for nearly a century, the canine pancreas secretes juice at a rate approaching 1 ml min^{-1} in response to ingestion of a meal. Measurement of the luminal pH in the duodenum during a meal indicates that only the proximal portion of duodenum is acidified below pH 5[132]. Studies using acidification of various lengths of the intestine[133, 134] have made it possible to estimate that a discrepancy exists between the length of bowel acidified during the meal in the dog and the pancreatic response. This difficulty is overcome if one assumes that the actual amount of secretin released during the digestion of the meal is small and would evoke only a slight pancreatic response if administered alone. Its action on pancreatic flow rate during digestion is augmented by vagal impulses and circulating gastrin and cholecystokinin. Proof of the importance of this effect in the dog and other species awaits application of accurate methods for measuring circulating levels of secretin. Until such measurements are available, speculation on the relative importance of the various excitatory mechanisms in response to a meal is futile.

8.5.5 Long-term regulation

The synthesis, storage and secretion of pancreatic enzymes has been discussed with the assumption that the proportions of all pancreatic enzymes remained parallel throughout the process. This section considers the problem of dissociation between individual pancreatic enzymes and the evidence for a form of regulation of the proportions of these enzymes over the long term.

Marked species differences are apparent in the proportions of the various enzymes. Amylase predominates over trypsinogen in the pancreatic juice of rats, but the converse is true in the pig, cow, and horse[135, 136]. More trypsinogen is present than chymotrypsinogen in the pig and rabbit, but chymotrypsinogen predominates in the rat and cow[137-139].

Within individual species, as noted in Section 8.3.5, there is argument whether synthesis is constant[76] or may be increased by feeding or the administration of agents stimulating enzyme secretion[73-75, 140-143]. Given fixed proportions of the various enzymes at the stage of synthesis and evidence that the proportions of the enzymes in pancreatic juice accurately reflect the proportions of enzymes in zymogen granules[138], one could argue that fixed proportions of enzymes should be found at all stages of the intracellular transport process and under all conditions of stimulation. As pointed out by Wormsley and Goldberg[144], much earlier experimentation in this area was compromised by the absence of accurate, specific methods for enzyme assay. In fact, however, the most recent evidence remains contradictory[62, 91, 145, 146]. Rothman has observed that 'non-parallel' distribution of enzymes at various stages in the transport process must indicate either that zymogen granules exist which are homogeneous in enzyme content and can be preferentially excreted, or that the idea of one pathway for intracellular transport of enzyme protein must be modified[147, 148]. The notion that the inner workings of the pancreatic acinar cell might be within the grasp of our understanding now appears a little more remote.

Studies in chick embryos, neonatal rats and human infants indicate that during development of the exocrine pancreas the proportions of the various enzymes in pancreatic tissue or juice may not remain constant[149-151]. The evidence suggests that these changes are only partially related to the dietary changes in the newborn and predominantly reflect intrinsic properties of the growing gland.

In general, long-term alterations in diet are reflected by changes in the proportions of pancreatic enzymes which appear to involve alterations at the level of synthesis. In rats, a carbohydrate-rich diet causes an increase in pancreatic tissue and juice amylase, and a high-protein diet causes an increase in proteases[152-156]. Identical results are available in other species, but no convincing evidence exists that similar changes occur in man[144, 157]. The pattern of these results appears purposeful, and, therefore, can be said to involve a form of feed-back regulation, but the nature of this regulation is unclear. Parenteral administration of glucose is associated with increased pancreatic amylase content and administration of insulin decreases amylase content, suggesting that regulation functions at the level of the acinar cell[144, 158, 159]. Studies of individual amino acids indicate, however, that regulation might be achieved by other pathways, perhaps involving the intestines[153-156].

References

1. Janowitz, H. D. (1967). Pancreatic secretion of fluid and electrolytes. *Handbook of Physiology, Section 6, vol II*, 925 (C. F. Code, editor) (Washington D.C.: American Physiol. Soc.)
2. Hokin, L. E. (1967). Metabolic aspects and energetics of pancreatic secretion. *Handbook of Physiology, Section 6, vol II*, 935 (C. F. Code, editor) (Washington D.C.: Amer. Physiol. Soc.)
3. Thomas, J. E. (1967). Neural regulation of pancreatic secretion. *Handbook of Physiology, section 6, vol II*, 955 (C.F. Code, editor) (Washington D.C: Amer. Physiol. Soc.)
4. Harper, A. A. (1967). Hormonal control of pancreatic secretion. *Handbook of Physiology, Section 6, vol II*, 969 (C. F. Code, editor) (Washington D.C: Amer. Physiol. Soc.)

5. Preshaw, R. M. (1967). Integration of nervous and hormonal mechanisms for external pancreatic secretion. *Handbook of Physiology. Section 6, vol II*, 997 (C. F. Code, editor) (Washington D.C: Amer. Physiol. Soc.)

6. Hallenbeck, G. A. (1967). Biliary and pancreatic intraductal pressures. *Handbook of Physiology, Section 6, vol II*, 1007 (C. F. Code, editor) (Washington D.C: Amer. Physiol. Soc.)

7. Lagerlöf, H. O. (1967). Pancreatic secretion: pathophysiology. *Handbook of Physiology Section 6, vol II*, 1027 (C. F. Code, editor) (Washington D.C: Amer. Physiol. Soc.)

8. Beck, I. T. and Sinclair, D. G. (1971). (editors) *The Exocrine Pancreas*, (London: J. and A. Churchill)

9. Harper, A. A. (1972). Progress report. The control of pancreatic secretion. *Gut*, 13, 308

10. Ham, A. W. (1969). *Histology*, 6th ed., 706 (Philadelphia: J. B. Lippincott)

11. Ekholm, R. and Edlund, Y. (1959). Ultrastructure of the human exocrine pancreas. *J. Ultrastruct. Res.*, 2, 453

12. Zimmerman, K. W. (1927). Die Speicheldrüsen der Mundhöhle und die Bauch-speicheldrüse. *Handbuch der Mikroscopischen Anatomie des Menschen, Vol 5 part I*, 61 (W. V. Möllendorf, editor) (Berlin: Springer)

13. Diamond, J. M. (1971). Water–solute coupling and ion selectivity in epithelia. *Phil. Trans. Roy. Soc. London B*, 262, 141

14. Tormey, J. M. and Diamond, J. M. (1967). The ultrastructural route of fluid transport in rabbit gall bladder. *J. Gen. Physiol.*, 50, 2031

15. Diamond, J. M. (1971). Standing-gradient model of fluid transport in epithelia. *Fed. Proc.*, 30, 6

16. Diamond, J. M. and Brossert, W. H. (1967). Standing-gradient osmotic flow. A mechanism for coupling of water and solute transport in epithelia. *J. Gen. Physiol.*, 50, 2061

17. Lenninger, S. (1972). The motility of the pancreatic duct of the cat; an *in vitro* study. *Acta Physiol. Scand.*, 84, 134

18. Swanson, C. H. and Solomon, A. K. (1970). Micropuncture study of the electrolyte secretion of the *in vitro* rabbit pancreas. *Fed. Proc.*, 29, 845 (abstr)

19. Reber, H. A., Wolf, C. J. and Lee, S. P. (1969). Rôle of the main duct in pancreatic electrolyte secretion. *Surg. Forum*, 20, 382 (abstr)

20. Schulz, I., Yamagata, A. and Weske, M. (1969). Micropuncture studies of the pancreas of the rabbit. *Pflüg. Arch.*, 308, 277

21. Way, L. W. and Diamond, J. M. (1970). The effect of secretin on electrical potential differences in the pancreatic duct. *Biochim. Biophys. Acta.*, 203, 298

22. Swanson, C. H. (1969). Micropuncture studies of the electrolyte secretion of the rabbit pancreas *in vitro*. *IUPAB, 3rd Int Congress, Cambridge, Mass.*, 5 (abstr)

23. Rothman, S. S. and Brooks, F. P. (1965). Pancreatic secretion *in vitro* in 'Cl⁻-free', 'CO₂-free', and low-Na⁺ environments. *Amer. J. Physiol.*, 209, 790

24. Swanson, C. H. and Solomon, A. K. (1972). Evidence for Na–H exchange in the rabbit pancreas. *Nature New Biology*, 236, 183

25. Case, R. M., Harper, A. A. and Scratcherd, T. (1968). Water and electrolyte secretion by perfused pancreas of the cat. *J. Physiol. (London)* 196, 133

26. Ridderstap, A. S. and Bonting, S. L. (1969). Na-K-activated adenosine triphosphatase and pancreatic secretion in the dog. *Amer. J. Physiol.*, 216, 547

27. Ridderstap, A. S. and Bonting, S. L. (1969). Na⁺-K⁺-activated ATPase and exocrine pancreatic secretion *in vitro*. *Amer. J. Physiol.*, 217, 1721

28. Kuriaki, R. and Magee, D. F. (1964). On the carbonic anhydrase activity of the alimentary canal and pancreas. *Life Sci.*, 3, 1377

29. Dreiling, D. A., Janowitz, H. D., and Halpern, M. (1955). The effect of a carbonic anhydrase inhibitor, Diamox, on human pancreatic secretion. *Gastroenterology*, 29, 262

30. Case, R. M., Harper, A. A. and Scratcherd, T. (1969). The secretion of electrolytes and enzymes by the pancreas of the anaesthetized cat. *J. Physiol. (London)*, 201, 335

31. Birnbaum, D. and Hollander, F. (1953). Inhibition of pancreatic secretion by the carbonic anhydrase inhibitor 2-acetylamino-1,3,4-thiadiazole-5-sulfonamide, Diamox (♯6063). *Amer. J. Physiol.*, 174, 191

32. Maren, T. H. (1967). Carbonic anhydrase: chemistry, physiology, and inhibition. *Physiol. Rev.*, 47, 595

33. Manzke, E. (1959). Inaugural dissertation, Kiel
34. Muther, T. F. (1966). On the non-specificity of histochemical methods for carbonic anhydrase. *Fed. Proc.*, **25**, 320 (abstr)
35. Rawls, J. A., Wistrand, P. J. and Maren, T. H. (1963). Effects of acid–base changes and carbonic anhydrase inhibition on pancreatic secretion. *Amer. J. Physiol.*, **205**, 651
36. Simon, B, Kinne, R. and Sachs, G. (1972). The presence of a HCO_3^--ATPase in pancreatic tissue. *Biochim. Biophys. Acta*, **282**, 293
37. Slegers, J. F. G. and Moons, W. M. (1968). Effect of acetazolamide on the chloride shifts and the sodium pump in secretory cells. *Nature (London)*, **220**, 181
38. Kitahara, S., Fox, K. R. and Hogben, C. A. (1967). Depression of chloride transport by carbonic anhydrase inhibitors in the absence of carbonic anhydrase. *Nature (London)*, **214**, 836
39. Ball, E. G., Tucker, H. F., Solomon, A. K. and Vennesland, B. (1941). The source of pancreatic juice bicarbonate. *J. Biol. Chem.*, **140**, 119
40. Case, R. M., Scratcherd, T. and Wynne, R. D. (1970). The origin and secretion of pancreatic juice bicarbonate. *J. Physiol. (London)*, **210**, 1
41. Davies, R. E. (1949). The rôle of carbon dioxide in the secretion of hydrogen and bicarbonate ions. *J. Physiol. (London)*, **108**, 25P (abstr)
42. Edsall, J. T. and Wyman, J. (1958). Carbon dioxide and carbonic acid. *Biophysical Chemistry*, 550 (New York: Academic Press)
43. Roughton, F. J. W. (1941). The kinetics and rapid thermochemistry of carbonic acid. *J. Amer. Chem. Soc.*, **63**, 2930
44. Schulz, I., Ströver, F. and Ullrich, K. J. (1971). Lipid soluble weak organic acid buffers as 'substrate' for pancreatic secretion. *Pflüg. Arch.*, **232**, 121
45. Schulz, I. (1971). Influence of bicarbonate-CO_2 and glycodiazine buffer on the secretion of the isolated cat's pancreas. *Pflüg. Arch.*, **329**, 283
46. Swanson, C. H. and Solomon, A. K. (1971). Secretion of HCO_3^- and weak acid anions by the *in vitro* rabbit pancreas. *Fed. Proc.*, **30**, 605 (abstr)
47. Reber, H. A. and Wolf, C. J. (1968). Micropuncture study of pancreatic electrolyte secretion. *Amer. J. Physiol.*, **215**, 34
48. Mangos, J. A. and McSherry, N. R. (1971). Micropuncture study of excretion of water and electrolytes by the pancreas. *Amer. J. Physiol.*, **221**, 496
49. Mangos, J. A., McSherry, N. R. and Nousia-Arvanitakis, S. (1973). Transductal fluxes of anions in the rat pancreas. *Amer. J. Physiol.*, **225**, 683
50. Wormsley, K. G. (1968). Response to secretin in man. *Gastroenterology*, **54**, 197
51. Palade, G. E., Siekevitz, P. and Caro, L. G. (1962). Structure, chemistry and function of the pancreatic exocrine cell. *CIBA Foundation Symposium: The Exocrine Pancreas*, 23 (A. V. S. de Reuck and M. P. Cameron, editors) (London, J. and A. Churchill)
52. Palade, G. E. (1959). Functional changes in the structure of cell components. *Subcellular Particles*, 64 (T. Hayashi, editor) (New York: Ronald Press Co.)
53. Caro, L. G. and Palade, G. E. (1964). Protein synthesis, storage, and discharge in the exocrine cell: an autoradiographic study. *J. Cell. Biol.*, **20**, 473
54. Redman, C. M., Siekevitz, P. and Palade, G. E. (1966). Synthesis and transfer of amylase in pigeon pancreatic microsomes. *J. Biol. Chem.*, **241**, 1159
55. Redman, C. M. and Sabatini, D. D. (1966). Vectorial discharge of peptides released by puromycin from attached ribosomes. *Proc. Nat. Acad. Sci.*, **56**, 608
56. Jamieson, J. D. and Palade, G. E. (1967). Intracellular transport of secretory proteins in the pancreatic exocrine cell. I. Rôle of the peripheral elements of the Golgi complex. *J. Cell. Biol.*, **34**, 577
57. Jamieson, J. D. and Palade, G. E. (1967). Intracellular transport of secretory proteins in the pancreatic exocrine cell. II Transport to condensing vacuoles and zymogen granules. *J. Cell. Biol.*, **34**, 597
58. Jamieson, J. D. and Palade, G. E. (1968). Intracellular transport of secretory proteins in the pancreatic exocrine cell. III. Dissociation of intracellular transport from protein synthesis. *J. Cell. Biol.*, **39**, 580
59. Jamieson, J. D. and Palade, G. E. (1968). Intracellular transport of secretory proteins in the pancreatic exocrine cell. IV. Metabolic requirements. *J. Cell. Biol.*, **39**, 589
60. Jamieson, J. D. and Palade, G. E. (1971). Condensing vacuole conversion and zymogen granule discharge in pancreatic exocrine cells: metabolic studies. *J. Cell. Biol.*, **48**, 503

61. Jamieson, J. D. and Palade, G. E. (1971). Synthesis, intracellular transport, and discharge of secretory proteins in stimulated pancreatic exocrine cells. *J. Cell. Biol.*, **50**, 135
62. Vandermeers-Piret, M. C., Camus, J., Rathé, J., Vandermeers, A. and Christophe, J. (1971). Distribution of hydrolases in the rat pancreas: some properties of the zymogen granules. *Amer. J. Physiol.*, **220**, 1037
63. Hokin, L. E. (1955). Isolation of the zymogen granules of the dog pancreas and a study of their properties. *Biochim. Biophys. Acta*, **18**, 379
64. Burwen, S. J. and Rothman, S. S. (1972). Zymogen granules: osmotic properties, interactions with ions, and some structural implications. *Amer. J. Physiol.*, **222**, 1177
65. Hokin, L. E. and Hokin, M. R. (1962). The synthesis and secretion of digestive enzymes by pancreas tissue *in vitro*. *CIBA Foundation Symposium: The Exocrine Pancreas*, 186 (A. V. S. de Reuck and M. P. Cameron, editors) (London: J. and A. Churchill)
66. Schramm, M. (1967). Secretion of enzymes and other macromolecules. *Ann. Rev. Biochem.*, **36**, 307
67. Amsterdam, A., Ohad, I. and Schramm, M. (1969). Dynamic changes in the ultrastructure of the acinar cell of the rat parotid gland during the secretory cycle. *J. Cell. Biol.*, **41**, 753
68. Redman, C. M. and Hokin, L. E. (1959). Phospholipid turnover in microsomal membranes of the pancreas during enzyme secretion. *J. Biophys. Biochem. Cytol.*, **6**, 207
69. Lin, T. M. and Grossman, M. I. (1956). Dose response relationship of pancreatic enzyme stimulants pancreozymin and methacholine. *Amer. J. Physiol.*, **186**, 52
70. Dickman, S. R., Holtzer, R. L. and Gazzinelli, G. (1962). Protein synthesis by beef pancreas slices. *Biochemistry*, **1**, 574
71. Webster, P. D. (1969). Effect of stimulation on pancreatic amylase secretion and nuclear RNA synthesis. *Proc. Soc. Exp. Biol. Med.*, **132**, 1072
72. Amsterdam, A. and Jamieson, J. D. (1972). Structural and functional characterisation of isolated pancreatic exocrine cells. *Proc. Nat. Acad. Sci.*, **69**, 3028
73. Farber, E. and Sidransky, H. (1956). Changes in protein metabolism in the rat pancreas on stimulation. *J. Biol. Chem.*, **222**, 237
74. Webster, P. D. (1968). Effect of methacholine on pancreatic amylase synthesis. *Gastroenterology*, **55**, 375
75. Webster, P. D. and Tyor, M. P. (1967). Effects of fasting and feeding on uridine-^{3}H incorporation into RNA by pancreas slices. *Amer. J. Physiol.*, **212**, 203
76. Poort, C. F. and Kramer, M. F. (1969). Effect of feeding on the protein synthesis in mammalian pancreas. *Gastroenterology*, **57**, 689
77. Morisset, J. A. and Webster, P. D. (1971). *In vitro* and *in vivo* effects of pancreozymin Urecholine, and cyclic AMP on rat pancreas. *Amer. J. Physiol.*, **220**, 202
78. Robison, G. A., Butcher, R. W. and Sutherland, E. W. (1971). *Cyclic AMP* (New York: Academic Press)
79. Case, R. M., Johnson, M., Scratcherd, T. and Sherratt, H. S. A. (1972). Cyclic adenosine 3',5'-monophosphate concentration in the pancreas following stimulation by secretin, cholecystokinin-pancreozymin and acetylcholine. *J. Physiol. (London)*, **233**, 669
80. Kukla, R. G. and Sternlicht, E. (1968). Enzyme secretion in mouse pancreas mediated by adenosine-3',5'-monophosphate and inhibited by adenosine-3',5'-phosphate. *Proc. Nat. Acad. Sci.*, **61**, 1123
81. Knodell, R. G., Toskes, P. P., Reber, H. A. and Brooks, F. P. (1970). Significance of AMP in the regulation of exocrine pancreas secretion. *Experientia*, **26**, 515
82. Ridderstap, A. S. and Bonting, S. L. (1969). Cyclic AMP and enzyme secretion by isolated rabbit pancreas. *Pflüg. Arch.*, **313**, 62
83. Baudoin, H., Rochus, L., Vincent, D. and Dumont, J. E. (1971). Rôle of cyclic 3',5'-AMP in the action of physiological secretagogues on the metabolism of rat pancreas *in vitro*. *Biochim. Biophys. Acta*, **252**, 171
84. Case, R. M. and Scratcherd, T. (1972). The actions of dibutyryl cyclic adenosine 3',5'-monophosphate and methyl xanthines on pancreatic exocrine secretion. *J. Physiol. (London)*, **223**, 649

85. Pederson, R. A., Pearson, J. A. and Brown, J. C. (1970). The effect of theophylline on the actions of pancreozymin and secretin. *Experientia*, **26**, 961
86. Birnbaumer, L. and Rodbell, M. (1969). Adenyl cyclase in fat cells. II. Hormone receptors. *J. Biol. Chem.*, **244**, 3477
87. Rodbell, M., Birnbaumer, L. and Pohl, S. L. (1970). Adenyl cyclase in fat cells. 3. Stimulation by secretin and the effects of trypsin on the receptors for lipolytic hormones. *J. Biol. Chem.*, **245**, 718
88. Rasmussen, H. (1970). Cell communication, calcium ion, and cyclic adenosine monophosphate. *Science*, **170**, 404
89. Case, R. M. and Clausen, T. (1971). Stimulus–secretion coupling in exocrine pancreas. II. The rôle of calcium ions. *5th Scandinavian Conference on Gastroenterology: Gastrointestinal Hormones and Other Subjects*, 67 (E. H. Thaysen, editor) (Aalborg, Denmark: Munksgaard)
90. Hokin, L. E. (1966). Effects of calcium omission on acetylcholine-stimulated amylase secretion and phospholipid synthesis in pigeon pancreas slices. *Biochim. Biophys. Acta*, **115**, 219
91. Robberecht, P. and Christophe, J. (1971). Secretion of hydrolases by perfused fragments of rat pancreas: effect of calcium. *Amer. J. Physiol.*, **220**, 911
92. Rasmussen, H., Goodman, D. B. P. and Tenenhouse, A. (1972). The rôle of cyclic AMP and calcium in cell activation. *CRC Critical Rev. Biochem.*, **1**, 95
93. Annis, D. and Hallenbeck, G. A. (1951). Effect of excluding pancreatic juice from duodenum on secretory response of pancreas to a meal. *Proc. Soc. Exp. Biol. Med.*, **77**, 383
94. Skinner, B. F. (1963). Behaviourism at fifty. *Science*, **140**, 951
95. Rothman, S. S. and Brooks, F. P. (1965). Electrolyte secretion from rabbit pancreas *in vitro*. *Amer. J. Physiol.*, **208**, 1171
96. Davies, R. E., Harper, A. A. and Mackay, I. F. S. (1949). A comparison of the respiratory activity and histological changes in isolated pancreatic tissue. *Amer. J. Physiol.*, **157**, 278
97. Solberg, L. I. and Brooks, F. P. (1969). Cholinergic control of rabbit pancreatic secretion. *Amer. J. Dig. Dis.*, **14**, 782
98. Puppi, A., Montskó, T., Komáromy, L. and Tigyi, A. (1971). Acetylcholine and the exocrine activity of the frog pancreas. *Acta Physiol. Acad. Sci. Hung.*, **40**, 79
99. Lenninger, S. (1971). Effects of parasympathomimetic agents and vagal stimulation on the flow in the pancreatic duct of the cat. *Acta Physiol. Scand.*, **82**, 345
100. Hickson, J. C. D. (1970). The secretion of pancreatic juice in response to stimulation of the vagus nerves in the pig. *J. Physiol. (London)*, **206**, 275
101. Dean, P. M. and Matthews, E. R. (1972). Pancreatic acinar cells. Measurement of membrane potential and miniature depolarisation potentials. *J. Physiol. (London)*, **225**, 1
102. Coupland, R. E. (1958). The innervation of pancreas of the rat, cat, and rabbit as revealed by the cholinesterase technique. *J. Anat.*, **92**, 143
103. Hickson, J. C. D. (1970). The secretory and vascular response to nervous and hormonal stimulation in the pancreas of the pig. *J. Physiol. (London)*, **206**, 299
104. Brown, J. C., Harper, A. A. and Scratcherd, T. (1967). Potentiation of secretin stimulation of the pancreas. *J. Physiol. (London)*, **190**, 519
105. Lenninger, S. and Ohlin, P. (1971). The flow of juice from the pancreatic gland of the cat in response to vagal stimulation. *J. Physiol. (London)*, **216**, 303
106. Preshaw, R. M., Cooke, A. R. and Grossman, M. I. (1966). Sham feeding and pancreatic secretion in the dog. *Gastroenterology*, **50**, 171
107. Orahood, R. C., Belsley, W. H., Dutta, P., Yanagisawa, T. and Eisenberg, M. M. (1972). The critical nature of gastrin in pancreatic exocrine secretion in dogs. *Surgery*, (*St. Louis*), **72**, 42
108. Sarles, H., Dani, R., Prezelin, G., Souville, C. and Figarelli, C. (1968). Cephalic phase of pancreatic secretion in man. *Gut*, **9**, 224
109. Novis, B. H., Banks, S. and Marks, I. N. (1971). The cephalic phase of pancreatic secretion in man. *Scand. J. Gastro.*, **6**, 417
110. Harper, A. A., Kidd, C. and Scratcherd, T. (1959). Vago-vagal reflex effects of gastric and pancreatic secretion and gastro-intestinal motility. *J. Physiol. (London)*, **148**, 417
111. White, T. E., Lundh, G. and Magee, D. F. (1960). Evidence for the existence of a gastropancreatic reflex. *Amer. J. Physiol.*, **198**, 725

112. Vagne, M. and Grossman, M. I. (1969). Gastric and pancreatic secretion in response to gastric distension in dogs. *Gastroenterology*, **57**, 300
113. Barlow, T. E., Greenwell, J. R., Harper, A. A. and Scratcherd, T. (1971). The effect of adrenaline and noradrenaline on the blood flow, electrical conductance and external secretion of the pancreas. *J. Physiol. (London)*, **217**, 665
114. Hubel, K. A. (1970). Response of rabbit pancreas *in vitro* to adrenergic agonists and antagonists. *Amer. J. Physiol.*, **219**, 1590
115. Henriksen, F. W. and Möller, S. (1971). Effect of secretin on the pancreatic secretion of protein. *Scand. J. Gastro.*, **9**, 181
116. Brown, J. C., Johnson, L. P. and Magee, D. F. (1966). Effect of duodenal alkalinisation on gastric motility. *Gastroenterology*, **50**, 333
117. Trimmer, J. D. (1950). *Response of Physical Systems*, 174 (New York: Wiley and Sons)
118. Magee, D. F., Nakajima, S. and Odori, Y. (1968). On potentiation. *Gastroenterology*, **55**, 648
119. Grossman, M. I. (1969). Potentiation, a reply. *Gastroenterology*, **56**, 815
120. Way, L. W. (1969). Comment on potentiation. *Gastroenterology*, **57**, 619
121. Henriksen, F. W. and Worning, H. (1967). The interaction of secretin and pancreozymin on the external pancreatic secretion in dogs. *Acta Physiol. Scand.*, **70**, 241
122. Wormsley, K. G. (1969). A comparison of the response to secretin, pancreozymin and a combination of these hormones in man. *Scand. J. Gastro.*, **4**, 413
123. Wormsley, K. G. (1971). Further studies on the response to secretin and pancreozymin in man. *Scand. J. Gastro.*, **6**, 343
124. Way, L. W. and Grossman, M. I. (1970). Pancreatic stimulation by duodenal acid and exogenous hormones in conscious cats. *Amer. J. Physiol.*, **219**, 449
125. Konturek, S. J., Radecki, T., Mikos, E. and Thor, J. (1971). The effect of exogenous and endogenous secretin and cholecystokinin on pancreatic secretion in conscious cats. *Scand. J. Gastro.*, **6**, 423
126. Meyer, J. H., Spingola, J. L. and Grossman, M. I. (1971). Endogenous cholecystokinin potentiates exogenous secretin on pancreas of dog. *Amer. J. Physiol.*, **221**, 742
127. Henriksen, F. W. (1969). Effect of vagotomy or atropine on the canine, pancreatic response to secretin and pancreozymin. *Scand. J. Gastro.*, **4**, 137
128. Moreland, H. J. and Johnson, L. R. (1971). Effect of vagotomy on pancreatic secretion stimulated by endogenous and exogenous secretin. *Gastroenterology*, **60**, 425
129. Wormsley, K. G. (1972). The effect of vagotomy on the human pancreatic response to direct and indirect stimulation. *Scand. J. Gastro.*, **7**, 85
130. Konturek, S. J., Radecki, T., Biernat, J. and Thor, P. (1972). Effect of vagotomy on pancreatic secretion evoked by endogenous and exogenous cholecystokinin and caerulein.
131. Konturek, S. J., Tasler, J. and Obtulowicz, W. (1971). Effect of atropine on pancreatic responses to endogenous and exogenous secretin. *Amer. J. Dig. Dis.*, **16**, 385
132. Brooks, A. M. and Grossman, M. I. (1970). Postprandial pH and neutralising capacity of the proximal duodenum in dogs. *Gastroenterology*, **59**, 85
133. Meyer, J. H., Way, L. W. and Grossman, M. I. (1970). Pancreatic bicarbonate response to various acids in duodenum of the dog. *Amer. J. Physiol.*, **219**, 964
134. Meyer, J. H., Way, L. W. and Grossman, M. I. (1970). Pancreatic response to acidification of various lengths of proximal intestine in the dog. *Amer. J. Physiol.*, **219**, 971
135. Marchis-Mouren, G. (1965). Étude comparée de l'equipment enzymatique du suc pancréatique de diverses espèces. *Bull. Soc. Chim. Biol. (Paris)*, **47**, 2207
136. Comline, R. S., Hall, L. W., Hickson, J. C. D., Murillo, A. and Walker, R. G. (1969). Pancreatic secretion in the horse. *J. Physiol. (London)*, **204**, 10P (abstr)
137. Rothman, S. S. (1966). Trypsin and chymotrypsin secretion from rabbit pancreas *in vitro*. *Amer. J. Physiol.*, **211**, 777
138. Keller, P. J., Cohen, E. and Neurath, H. (1958). The proteins of bovine pancreatic juice. *J. Biol. Chem.*, **223**, 344
139. Pelot, D. and Grossman, M. I. (1962). Distribution and fate of pancreatic enzymes in small intestine of the rat. *Amer. J. Physiol.*, **202**, 285
140. Meldolesi, J. (1970). Effect of caerulein on protein synthesis and secretion in the guinea-pig pancreas. *Brit. J. Pharmacol.*, **40**, 721
141. Reggio, H., Cailla-Deckmyn, H. and Marchis-Mouren, G. (1971). Effect of pancreozymin on rat pancreatic enzyme biosynthesis. *J. Cell. Biol.*, **50**, 333

142. Leroy, J., Morisset, J. A. and Webster, P. D. (1971). Dose-related response of pancreatic synthesis and secretion to cholecystokinin-pancreozymin. *J. Lab. Clin. Med.*, **78**, 149

143. Morisset, J. A. and Webster, P. D. (1972). Effects of fasting and feeding on protein synthesis by the rat pancreas. *J. Clin. Invest.*, **51**, 1

144. Wormsley, K. G. and Goldberg, D. M. (1972). The interrelationships of the pancreatic enzymes. *Gut*, **13**, 398

145. Rothman, S. S. (1967). Non-parallel transport of enzyme protein by the pancreas. *Nature (London)*, **213**, 460

146. Sarles, H., Figarella, C., Prezelin, G. and Souville, C. (1966). Comportement différent de la lipase, de l'amylase et des enzymes protéolytique pancréatiques après différents modes d'excitation du pancréas humain. *Bull. Soc. Chim. Biol. (Paris)*, **48**, 951

147. Rothman, S. S. and Wells, H. (1969). Selective effects of dietary egg white trypsin inhibitor on pancreatic enzyme secretion. *Amer. J. Physiol.*, **216**, 504

148. Rothman, S. S. (1970). Subcellular distribution of trypsinogen and chymotrypsinogen in rabbit pancreas. *Amer. J. Physiol.*, **218**, 372

149. Marchaim, U. and Kukla, R. G. (1967). The non-parallel increase of amylase, chymotrypsinogen and procarboxypeptidase in the developing chick pancreas. *Biochim. Biophys. Acta*, **146**, 553

150. Hadorn, B., Zoppi, G., Shmerling, D. H., Prader, A., McIntyre, I. and Anderson, C. M. (1968). Quantitative assessment of exocrine pancreatic function in infants and children. *J. Pediat.*, **73**, 39

151. Snook, J. T. (1971). Effect of diet on development of exocrine pancreas of the neonatal rat. *Amer. J. Physiol.*, **221**, 1388

152. Grossman, M. I., Greengard, H. and Ivy, A. C. (1942). The effect of dietary composition on pancreatic enzymes. *Amer. J. Physiol.*, **138**, 676

153. Hong, S. S. and Magee, D. F. (1957). Influence of dietary amino acids on pancreatic enzymes. *Amer. J. Physiol.*, **191**, 71

154. Ben Abdeljlil, A., Visani, A. M. and Desnuelle, P. (1963). Adaptation of the exocrine secretion of the rat pancreas to the composition of the diet. *Biochim. Biophys. Res. Comm.*, **10**, 112

155. Ben Abdeljlil, A. and Desnuelle, P. (1964). Sur l'adaptation des enzymes exocrines du pancréas a la composition du régime. *Biochim. Biophys. Acta*, **81**, 136

156. Snook, J. T. (1971). Dietary regulation of pancreatic enzymes in the rat with emphasis on carbohydrate. *Amer. J. Physiol.*, **221**, 1383

157. Véghelyi, P. V. (1949). Pancreatic enzymes: normal output and comparison of different methods of assay. *Pediatrics*, **3**, 749

158. Grossman, M. I., Greengard, H. and Ivy, A. C. (1944). On the mechanism of the adaptation of pancreatic enzymes to dietary composition. *Amer. J. Physiol.*, **141**, 38

159. Morisset, J. A. and Dunnigan, J. (1971). Effects of glucose, amino acids, and insulin on adaptation of exocrine pancreas to diet. *Proc. Soc. Exp. Biol. Med.*, **136**, 231

9
Absorption of Water Soluble Substances

R. LEVITAN and D. E. WILSON
University of Illinois

9.1 INTRODUCTION

The development of new experimental techniques during the past 10 years has
generated a mass of literature describing intestinal absorption and transport
of water, electrolytes, and other water-soluble substances. We have reviewed
some of the accumulated material, emphasising human data. We have made
no attempt to provide an encyclopaedic review, but we have highlighted
points that seem important to us in understanding the current concepts of
absorption.

9.2 EMBRYOLOGY

The intestine originates from a two-layered structure, the splanchnopleure,
whose endodermal layer gives rise to the intestinal epithelial components[1-4].
During the early stages of foetal development, the small intestine is lined by
two to four layers of stratified epithelium. The multilayered epithelium is
later reduced to a single layer of columnar cells. At an embryonic length of
approximately 20 mm, villi are usually differentiated. The ratio of villus
height to width is about 0.1 in the embryo, whereas this ratio is reversed to
approximately 3.5 in the neonate. In the adult intestine, cellular division is
limited to the crypt area. Only during embryonic formation are epithelial
cells in all areas capable of cellular division.

An active transport mechanism for the absorption of glucose in the intestine exists late in the first trimester of pregnancy in the human embryo[5].
Foetal and neonatal energy sources for supporting active transport differ
somewhat from those seen in adult intestinal tissues. Before birth, the foetal
rabbit gut transports L-histidine both anaerobically and aerobically[6]. This
ability to support anaerobic transport decreases during the first week of
life; 35 days after birth the rabbit intestine is unable to maintain anaerobic
activity transport. A sodium-potassium-activated ATPase, thought to provide
the energy for active transport, has been demonstrated at about the 40th
day of gestation in the small intestine of the foetal guinea-pig, paralleling the
development of intestinal transport of L-lysine in this species[7]. The absorptive
and transport changes in the developing gut cannot be explained merely
by an increased absorptive capacity due to developing villi and microvilli.
They are partly due to the appearance of several active transport systems and
the disproportionate increases in intestinal enzymes[8]. In the human neonate,
both α-glucosidase and β-glucosidases are active; the α-glucosidases reach
their peak levels earlier, during gestation[9-11].

9.3 MORPHOLOGY

The mucosa of the small intestine consists of three layers, the absorptive layer, the lamina propria, and the muscularis mucosae. The muscle coat separates the mucosa from the underlying submucosa (Figure 9.1). The middle layer, the lamina propria, is heterogeneous in composition and contains various cell types. In addition to its structural function, the lamina propria produces immunoglobulins. The absorptive layer consists of a single sheet of columnar epithelium attached directly to the underlying lamina propria. In the duodenum and jejunum of man, the villi range from 0.5 to 1.0 mm in height and increase the absorptive surface of the gut nearly eightfold[4].

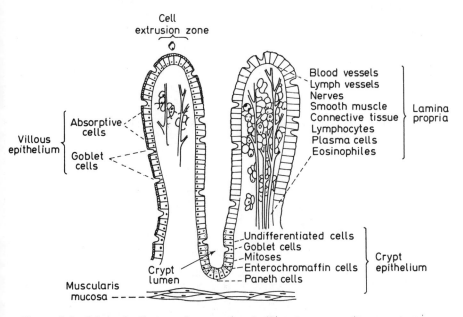

Figure 9.1 Schematic diagram of two sectioned villi and a crypt to illustrate the histologic organisation of the small intestinal mucosa. (From Trier[259], by courtesy of American Physiological Society)

Both the morphology and the function of the superficial epithelium vary with its location. The surface of the villi contains absorptive, goblet, and enterochromaffin cells (Figure 9.1). The crypts contain undifferentiated cells and are the region where cells multiply. As cells migrate toward the villus tip, they differentiate into specific cell types. The time required for cells to migrate from the crypt to the villus tip is 5–7 days in the duodenum and jejunum[12,13] and about 3 days in the ileum[14].

Microvilli (Figure 9.2) further increase the absorptive surface of the intestine about 30- to 40-fold[15]. Attached to the outer leaflet of the apical plasma

296

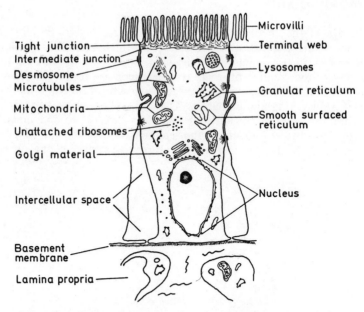

Microvilli
Tight junction
Intermediate junction
Desmosome
Microtubules
Mitochondria
Unattached ribosomes
Golgi material
Intercellular space
Basement membrane
Lamina propria

Terminal web
Lysosomes
Granular reticulum
Smooth surfaced reticulum
Nucleus

Figure 9.2 Schematic diagram of an intestinal absorptive cell. (From Trier[259], by courtesy of American Physiological Society)

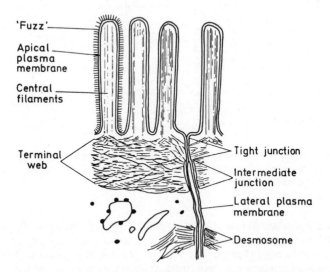

'Fuzz'
Apical plasma membrane
Central filaments
Terminal web

Tight junction
Intermediate junction
Lateral plasma membrane
Desmosome

Figure 9.3 Schematic illustration of the specialisation of the apical cytoplasm of the plasma membrane of intestinal absorptive cells. (From Trier[259], by courtesy of American Physiological Society)

membrane covering the microvillus is a coating of fine filaments, called the fuzzy coat (Figure 9.3). Histochemical studies have indicated that the fuzzy coat consists of glycoprotein, differs from mucus, is weakly acidic and sulphated, and reacts positively to the periodic acid-Schiff test[16]. Studies have suggested that this coat is synthesised by the epithelial cell to which it is attached[17]. Although the surface coat may function as a barrier against the penetration of epithelial cells by foreign materials, it may also serve an important function in starting absorption; i.e., it may selectively adsorb certain substances before absorption and may activate digestion[18-21]. The microvilli (brush border) have been isolated intact from the rest of the epithelium and found to contain high concentrations of disaccharidases[22]. Other studies have demonstrated that disaccharides are digested to monosaccharides, probably at the level of the microvilli[23]. Further fractionation of the brush border to obtain purified preparations of the plasma membrane coats has shown that up to 90% of the enzyme activity of disaccharidases and alkaline phosphatase is localised in the plasma membrane fractions. This, too, suggests that the apical membrane plays a role not only in absorption but in carbohydrate digestion[24]. In addition, other enzymes are probably present in high concentrations in this cellular fraction[25]. The ultrastructure of the absorptive cell resembles that of other epithelial cells (Figure 9.2).

Goblet cells, so named because of their shape, are readily distinguishable from other secretory epithelial cells by the mucous granules that fill the cytoplasm between the nucleus and the cellular apical border. This cell has an apical striated border morphologically similar to that seen on the surface of the absorptive epithelial cell[26]. The exact functions of the secreted mucous remain undefined.

Enterochromaffin cells, also known as argentaffin or Kultschitzky cells, are most abundant in the intestinal crypts, becoming less numerous towards the villus tip. The secretory granules of these cells are located in the basal portion of the cell (as opposed to the apical portion), adding to the speculation that these cells may secrete in an endocrine rather than an exocrine fashion. The ability of enterochromaffin cells to reduce silver and osmium to their metallic form makes them easy to identify in histologically prepared tissue secretions[27]. Although these cells are known to contain significant amounts of serotonin, the function of this compound in gut physiology remains speculative[28]. They may secrete a kallikrein-like enzyme that facilitates kinin liberation, suggesting that they may help control intestinal motility[29]. Paneth cells abound in the intestinal epithelium of man and some other species, such as monkeys, mice and rats. However, many mammals (e.g. cats, dogs and pigs) have few or no Paneth cells in the intestinal epithelium[30-31]. The morphology of these cells suggest that they are highly differentiated secretory cells similar to the zymogenic cells of the pancreas and parotid glands.

Undifferentiated cells are the predominant cell type in the crypts, and are generally confined to these areas. They secrete a glycoprotein substance, although the function of their secretions and the factors controlling release are unknown. As these cells migrate from the crypt onto the villus, they differentiate into absorptive cells, losing all morphologic evidence of secretory activity and the ability to divide. By the time these cells arrive at the base of the villus, they show histochemical evidence of enzyme activity[32].

9.4 METHODOLOGY

Intestinal absorption has been studied extensively during the last 20 years. The increased and widespread interest in the subject has resulted partly from many technical advances.

9.4.1 *In vivo* studies

The simplest and most indirect method of defining the intestinal absorption of a particular substance is to measure the increased blood level of the material after its instillation into the gut. Tolerance tests introduced as early as 1930 to study carbohydrate absorption in man[33] are examples of this technique. While these methods do not directly measure intestinal absorption, they do give semiquantitative information about the rate of appearance of the substance in the blood or urine and can thereby be used in a limited way clinically to evaluate absorption. The d-xylose excretion test[33], glucose tolerance test[34], and lactose tolerance test[35] are common examples of this approach. Radioisotopic scanning of organs is also used to indirectly indicate intestinal absorption of various radiolabelled materials.

Balance studies have been used for some time to give gross information about intestinal absorptive rates. These studies are based on the assumption

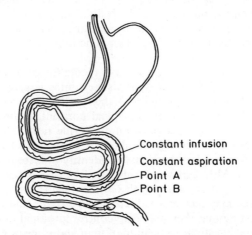

Constant infusion
Constant aspiration
Point A
Point B

Figure 9.4 Diagram of triple-lumen tube positioned in the intestine. (From Cooper *et al.*[40], by courtesy of *Gastroenterology* and Williams and Wilkins Co.)

that during steady-state conditions, with maintenance of a constant intestinal input of the measured substance, the difference between the oral input and the faecal output of the substance represents its absorption.

In animals, isolated intestinal loops have been surgically constructed to provide for more direct measurements of intestinal absorption. Thiry introduced this technique in 1864[36], and since then several modifications have been described.

In 1934, Miller and Abbott[37] described the technique of introducing a long double-lumen tube with a balloon on the end into the intestinal tract of man to study absorption. They later modified this approach, using a triple-lumen tube with two attached balloons in order to 'isolate' a segment of bowel and sample contents from the 'isolated' segment[38]. This technique, however, introduced several problems. One could not gather information during the normal emptying of loops, making the calculations of absorption only approximate. Moreover, it was difficult to effectively establish isolated intestinal segments using balloons. The local stimulation of segment motility and secretion induced by the balloons also affected the accurate measurement of substrate absorption. Furthermore, the balloons caused the study subject a great deal of physical discomfort.

In 1955, Blankenhorn et al.[39] attempted to avoid some of the problems of the balloon tubes by intubating the bowel with a thin polyethylene tube through which one could sample intestinal contents throughout the length of the bowel. Over the years, this technique has been modified in various ways, and in 1966 Cooper et al.[40] modified a double-lumen perfusion system previously introduced by that group[41] to provide a triple-lumen tube system (Figure 9.4). This currently used method allows measurement of absorption or secretion of water and solutes within a specific test segment of intestine. The use of a non-absorbable water-soluble marker, polyethylene glycol (PEG), allows calculation of any volume changes during the perfusion period.

9.4.2 *In vitro* studies

In 1892, Reid showed that the intestine could be used to study absorption *in vitro*[42]. Little note was taken of his work, however, and over 50 years passed before investigators returned to the isolated intestine as a model to study the physiology of intestinal absorption. While a number of modifications are available, the technique basically consists of using isolated intestinal segments immersed in a reservoir chamber, usually containing an oxygenated solution of the Krebs–Ringer type. A similar solution containing the substrate is circulated through the lumen of the isolated segment, and intestinal absorption is calculated by measuring the changes in substrate concentrations in the intraluminal and extraluminal bathing fluids with time.

In 1954, a similar but somewhat simpler method was introduced by Wilson and Wiseman[43]. They everted segments of intestine, thereby exposing the absorbing mucosal surface to a large volume of solution containing the substrate. The transport of substrate into the everted sac (serosal fluid) was then measured without the need to circulate fluid through the intestinal lumen.

In 1951, Ussing and Zerahn[44] noted the importance of relating the ionic movements across a membrane to the transmembrane short-circuit current. Several methods have been described to measure substrate uptake and transport in various preparations of intestinal mucosa[45-48] and even isolated epithelial cells[49].

Our information about intestinal absorption and transport is limited by the ability of the models to reflect accurately the true kinetics of substrate absorption. Much of the contradictory data in the literature may reflect differences in experimental design more than differences in true transport kinetics. One cannot yet unequivocally transpose observations on various isolated intestinal preparations in various animals to the sequence of absorptive events in man.

9.5 TRANSPORT MECHANISMS

Specific mechanisms of intestinal absorption and membrane transport will not be covered in detail in this section. The electrophysiology and energetics of intestinal transport are discussed at length in Chapter 3. Some general principles will be outlined, however, with more detailed discussion given when the absorption of specific substances is considered.

Intestinal absorption is assumed to mean the passage of a substance through the intestinal epithelium and into the blood, lymphatics, or subcellular tissue space. Absorption is divided into at least two components: (1) the movement of a substrate from the intestinal lumen into the absorbing cell, and (2) the movement from the absorbing cell into the subcellular space. This division becomes more complex when one realises that a particular substance entering the absorbing cell need not come out the other side, but may be metabolised or may appear in the subcellular space as a different substance. In addition, substrate movement across the absorbing cell is bidirectional. The net movement of a particular substrate therefore becomes the difference between movement into (influx) and movement out of (efflux) the cell. To measure intestinal absorption and transport accurately, one must deal with bidirectional fluxes at the apical and basilar surfaces of the cell, a formidable task at this time.

A characteristic of most living cells is their ability to maintain an internal environment different from the external environment. This function is related to the presence of the cellular plasma membrane which possesses specialised permeability and transport properties, allowing it to influence the rate at which molecules enter and leave the cell[50-52]. Differences between the function of the plasma membrane at the apical and basilar portions of the cell create the net movement of molecules and an electrical potential difference (p.d.) across an intact layer. Within the cell are energy-requiring systems (pumps) that regulate the intracellular concentration of diffusable ions such as Na^+ and maintain an intracellular–extracellular Na^+ concentration gradient accounting for most of the observed electrical p.d. noted across the cellular layer in some cells.

9.6 ABSORPTION OF SUGARS

Sugars are absorbed in the small intestine almost entirely in the form of monosaccharides. Some hexoses, such as glucose, which are rapidly absorbed and can move against a concentration gradient were classically considered to be absorbed by active transport. Other sugars, absorbed slowly, were felt to move across the membrane by passive diffusion. Before the absorption of specific sugars is reviewed, a look at some of the current thoughts on the mechanics of sugar transport is in order.

The finding both *in vivo* and *in vitro* that glucose is absorbed against a concentration gradient indicates that the mechanics of glucose absorption involves active membrane transport. Accumulated evidence further indicates that the concentration gradient is established and maintained by the brush border of the epithelial cell[53-55]. Disaccharidase activity has been localised to the brush border[56], and pure plasma membrane fractions of disrupted brush borders have also been found to contain both disaccharidase and alkaline phosphatase[24,57]. Further evidence that the brush border is, indeed, the site of sugar transport was suggested by the fact that phlorizin (diphenylglycoside) inhibited the entry of sugar into the epithelial cell in both high and low concentrations[53-55,58]. In low concentrations, it behaved as a competitive inhibitor of sugar entry but did not penetrate the cell itself in measurable quantities. However, studies using phlorizin to inhibit sugar transport probably need re-evaluation. Recent evidence[59] indicates that the brush border contains an enzyme which hydrolyses phlorizin, yielding phloretin. This substance is lipid-soluble and may be the actual inhibitor of sugar transport.

The mobile-carrier concept has been invoked to explain the membrane transport of sugar. The demonstration of counterflow has supported this concept. Counterflow[60] is the movement of a previously accumulated substrate out of the cell when a different substrate is added to the medium. The existence of counterflow rests on the assumptions that (1) the second substrate entering the cell uses the same carrier as the first, and (2) if an added compound is not a substrate but just an inhibitor, the accumulation rate of the initial substrate will diminish without the occurrence of counterflow. The mobile carrier would then be expected to move freely between the lipid–water interfaces and to have specific binding sites for a group of related substrates. It would not, however, react with the substrates other than to transport them through the membrane.

Although numerous observations had previously been made alluding to a role for sodium in glucose absorption, Riklis and Quastel[61] first concluded that Na^+ must be present for glucose absorption to occur. Further studies, *in vivo*[62] and *in vitro*[63], indicated that sugar absorption could be enhanced or diminished depending upon the presence or absence of Na^+. The idea was proposed that sugars undergoing active membrane transport entered the cells by Na^+-requiring carriers. The entry of sugars in the absence of Na^+ and the of entry sugars not actively transported occurred by diffusion instead. Studies by Bihler[64-65], using three sugars classically accepted as undergoing active transport (3-methyl-D-glucose, D-galactose, and a-methyl-D-glucoside) and two sugars thought not to undergo active transport (L-rhamnose and L-arabinose), showed that, in the presence of Na^+, the K_m for the actively transported sugars was low and for the non-transported sugars it was high. The V_{max}, however, was the same for both the actively and non-actively transported sugars. In the absence of Na^+, the K_m increased (indicating lower affinity) for the three actively transported sugars but did not change significantly for two non-actively transported sugars. Again, the V_{max} was identical for all sugars. Bihler further used these kinetic studies to indicate the presence or absence of active transport for other sugars. His studies suggested that both actively and non-actively transported sugars share a common entry process having the same V_{max} in the presence or absence of Na^+. To some extent, these studies supported the proposal of Crane[66] that sodium acts at the brush border to stimulate an energy-independent influx of sugar, the influx of Na^+ being coupled to the influx of sugar molecules across the brush border.

Caspary[67] suggests that two transport pathways exist for glucose in the small intestine: one is the Na^+-dependent system and the other, close to where hydrolysis occurs, transports glucose independent of Na^+ activity.

In contrast, Goldner et al.[68], using the rabbit ileum, found that changing the sodium concentration decreased the influx capacity of sugars but did not change the sugar-carrier affinity (K_t). They proposed that the carrier combined with sugar and Na^+ to form a ternary complex in order to cross the membrane. Binary complexes could be formed and also cross the membrane, but much more slowly.

Many of the data differences between different species and between in vitro and in vivo studies may be due to methodology. Parsons and Prichard[69] pointed out that K_m values for intestinal sugar absorption were larger in vivo than in vitro. Olson and Ingelfinger[70] also noted a lower sodium dependency for sugar absorption in vivo than in vitro. However, agreement appears general that Na^+ is a co-substrate in the intestinal transport of both sugars and amino acids and that the ion gradient hypothesis of Crane[66] best explains most current observations. K^+ has been observed to serve as a competitor for Na^+[65]. Increasing extracellular K^+ from 0–10 mM stimulates sugar transport but a further increase in K^+ concentration inhibits transport. Semenza suggests[71] that the stimulatory effect of K^+ at low levels may be due to a stimulatory effect on intracellular metabolism or stimulation of the sodium–potassium pump, while the inhibitory effect at higher concentrations may be due to competition for the Na^+ site on the carrier. Using this model, the active transport of sugars across the epithelial cell membrane would not be directly attached to a metabolic reaction but would be coupled to the downhill flow of Na^+ and K^+. This coupling requires no energy. Indirectly, energy would be consumed, that being necessary to supply the pumps maintaining the intracellular–extracellular K^+ and Na^+ gradients.

Two distinct sugar-binding proteins have been isolated from the brush borders of small intestine. One protein is from the core area of the microvillus and requires no Na^+[72]. The other is isolated from the brush border membrane and is Na^+-dependent[73,74].

9.6.1 Disaccharide absorption

Most carbohydrates in the Western diet are ingested as starches or disaccharides. Pancreatic amylase initially attacks starch, breaking the molecules into oligosaccharides, which are further hydrolysed to maltose and maltotreose[75]. In addition to adsorbed pancreatic amylase, the intestinal microvilli contain a glycoamylase[76-77]. However, whether the cellular amylase normally participates in starch digestion remains uncertain.

Normally, disaccharides are only minimally absorbed in the intact form. Studies using a synthetic non-digestible disaccharide, lactulose, indicate negligible absorption in the intact form normally in man[78], only 1% of ingested lactulose being absorbed. Increased absorption of disaccharides can be seen, however, if unusually large concentrations of these sugars reach the intestinal mucosa or if mucosal disease is present (as in non-tropical sprue)[79]. Other conditions which may introduce large amounts of undiluted disaccharides into the gut, i.e. a gastroenterostomy, may cause increased absorption of intact disaccharide.

Except in the duodenum and the terminal ileum, disaccharidase activity seems to be evenly distributed throughout the small intestine [77,80,81]. Although the hydrolysis and absorption of disaccharides are intimately related, the exact characteristics of this relationship are unknown. The presence of disaccharidase activity in the brush border of the intestinal epithelial cell has been unequivocally determined[22]. In the case of sucrose, the intraluminal accumulation of the monosaccharide by-products suggests that hydrolysis of the sugar by mucosal enzymes proceed more rapidly than the absorption of the monosaccharides[82-83]. While this does not indicate whether hydrolysis occurs intraluminally or intracellularly, the finding of inadequate amounts of intraluminal disaccharidase to account for the hydrolysis of ingested diaccharides[77] implies that back-diffusion of monosaccharides is occurring and that absorption is the rate-limiting step for hydrolysis and absorption of sucrose. Lactose, however, appears to be absorbed more slowly than its monosaccharide components, suggesting that hydrolysis may be the rate-limiting step in lactose digestion[83].

A stimulatory effect of Na^+ on intestinal sucrase activity has been observed[84], suggesting that the disaccharidase and the hexose transport system share a similar or the same sodium interaction site[85].

The disaccharidases of the intestinal epithelium consist of at least six a-glycosidases and two β-glycosidases[22,86-88] (Table 9.1). The a-glycosidases catalyse the hydrolysis of sugars such as maltose, isomaltose, and

Table 9.1 Brush border disaccharidases

A. *a-Glycosidases*
   1. Maltase Ia (Isomaltase)
   2. Maltase Ib (Sucrase)
   3. Maltase II
   4. Maltase III
   5. Glucoamylase
   6. Trehalase

B. *β-Glycosidases*
   1. Lactase
   2. β-Glucosidase

---

sucrose, and limit dextrins, while the β-glycosidases catalyse the hydrolysis of lactose and synthetic β-glycosides. Much substrate crossover takes place within each class of enzymes.

9.6.2 Monosaccharide absorption

Glucose absorption from the stomach is virtually non-existent except when an extremely hypertonic solution is ingested and limited absorption occurs. When Shay et al.[89] measured glucose disappearance from the intraluminal contents as an indication of absorption. they found that by the time the ingested meal reaches the distal duodenum nearly 50% of the glucose has been absorbed when an isosmotic solution was used. Only 20% was absorbed when a highly concentrated solution was used. By the time the ileum was reached, approximately 90% of the glucose had been absorbed, regardless of the concentration in the ingested meal. In man, studies indicate that the relationship between glucose absorption and glucose concentration is linear until a point is reached where the load infused exceeds $10 \, g \, h^{-1}$ or the concentration of glucose infused exceeds 139 mM[89].

Galactose absorption in man apparently resembles that of glucose. Fructose is absorbed by a slightly different mechanism[90]. In man, approximately 90% of ingested fructose is absorbed from the upper small intestine[90]. Some fructose may be converted to glucose within the cell[91], but the significance of this conversion in terms of the mechanics of the intestinal absorption of fructose is unclear. The existence of a disorder termed 'monosaccharide malabsorption (in which glucose, galactose, and 3-0-methyl-D-glucose absorption is impaired while fructose absorption is normal) further suggests a common mechanism for glucose and galactose absorption and a different mechanism for fructose absorption[92-94]. In non-tropical sprue, the rate of monosaccharide absorption is diminished, presumably secondary to the diminution in the absorptive surface area[95], while the mechanics of the absorptive process remain unchanged[96].

Gracey and co-workers[97] have shown that fructose is actively transported in the rat gut. They showed transport of fructose against a concentration gradient in vitro, competitive inhibition of fructose transport by D-glucose, D-galactose, and 3-0-methyl-glucose (although the inhibition was less than that usually seen with other actively transported sugars), and some inhibition of fructose transport by amino acids. While fructose appears to be handled by the rat much as it is by man, these studies should be substantiated by human work, since they suggest that fructose is transported by a carrier-mediated system resembling that of glucose.

Crane[95] and Wilson and Landau[98] proposed some of the structural requirements for sugars to undergo active transport. Barnett and Munday[99] further defined these structural requirements for sugar in the hamster intestine. They substitute at various carbon positions the available hydrogen bonds with non-binding groups and measured the effect on sugar transport. In general, substitution at C-6 or C-3 diminished the active accumulation of sugars. Substitution at the C-1 and C-4 position also indicate the substrate-carrier binding occurs at those positions, but to a lesser extent. However, substitution at C-5 had no effect, indicating that hydrogen binding for D-glucose occurs at the C-1, C-2, C-4 and C-6 positions but not at the C-5 position.

Removal of the hydroxyl group at the C-2 position totally abolished sodium-dependent uptake, which differed quantitatively from the reduced uptake seen with sugars having two hydrogen substitution defects, such as

6-deoxy-D-galactose or 3-deoxy-D-galactose. Barnett and Munday[99] further found that none of the sugars modified at the C-2 position inhibited D-galactose transport. They concluded that the interaction between the sugar's C-2 hydroxyl group and the carrier takes the form of a covalent bond.

If one invokes the ion gradient hypothesis to explain the active transport of sugars, the concentration of sugar in equilibrium with the carrier would be related to Na$^+$ concentration, with the sugar binding strongly to the

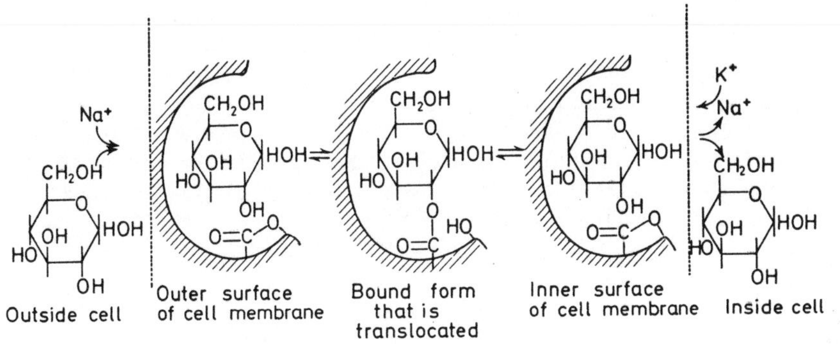

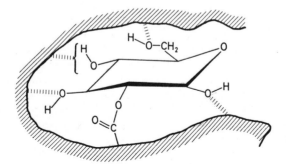

Figure 9.5 Possible mechanism for sugar transport. (From Barnett and Munday[99], by courtesy of Churchill Livingstone)

Figure 9.6 Hypothetical model for carrier-sugar bonding. (From Barnett and Munday[99], by courtesy of Churchill Livingstone)

carrier in the presence of Na$^+$ and weakly in its absence. The Na$^+$ concentration gradient and the K$^+$ concentration gradient would be maintained by intracellular pumps at the expense of ATP. A schematic model of this hypothesis is presented in Figure 9.5. Sugar is absorbed to the carrier in the presence of Na$^+$, with the hydroxyl group at C-2 cleaving an intramolecular ester on the membrane to form an ester bond between the sugar and the membrane. With the regeneration of the intramolecular ester the sugar is released in an area of low Na$^+$ concentration inside the cell. With this in mind, Barnett and Munday[99] presented a model for carrier transport of sugars (Figure 9.6).

This model indicates that while the configuration at the C-2 position remains the same as that for D-glucose, the sugar will be accumulated by the sodium-dependent carrier unless too many hydrogen binding sites are inhibited at other positions.

Little precise information is available concerning the role of various hormones on sugar absorption and transport in the small intestine. The increased glucose absorption associated with the diabetic state is not influenced by insulin and may well be secondary to the observed increase in sodium absorption[100]. Probably, too, the diminished glucose absorption observed in the adrenalectomised state is secondary to changes in sodium transport, since the low rate of glucose absorption can be corrcted or prevented in animals by adding sodium chloride to their drinking water[101]. Recently, prostaglandin E_1 has been reported to inhibit intestinal glucose absorption *in vivo* in rats. The kinetics of this inhibition are unclear, although the inhibition of absorption appears not to result from the known stimulatory effect of prostaglandins on intestinal adenylate cyclase. Administration of exogenous dibutyryl cyclic AMP does not inhibit glucose absorption but causes a slight increase[102].

9.7 ABSORPTION OF PROTEIN

Ingested protein is hydrolysed by digestive enzymes almost completely to amino acids or to peptide subunits. No evidence exists that intact protein is absorbed in man. In the past, a number of observations suggested that proteins were taken up by the intestinal epithelium only after intraluminal hydrolysis to amino acids. The finding of an increased intraluminal concentration of amino acids after protein administration[103-104], an increase in blood levels of amino acids after protein ingestion[105], and the absence of measurable peptide levels in the blood after protein ingestion[106] all suggested that complete hydrolysis to free amino acids was, in fact, the mode of protein absorption. Further studies[107] indicate that, while peptide complexes could be taken up by the intestinal epithelial cell, only trace amounts reached the subepithelial space. While 5% of ingested gelatin can be absorbed in normal man in the form of intact peptides[108], only minute amounts of intact peptide (except hydroxyproline peptides) have been found to reach the blood *in vivo* or the serosal fluid in everted sac studies *in vitro*. Newey and Smyth[109] noted that some intact peptides were absorbed from the intestine and proposed that one possible route for protein absorption is the partial intraluminal hydrolysis of protein to peptides, the entry of these peptides into the epithelial cells, and the further intracellular hydrolysis to amino acids, with the subsequent passage of the amino acids into the blood. Recent studies[105] suggest that dipeptide disappearance from the gut is primarily due to their uptake as dipeptides without intraluminal hydrolysis.

In man, protein absorption is nearly complete during passage through the duodenum and proximal jejunum[110]. The entire human small intestine appears capable of absorbing enough amino acids and dipeptides to maintain nutrition, although the intracellular hydrolysis of dipeptides is greater in the ileum than in the jejunum.

9.7.1 Peptide absorption

Additional support for the absorption of peptides in the intact form can be found in studies investigating peptide and amino acid absorption in patients with inborn errors of amino acid transport. In patients with Hartnup disease, plasma levels of histidine, phenylalanine, tryptophan, and tyrosine remain unchanged after the oral ingestion of these four amino acids. In contrast, the plasma concentrations of these amino acids normally increase when similar amounts of dipeptides, β-alanyl-histidine, phenylalanylphenylalanine, glycyl-tryptophan, and glycyltyrosine, are ingested[111]. The intestinal mucosa from a patient with Hartnup disease showed no mucosal evidence of histidine uptake during *in vitro* incubation, while incubation with glycylhistidine resulted in a mucosal histidine content greater than the sum of peptide and free histidine in the incubation medium[112].

Peters[113] reported that only 10% of the hydrolytic activity against dipeptides was present in the brush border of the intestinal epithelial cell, the rest existing within the cytosol. When tripeptides were used as substrates, however, he found significant hydrolytic activity within the cellular brush border. Further studies[114], measuring the differential hydrolysis of oligoglycines and oligoleucines from C-2 to C-6 in length, indicated that, except for the dipeptide, peptidase activity was concentrated within the brush border as compared to the cytosol homogenate. The greatest amount of activity was shown against the tripeptides. The incubation of guinea-pig brush border with polypeptides (mol. wt. 69 000 to 100 000) revealed no breakdown to shorter peptides or free amino acids.

Using starch-gel electrophoresis, Peters *et al.*[113] separated at least seven distinct peptidases which they designated as a, b, a, β-1, β-2, γ, and δ. These peptidases hydrolysed a wide range of substrates but did show some specificity.

These studies suggest that separate pathways exist for the uptake of amino acids and dipeptides in the intestinal mucosa. With transport systems existing for both amino acids and dipeptides in the brush border, proportionately little hydrolytic activity against dipeptides may be found within the brush border. On the other hand, the larger peptides probably have no specific transport system, and proportionately more hydrolysis of larger molecules occurs within the brush border (assuming that hydrolysis occurs before transport across the membrane). Hydrolytic activity against peptides with molecular weights below 225 may yield less brush border localisation than one finds with hydrolases against peptides of molecular weights above 230. (A molecular weight of about 225 is the upper limit for direct passage of peptide across the mucosal membrane[115]; it corresponds to a radius of approximately 4 Å, which is the estimated size of plasma membrane pores[52]). Many studies support the concept that gastric and pancreatic proteidases hydrolyse proteins to short peptides (up to six residues long). These peptides are further hydrolysed at the brush border to free amino acids or to shorter peptides with molecular weights below 250, allowing their entry to intestinal mucosa (probably by diffusion and active transport). Within the epithelial cell, the small peptides are hydrolysed completely to amino acids.

9.7.2 Amino acid transport

In 1951, Gibson and Wiseman[116] studied the disappearance of L and D forms of a number of amino acids from the rat small intestinal lumen and noted a more rapid uptake of L than D amino acids. L Amino acids were later shown to enter the blood more rapidly than D amino acids[117]. Wiseman[117-119] later reported that several amino acids in their L form were transported against concentration gradients, suggesting that L amino acids were also actively transported. Studies later showed that D-methionine also moved slowly against its concentration gradient[120]. A role for Na^+ in absorption of amino acids was demonstrated by the finding that a decline in extracellular sodium (by substitution with potassium, lithium, or choline) decreased the activity transport of several amino acids[120-123].

Several apparently distinct pathways have been described for amino acid transport which are type-specific[124-128]:

1. A pathway for monoamino-monocarboxylic (neutral) amino acids. Partial inhibition of this pathway occurs with other amino acids within the group, but neutral amino acid transport is unaffected by the presence of acidic or basic amino acids.

2. A pathway for dibasic (basic) amino acids. The neutral amino acids may also use this pathway, and its partial inhibition may be caused by some neutral amino acids.

3. An imino acid system specific for proline, hydroxyproline and N-methyl-substituted glycines. Except for proline and hydroxyproline, neutral amino acids have no inhibitory effect upon this pathway.

4. A pathway for dicarboxylic (acidic) amino acids.

In addition to the information that Na^+ concentration outside the mucosal membrane could affect amino acid uptake by the epithelial cell, other similarities exist between hexose transport and amino acid transport. Studies revealed that some actively transported sugars affected amino acid transport. Reiser[126] studied the effect of some sugars clasically felt to be actively transported (galactose, a-methyl-D-glucoside, and 3-O-methyl-D-glucose) and sugars considered to have a different transport system (fructose and 2-a-D-glucose) on amino acid uptake and transport in the rat intestine. The first group caused variable inhibition of transport of lysine, valine, and glycine, while the second group had no significant effect on amino acid uptake. Reiser concluded that since the actively transported sugars inhibited three distinct amino acid transport systems, the inhibitory effect was probably due to a competition between the sugars and amino acids for an energy source and not an interaction at the carrier level. This concept had been previously proposed[129], and other investigators had reported a direct relationship between the inhibitory ability of a specific sugar and that sugar's ability to maintain or synthesise ATP[130].

Alvarado[131], using guinea-pig intestine, took the opposite view, concluding that the interaction between sugars and amino acids occurred at the level of carrier-mediated influx and not at the level of energy-dependent accumulation. He based his conclusion on the following assumptions and experimental data:

1. The dual dependency for sugar and amino acid transport on Na^+

localised at the membrane level indicates that substrate binding sites are involved in the sugar–amino acid interaction.

2. The inhibitory effect of galactose on transport of the non-metabolisable amino acid cycloleucine occurs at the start of the incubation, suggesting that galactose acts on the outer surface of the membrane. Presumably galactose would have insufficient time to enter the plasma membrane.

3. The inhibitory effect of galactose after an elapse period of time during which galactose entered the plasma membrane was no different from its inhibitory effect at the start of the incubation. Alvarado[131] measured the effects of increasing concentrations of galactose on the transport of several concentrations of cycloleucine and found that as galactose concentration increased, the rate of cycloleucine transport decreased to a plateau, beyond which a further increase in galactose did not further inhibit cycloleucine uptake.

These data, plotted according to the criteria of Thorn[132], do not produce a straight line, suggesting that a single binding site would not explain the competition between galactose and cycloleucine transport. Alvarado suggested that these data indicate that the galactose binding site is different from but closely associated with the cycloleucine binding site and that the galactose inhibitory and transport sites are identical. His data support his concept of amino acid and hexose transport in the plasma membrane by means of a mosaic-type of polyfunctional unit[133]. This concept is inconsistent with the usual representation of carriers as structural components able to move back and forth across the plasma membrane. In addition, one must explain the failure of other investigators to support his findings in other systems. Alvarado presents two concepts of a polyfunctional unit in Figure 9.7A and B. Figure

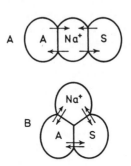

Figure 9.7 Possible polyfunctional units for amino acid transport. (From Alvarado[131], by courtesy of Charles C. Thomas)

9.7A shows his concept of a 'loosely coupled' system where sugar and amino acid binding sites are coupled to a sodium site but not to each other. In Figure 9.7B, his 'tightly coupled' system, there is not only substrate–sodium interaction but also substrate–substrate interaction. He suggests that either of these two systems may exist in various animal systems.

Munck[134] directly challenged the conclusion of Alvarado and his polyfunctional carrier system. Using isolated mucosal preparations of rat intestine, he found that the epithelial accumulation of leucine and proline was inhibited by galactose, but that influx across the brush border and influx across the total intestinal wall were unaffected by galactose. Efflux across the

total intestine wall was increased, suggesting that Alvarado may not have
been measuring true transport kinetics.

As in sugar transport, the ion gradient hypothesis has been used to explain
amino acid transport. Riggs et al.[135], in their original statement of the hypothesis, indicated that the carrier binding the amino acid must also be associated with Na^+ or K^+. Their observation in Ehrlich ascites cells indicated
that amino acid uptake required Na^+ and was inhibited by K^+ increases in
the extracellular fluid, resulting in a net gain of Na^+ and a loss of K^+ by the
cells. Studies of amino acid transport in mouse tumour cells[136] suggest that
energy inherent in the K^+ gradient might be coupled to amino acid transport. However, no evidence supports the importance of K^+ gradient in
amino acid uptake by intestinal epithelial cells. Potashner and Johnstone[137]
rejected the possible role of a K^+ gradient and focused upon the positive
correlation they noticed between cellular ATP content and the methionine
gradient, concluding that ATP hydrolysis was probably the primary energy
force supporting amino acid transport besides the ionic gradient. However,
it is difficult to transpose information on ATP hydrolysis in isolated tissue
where ionic constitutents of the media and time may affect ATP kinetics
differently than in the *in vivo* situation. The effect of ATP may be primarily to
maintain the Na^+ and R^+ gradients, which then affect an amino acid transport system. Resolution of the transport mechanism must await studies
technically suitable for transposition to *in vivo* conditions.

9.7.3 Effects of pH

Previous studies in the rat[138] indicated that lowering the pH diminished ileal
influx of amino acids across the brush border. In man, protein malabsorption
was observed in patients with increased gastric acid secretion[139]. Normally,
the pH of intraluminal fluid in the jejunum in man is neutral. Adibi et al.[140]
studied the effects of lowering intraluminal pH in man on leucine transport
using segmental perfusion studies. No significant change in leucine uptake
was seen until the pH reached 3. At that point, leucine uptake diminished and
net movement of Na^+, Cl^-, and water ceased. The presence of leucine in the
perfusion fluid stimulated Na^+ absorption when the pH was close to neutral,
but when the segment was acidified enough to affect absorption, the presence
or absence of leucine did not influence Na^+ absorption.

9.8 ABSORPTION OF WATER AND ELECTROLYTES FROM THE SMALL BOWEL

One of the major functions of the intestine is the absorption of water and
electrolytes. Each day, the human gut handles 5–10 l of endogenous secretions (salivary, gastric, biliary, pancreatic, intestinal) and ingested fluid.
Of this large volume, about 150 ml of fluid is lost in the faeces daily. Most
of the fluid conservation occurs in the small bowel. It is noteworthy that
80% of sodium chloride and 50% of the potassium and calcium handled by
the gut originates from endogenous secretions. Obviously, any derangement in

electrolyte or water absorption from the bowel will profoundly alter the fluid and electrolyte balance in the body.

The absorption or secretion of water and electrolytes taking place in the intestine is the end result of bidirectional movements of ions and water in opposite directions, namely from the mucosa to serosa (m→s flux) and from the serosa to mucosa (s→m flux). In man, these unidirectional fluxes exceed net movement by two to three times. Net absorption or secretion is a result of (m→s flux) − (s→m flux)[141].

The intestinal mucosal surface consists of a bimolecular lipid membrane of the mucosal cell, presumably containing small pores[142]. Water and solutes, according to this hypothesis, move through these pores only to enter the cell, while lipid-soluble substances can traverse the lipid cell membrane[143].

The simplest concept of pores is that they are water-filled channels through which water and hydrophilic substances can move into the cell according to existing concentration gradients. The main feature of transport into the cell via pores is that the molecular size of the penetrating substance is critical in determining the ability and rate of movement. Substances with more than four carbon atoms have difficulty entering the cell via the pores whose size in the human jejunum and ileum has been estimated to be 7.5 and 3.4 Å. respectively[144]. The relative paucity of the pores and their small size precludes their identification by electron microscopy or x-ray diffraction[142]. Electrical gradients exist between the mucosa of the gut and plasma. The plasma is positively charged and the mucosa is negatively charged, with a potential difference (p.d.) in the human small bowel of 0–10 mV[145], the p.d. transport of charged particles. The mechanisms of ionic transport across the intestinal mucosa have been reviewed in detail by Fordtran and Dietschy[142] and in Chapter 3 of this volume.

Certain ions, especially sodium, are transported actively by an energy-requiring mechanism against a combined electrochemical gradient. Passive movement of other ions result from diffusion down an electrochemical gradient due to bulk water flow and coupled exchange mechanisms.

Absorption of water is a passive phenomenon which cannot occur without solute movement. Water accompanies solute movement in isotonic proportions and moves across the intestinal mucosa in response to osmotic gradients. The rate of water absorption in any given region of the bowel is a function of solute transport in this area. All areas of the intestine absorb water. Visscher[141] originally considered the ileum and colon as absorbing sites for water, because water was absorbed from isotonic NaCl solutions from the ileum and colon but not from the duodenum and jejunum to any extent. When glucose is present in the duodenal and jejunal lumen, Na^+ and water are known to be absorbed in these areas even faster than in the ileum and colon. In fact, after man has ingested a meal, most of the water and electrolyte absorption occurs within a few hours in the upper small bowel[110].

Sodium can move against a chemical and electrical concentration gradient[142] in the small bowel. The sodium absorption processes, however, apparently differ in different parts of the small bowel. For example, isotonic saline solutions are absorbed from the dog and rat ileum but not from their jejunum or duodenum[141,146].

In man, salt and water can be absorbed from all levels of the small bowel at the same rate[41,144]. This does not necessarily mean, however, that the characteristics of the transport processes are also the same at all levels, especially since permeability in the human jejunum differs from that in the ileum[147,148]. The passive movement of salt and water resulting from the active sugar and amino acid absorption accounts for most salt and water absorption in the jejunum. By contrast, in the ileum most sodium and water movement is accounted for by active sodium absorption[147,148]. Using the triple-lumen perfusion technique, Fordtran et al.[145] showed that sodium absorption in the humen ileum occurs against a significant electrical (5–15 mV) and chemical gradient (110 mequiv.l^{-1}), while jejunal sodium absorption occurs in the presence of no electrical gradient (0 mV) and only a small chemical gradient (13 mequiv.l^{-1}).

In the jejunum, sodium movement is dramatically influenced by water movement and is markedly stimulated by addition of glucose, galactose, and bicarbonate. In the ileum, sodium movement is unaffected by rate direction of water flow and is unstimulated by the presence of glucose, galactose, or bicarbonate[145]. Apparently, the human ileum possesses an active, efficient sodium transport mechanism across the membrane and the ileum is relatively impermeable to sodium. The jejunum is different; only a small fraction of sodium absorption is mediated by active transport, coupled to either active absorption of bicarbonate or active secretion of hydrogen ions. Most sodium absorption in man, after ingestion of a meal, results from bulk water flow of solutions along osmotic pressure gradients[145]. Interestingly, sodium movement from the human jejunal lumen can occur when water movement is zero, namely when chloride concentration gradient is abolished by partial substitution with sodium sulphate in test solutions[149]. The conclusions from these jejunal perfusion studies are: (1) when net water flow is zero, sodium absorption is also zero if no concentration gradient exists to favour net NaCl diffusion, (2) the rate of sodium absorption is markedly influenced by bulk water flow, and (3) the p.d. between abraded skin and jejunal lumen is near zero when saline is perfused. These observations suggest that sodium absorption from saline is entirely passive in the human jejunum, but in the presence of sodium bicarbonate sodium is absorbed actively against electrochemical gradients[149].

When one considers bicarbonate absorption from the human jejunum, it appears that: (1) bicarbonate generates no potential difference between abraded skin and jejunal lumen, (2) it occurs against steep electrochemical gradients, (3) it generates high CO_2 tension in the jejunum, and (4) it is inhibited by acetazolamide (Diamox)[149]. These data suggest that bicarbonate absorption in the jejunum is mediated by active hydrogen secretion and that the link between sodium and bicarbonate transport is best explained by sodium hydrogen exchange (Figure 9.8).

Normal subjects absorb potassium as well as sodium and water from the jejunum, however, in contrast to patients suffering from non-tropical and tropical sprue who have diarrhoea and steatorrhoea and secrete water, sodium, and potassium into the intestinal lumen[147]. Important physiologic observations have been derived from the study of absorption in different diarrhoeal states. Thus, an interesting abnormality of electrolyte absorption was elucidated recently by the study of absorption in a patient who had congenital alkalosis with diarrhoea[150]. In this condition, it was found that: (1) chloride is not transported against electrochemical gradients, but is absorbed and secreted down an electrochemical gradient, (2) chloride secretion down an electrochemical gradient is increased by raising the bicarbonate concentration in the intestinal lumen, (3) sodium absorption occurs against electrochemical gradients and is associated with hydrogen ion secretion, (4) electrical potential difference is near zero between the lumen and blood when luminal sodium concentration is 140 mequiv.l^{-1}, (5) sodium diffusion potential is abnormal, and (6) potassium is transported passively in response to electrochemical gradients. The observed abnormalities of ileal electrolyte absorption is congenital alkalosis with diarrhoea were reproduced in healthy subjects by perfusing their ileum with a test solution in which chloride was replaced with poorly absorbed phosphate or sulphate. This study is important, since the findings can be explained by a single defect in the double-ion

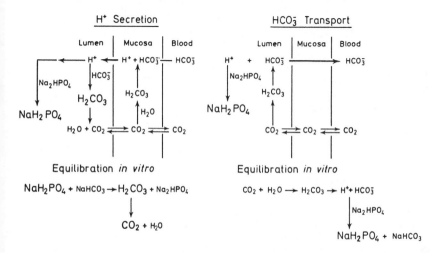

Figure 9.8 Two mechanisms for bicarbonate absorption in the jejunum. Hydrogen secretion, depicted on the left, generates a high CO_2 tension in luminal fluid. By contrast, HCO_3^- absorption acidifies luminal contents without generating excess CO_2. (From Turnberg et al.[149], by courtesy of *J. Clin. Invest.* and Rockefeller University Press)

exchange model in the ileum: $Na^+ \rightleftarrows H^+$, and $Cl^- \rightleftarrows HCO_3^-$ (Figure 9.9). In congenital alkalosis with diarrhoea, the chloride–bicarbonate exchange is incapable of transporting Cl^- against an electrochemical gradient, and yet it continues to transport anions passivley. The findings appear incompatible with the concept of an ileal electrogenic sodium transport.

In infants with acute diarrhoea (due to pathogenic *Escherichia coli* or non-specific causes), absorption of glucose from the jejunum is impaired[151]. In normal infants, infants with diarrhoea, and adults[147,148] net absorption of water and salt from the jejunum depends upon the proportion of glucose absorbed[151]. Thus, when the amount of non-absorbed glucose is high, salt and water moves into the bowel lumen according to osmotic gradients instead of being absorbed, thus creating the diarrhoeal state. Probably, then in diarrhoeal disease of infancy, impaired absorption of glucose or other sugars explains the mechanism of diarrhoeal stool production.

In cholera and other diarrhoeal illnesses, the situation is quite different. In cholera, the absorption of glucose and glucose-associated sodium and water absorption from the jejunum remains normal[152] while large amounts of fluid are secreted from an apparently normal mucosa. The observation has therapeutic significance, since fluid replacement can be either accomplished or assisted by oral administration of glucose-electrolyte solutions. The diarrhoea in cholera results from excessive secretion induced by the exotoxin released from *Vibrio cholerae*. The exotoxin, a macromolecule with a molecular weight of about 84 000, binds to the mucosa with an exposure as short

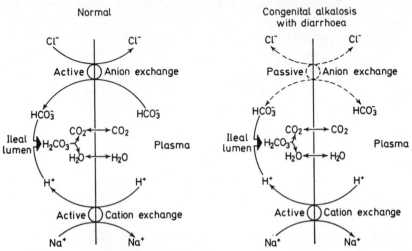

Figure 9.9 Model representing ileal electrolyte transport in normal subjects and in patient R.A. In normal subjects, both ion exchanges are active. In the patient with congenital alkalosis with diarrhoea, the cation exchange is active but the anion exchange is passive. (From Bieberdorf *et al.*[150], by courtesy of *J. Clin. Invest.* and Rockefeller University Press)

as 5 min. It stimulates secretion for more than 12 h. Cholera toxin increases the short-circuit current across isolated rabbit ileal mucosa and promotes net chloride movement from serosa to mucosa[153,154]. Whether the exotoxin stimulates the secretory cells directly or indirectly via local humoral mechanisms is unclear. Thus, evidence exists that the exotoxin activates adenylate cyclase in the cell wall of the secretory epithelium with a consequent increase in the levels of cyclic AMP (cAMP)[155]. From recent studies in rabbits, cholera toxin appears to contact the luminal side of the epithelial cells, but exerts its effect on the opposite side of the cell, namely the basal and lateral sides. After exposure to the toxin, adenylate cyclase activity at such sites increases, and Na^+, K^+-ATPase activity falls[156]. Intestinal secretion *in vivo* can be blocked by cycloheximide, an inhibitor of protein synthesis, in the rabbit model[157].

The triple-lumen perfusion technique was used to study the mechanisms of diarrhoea in nine patients with cholera and three with *E. coli*-induced diarrhoea[158]. All patients demonstrate net water and sodium secretion both in the jejunum and ileum. Both serosal-to-mucosal and mucosal-to-serosal unidirectional fluxes of sodium and water were increased, although the change in serosal-to-mucosal fluxes primarily accounted for the changes observed in producing the secretory state[158]. Fluid secretion was more pronounced in the jejunum than in the ileum.

The secretory mechanism in cholera is probably not unique. Apparently other bacterial toxins produced by many enteric bacteria act similarly. In addition, certain hormones such as glucagon and prostaglandins and other humoral factors produced by various neoplasms associated with diarrhoea (medullary thyroid carcinomas, carcinoids, non-gastrin-secreting adenomas of the pancreas, tumours of the sympathetic nervous system) may act via the same secretory mechanism[159].

Bile salts also influence absorption from the small bowel. Their mechanism of action is still unclear. Thus, it has been shown that free dihydroxy bile salts inhibit the absorption of water and electrolytes and, at higher concentrations, even induce secretion. The described effects depend on the intraluminal concentration of bile salts and are associated with mucosal damage only at high concentrations of bile salts[160]. A trihydroxy bile acid, cholic acid, fails to produce secretion whether present in the free of conjugated form. Nor do taurine conjugates of bile acids change fluid and electrolyte absorption. Specifically, deoxycholate in concentrations of 2.5–5 mM induce secretion of water and electrolytes and impair jejunal absorption of glucose and galactose. Cholate, taurocholate, and taurodeoxycholate, each at a concentration of 5 mM, are less effective inhibitors of glucose transport than deoxycholate and chenodeoxycholate. These observations may be relevant to the pathogenesis of diarrhoea in the blind-loop syndrome, since concentrations of unconjugated bile salts close to those used in the above study have been found in the bowel lumens of such patients[160].

The small intestinal absorption of sodium is influenced by many hormones such as ADH[167], pentagastrin[161-164], prostaglandins[154,165] secretin, and cholecystokinin[166]. ADH is man caused a decrease in net absorption of sodium and water[167]. The effect involves no changes in motility. Gastrin and pentagastrin have been found to decrease water, electrolyte, and glucose absorption in the canine jejunum and ileum[161], but the results in man appear controversial since decreases in absorption have been reported by some authors[162] but not by others[163]. However, the observations in patients with Zollinger–Ellison syndrome suggest that gastrin does affect the water and electrolyte absorption[164].

The effect of prostaglandins on absorption is interesting. PGE_1, when given intrajejunally during perfusion experiments in man ($40 \, \mu g \, kg^{-1} \, 45 \, min^{-1}$), produces a significant net secretion of water, sodium, chloride, bicarbonate, and potassium. In addition, glucose absorption decreases by about 25%. These changes in absorption could not be ascribed to accelerated transit time of the test solution via the test segment. Like cholera toxin, PGE_1 augments the plasma-to-lumen flux of water and electrolytes, but unlike cholera toxin, it decreases glucose absorption[165]. These findings in man resemble some previous observations in dogs[154].

While the experiments cited clearly indicate that hormones and certain toxins such as cholera promote a secretory mechanism in the small bowel which may be mediated by cyclic AMP, we do not know what regulatory mechanism, if any, these substances have under physiologic circumstances. However, one can reasonably speculate that certain hormones contribute significantly to the regulation of net fluid and electrolyte absorption from the bowel.

9.9 WATER SOLUBLE VITAMINS

The water-soluble vitamins contain widely different compounds. The general principles applying to the absorption of other compounds apply to this group of substances as well; namely, un-ionised compounds, weak acids, and weak bases (especially those of low molecular weight) are steadily absorbed, while strong electrolytes or large molecules are poorly absorbed[128]. Vitamin B_{12} and choline are two exceptions. The low-molecular weight compounds such as pyridoxine hydrochloride (mol. wt. 205), riboflavin (mol. wt. 376), nicotinamide, inositol, p-aminobenzoic acid, ascorbic acid, and biotin diffuse readily across the intestinal barrier.

With riboflavin, no evidence of saturation of the absorption mechanism exists with doses up to 20 mg. It is readily absorbed from the upper small bowel of man despite the fact that in the rat its main site of absorption is the ileum[168]. Pyridoxine is rapidly absorbed from the proximal small bowel in man and rats; the linear relationship between dose given and absorption is compatible with the mechanism of simple diffusion[168]. Biotin is actively transported in some species but not in others. Choline is a strong base and fairly well absorbed, suggesting its absorption by an active transport system in the small bowel[128]. Ascorbic acid (mol. wt. 176) is rapidly absorbed from the proximal small intestine in humans. No active transport of ascorbic acid is evident in the rat or hamster. Current data suggest that the water-soluble vitamins (except for vitamin B_{12}, folic acid, and choline) are absorbed by passive diffusion[169] in the upper small bowel.

9.9.1 Absorption of thiamine

Thiamine, a large and highly basic molecule, is poorly absorbed, 5 mg day^{-1} being the maximal oral intake for man without faecal loss. Recent studies indicate that two processes, one active and one passive, are involved in the transport of thiamine across the small intestine in many animal species[170]. In humans, the maximal absorptive capacity was found to be limited[171]. At high luminal concentrations thiamine is absorbed by passive diffusion, whereas at low concentrations, it is absorbed both *in vivo* and *in vitro* by an active process[170]. Diffusion and a carrier-mediated mechanism have both been proposed to explain entry of thiamine into the intestinal cell. Diffusion occurs down a concentration gradient from higher levels in the mucosal fluid to lower levels in mucosal cells. Concentrations of thiamine inside the cells reach an equilibrium with that of the mucosal fluid. Simple diffusion does not explain entry of thiamine into the cell, because metabolic inhibitors, thiamine analogues, and lack of sodium all depress thiamine content in mucosal cells[170,172].

Carrier-mediated entry of thiamine into the cell is the principal mechanism for thiamine absorption when the vitamin is present in small amounts in the intestinal lumen. This carrier-mediated mechanism depends either on thiamine phosphorylation–dephosphorylation coupling or on some metabolic–energetic mechanism, possibly activated by Na^+. Similar conclusions were reached after studies of thiamine uptake by *E. coli*[173].

An active mechanism for transport of thiamine out of intestinal cells exists because the concentration of thiamine in the mucosal cell is always lower than in the serosal fluid. The presence of Na^+ is necessary, both for the entry and exit of thiamine from the cell[172]. Exit of thiamine is linked to normal function of ATPase at the serosal pole of mucosal cells[170].

Several other substances, including basic amino acids[174], pyrimidines[175], d-xylose[176], vitamin B_{12}[177], choline[178] and folic acid[179], share with thiamine the dual mechanism of absorption, namely: (1) an active process that operates at low physiological concentrations, and (2) passive diffusion that takes place in the presence of high luminal concentrations.

9.9.2 Folic acid

Folic acid (pteroylglutamic acid) contains two carboxyl groups and has a molecular weight of 441. The molecule contains glutamic acid, p-aminobenzoic acid, and pteridine components. The polyglutamic form of folate, for example, has a molecular weight of 1215, has a large molecular radius, and is strongly electronegative and highly water-soluble at a physiological pH. It cannot be absorbed intact and therefore must undergo enzymatic conversion by intestinal conjugase γ-glutamyl carboxidase (located in the mitochrondrial lysosomal fraction of intestinal cells) to the monoglutamic form before absorption takes place[180]. The site of hydrolysis, whether at the brush border, within the intestinal cell, or in the lumen, is undetermined. The mode of folate transport across the cell membrane is unclear. Folate appears to be absorbed throughout the small intestine, most being absorbed in the duodenum and upper jejunum. Folate in the monoglutamic form is more soluble at a pH above 7, a fact which is probably important in absorption, since a slightly faster rate of folate absorption was found in patients with achlorhydria[181]. After absorption, folic acid can be found in the serum in the monoglutamic form. During active absorption, the serum folate is actually a mixture of recently absorbed folate and folate originating from the tissues[182]. About 60% to 70% of serum folate is losely bound to serum protein. Cellular folate exists mostly in the polyglutamic form; usually up to seven glutamic acid molecules are added to each folate molecule. This form of folate is trapped in the cell until it is destroyed or the glutamic acid is split off to return the folate to its monoglutamine form. There is reason to believe that, of the available folate for absorption, as much as 50% cannot be absorbed because of the 'inefficiency' of conversion of polyglutamic folate to the monoglutamic form.

In the rat, small physiological quantities of folate are absorbed by an active energy-requiring process which can function against a concentration gradient in the upper third of the intestine[183-184]. Large quantities of folate can be absorbed by mass action along the entire length of the rat small bowel[183]. In the everted rat intestine, folate absorption is inhibited by 2,4-dinitrophenol and decreased by irradiation. Addition of ATP reverses the irradiation-induced inhibition, suggesting that ATP is required for folate transport[185]. When a double-lumen tube perfusion technique is used in man, folic acid is actively transported in the duodenum and jejunum[186].

9.9.3 Vitamin B_{12} absorption

Vitamin B_{12} is a water-soluble vitamin with a molecular weight of 1355 and a molecular radius of 8 Å. It is synthesised almost exclusively by micro-organisms. The absorption of physiological doses (2 µg or less) of vitamin B_{12} requires the presence of intrinsic factor (IF), a carrier glycoprotein-Castle's factor. Physiological vitamin B_{12} absorption requires three major steps: (1) IF combines with free vitamin B_{12} to form the IF–B_{12} complex, (2) IF–B_{12} complex is absorbed in the ileum by attaching to receptors on the brush border (the attachment being aided by divalent cations, especially calcium or magnesium at alkaline pH), and (3) B_{12} enters the absorptive cells in the ileum. Large non-physiological doses of vitamin B_{12} can be absorbed from the mucosa without intrinsic factor by so called 'mass action'[179,187].

Experiments in man during surgery suggest that IF is present in the small intestine. Whether IF is present in a free form, however, or whether it is attracted there to receptors remains unclear[188]. EDTA instilled via a jejunal tube in man markedly reduces the absorption of physiological doses of vitamin B_{12}, while the administration of calcium, magnesium, or strontium counteracts this effect[189-190].

How B_{12} is absorbed after the attachment of B_{12}–IF complex to the receptor remains largely unknown. In that respect, experiments on the mechanism of vitamin B_{12} deprivation by *Diphyllobothrium latum* are of interest. Evidently, this tapeworm has a factor that liberates B_{12} from the IF[191] more efficiently than high concentrations of cyanocobalamin[191]. Perhaps, a 'releasing factor' is also present in the intestinal lumen or at the mucosal surface, resembling that found in the tapeworm.

The nature of the so-called receptor to which the B_{12}–IF complex is absorbed has thus far defied biochemical characterisation. After absorption, labelled vitamin B_{12} appears in the mitochondria[192]. The radioactivity later decreases with a concomitant rise in hepatic radioactivity, suggesting the release of B_{12} from the mitochondria for transport to the liver. The role of the pancreas in vitamin B_{12} absorption has attracted attention since both experimental and clinical evidence suggests a role for 'a pancreatic factor' in B_{12} absorption[193]. Toske *et al.*[193] found B_{12} malabsorption in 9 of 22 patients with pancreatic insufficiency. None of these patients had IF deficiency, nor was the B_{12} malabsorption related to pH or calcium content of aspirated ileal contents. Administration of pancreatic extracts and bicarbonate improved the B_{12} absorption. Malabsorption of vitamin B_{12} may occur with any condition that damages gastric parietal cells, IF action, and/or ileal mucosal cells. These conditions include pernicious anaemia, chronic atrophic gastritis, total and subtotal gastrectomy, ileal resections, tropical and non-tropical sprue, fish-tapeworm infestation, and so-called selective B_{12} malabsorption states. Why IF secretion is absent in pernicious anaemia remains unknown. Selective vitamin B_{12} malabsorption has been described previously[187].

9.10 IRON

Recently, authors ably summarised information about iron absorption[194-196]. Each day, 1–2 mg of iron is absorbed, an amount equal to the daily loss. The absorbed iron travels to the portal circulation with significant uptake by the lymphatics. According to classical concepts, the ferrous ion passes from the intestinal lumen into the mucosal cell where it oxidised to the ferric form. The ferric ion as ferric hydroxide phosphate combines with apoferritin, leading to the formation of ferritin. The ferritin ion is reduced to the ferrous form at the vascular surface of the mucosal cell, and after entering the bloodstream, combines with a globulin called transferrin. If the iron concentration is high in the intestinal contents, iron is absorbed directly into the plasma, by-passing the ferritin-forming step. Iron equilibrium is maintained by a balance between iron loss and iron absorption. Iron absorption is more active than excretion in regulating the iron equilibrium. The simplest model for iron absorption should explain the mucosal uptake of dietary iron and the transfer of iron from the intestinal cells into the body. A model that provides anatomic localisation for studying regulatory factors in intraluminal, absorptive cell, and corporeal sites is shown in Figure 9.10.

The intraluminal factors are listed in Table 9.2 dietary iron content being

Table 9.2 Intraluminal factors affecting iron absorption

Increase absorption	Decrease absorption
Dietary	*Chelates*
Dose	Oxalate
Absorption proportional to amount	Phytate
Valency	Phosphate
Ferrous is better absorbed than ferric	
Reducing compounds	
Amino acids	
Sugars	
Alcohol	
Ascorbic acid	
Succinic acid	
Gastric factors	*Gastroferrin*
HCl	
Intrinsic factor	
Stabilising factor	
Pancreas	*Bicarbonate*
Secretions	
Other than bicarbonate	
Intestinal enzymes	

the most important. Dietary ingredients and intestinal secretions that precipitate iron or cause macromolecular aggregations of iron decrease absorption. Haemoglobin iron is absorbed more efficiently from food than inorganic iron[195-196]; more ferrous iron is absorbed than ferric iron; dietary constituents that solubilise iron enhance absorption. EDTA (ethylenediaminetetra-acetate) is a sequestering agent for metal, forming a stable water-soluble iron chelate which inactivates the metal ion and decreases absorption. In contrast, certain amino acids and sugars form less stable complexes that hold iron in solution even at weakly alkaline or neutral pH. These ligands facilitate the absorption of iron from alkaline duodenum. Actually, certain amino acids and sugars

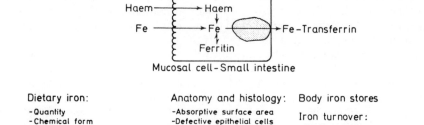

Luminal   Mucosal   Corporeal

Mucosal cell-Small intestine

Dietary iron:
- Quantity
- Chemical form
- Physical form

Chelation and precipitation:
- Dietary composition
- Intestinal secretions

Intestinal motility

Anatomy and histology:
- Absorptive surface area
- Defective epithelial cells
- Blood flow
- Mucosal lifespan

Mucosal iron content:
- Quantity
- Chemical form

Body iron stores

Iron turnover:
- Erythropoiesis
- Sideroblastic disorders
- Anabolism-catabolism
- Reticuloendothelial block

Hypoxia

Idiopathic haemochromatosis

Figure 9.10 Dietary iron is absorbed primarily in the proximal small intestine either as inorganic iron or haem. Iron is split from haem. within intestinal epithelial cells and is transferred into the body in an inorganic form. Many factors affect iron absorption. They are listed above according to the anatomic area where they exert an effect. (From Conrad[261], by courtesy of *Gastroenterology*)

depolymerise and solubilise iron to enhance absorption. All metal-precipitating agents, such as oxalates and phosphates, form insoluble salts with iron which are poorly absorbed. Gastrointestinal enzymes aid iron absorption indirectly by releasing sugars and amino acids from dietary sources. However, it is unclear whether individual enzymes directly affect iron absorption. Gastric juice contains a 'stabilising factor' which solubilises iron at the duodenal pH. This may be either a B_{12}-binding protein or endogenous ascorbic acid secreted into the stomach. Another substance that binds iron and decreases iron absorption is found in gastric juice and is called gastroferrin Gastrectomy and pernicious anaemia are associated with decreased absorption of dietary iron. Alcohol ingestion enhances the absorption of ferric but not ferrous iron. Ligation of bile ducts of normal rats lead to a significant decrease in iron absorption from ferrous and ferric chloride. In iron-deficient rats, however, the absorption is decreased from ferric chloride but not from ferrous chloride.

The exocrine pancreas plays a controversial role in iron absorption. In experimental animals, destruction of the acinar pancreas enhances iron absorption. An analogous situation occurs in patients with pancreatic insufficiency secondary to chronic pancreatitis and cystic fibrosis. The addition of sodium bicarbonate to solutions of ferrous sulphate markedly enhances the formation of macromolecular iron and reduces the absorption of iron by animals and man. Secretin stimulation has similar effects. The findings explain the elevated iron absorption in conditions where bicarbonate secretion is low (e.g. pancreatic insufficiency and experimental destruction of the pancreas). In the absence of HCl and bile, iron-depleted animals can still absorb increased quantities of iron; the same is true when bicarbonate is increased. These findings suggest that intraluminal factors are less important regulators of iron absorption than the body's iron requirements.

The absorptive cells in the duodenum act as an iron pool located between the plasma and intestinal lumen. The mucosal cell iron content seems to regulate, within limits, the quantity of iron entering these cells from the intestinal lumen. However, this does not regulate the transfer of iron from the mucosal cells into the plasma. How the absorptive cells are informed of corporeal iron requirements remains unclear, as well as how the mucosal content of iron influences its serosal transfer. The concept of control of iron absorption by the cells is depicted in Figure 9.11.

The corporeal iron needs determining iron absorption are the size of the iron stores and the activity of the erythroid marrow. For example, iron absorption rises in iron-deficiency anaemia and in non-anaemic subjects with decreased iron stores, while it drops in persons with excess iron stores. Other factors stimulating erythropoiesis also increase iron absorption, e.g. acute haemorrhage, haemolysis, and ascent to high altitudes. Factors that depress the erythroid marrow (e.g. radiation, starvation, hypertransfusion, and return to a normal environment after oxygen lack) also depress iron absorption. In certain cirrhotic individuals and patients with sideroclastic hypochromic anaemia, iron absorption may increase without iron stores being depleted, erythropoiesis becoming accelerated. Perhaps the increased iron turnover in these patients is related to enhanced iron absorption.

Orally ingested iron is taken up largely in the duodenum and upper jejunum, but any segment of small bowel can take up reduced iron placed in contact with the mucosa. The duodenum performs somewhat better than the rest of the gut in isolated gut preparations and also *in vivo*. Luminal pH and the redox potential may particularly influence iron absorption in this area[194]. However, *in vitro* experiments on everted sacs of rats showed that iron absorption was maximal in the duodenum and decreased progressively toward the ileum[197], showing that the duodenal ability for increased absorption is not only pH-dependent. In these experiments, transport of iron against a concentration gradient occurred nowhere in the intestine[197]. These findings contrast with data from previous experiments performed mostly with intestinal sacs prepared from dead animals and from experiments involving incubation periods longer than 90 min. Iron deficiency enhanced iron absorption both *in vivo* and *in vitro*[197]. Apparently the iron content of the intestinal epithelial cells regulates the rate of iron uptake by the enterocyte. Iron transport across the proximal small intestine of the rat may involve

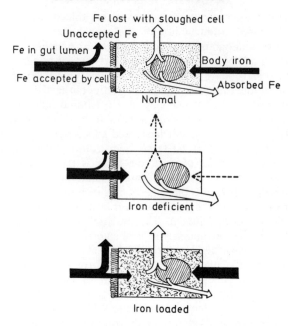

Fe lost with sloughed cell

Unaccepted Fe

Fe in gut lumen

Fe accepted by cell

Body iron

Absorbed Fe

Normal

Iron deficient

Iron loaded

Figure 9.11 A concept of control of iron by the intestinal mucosa. It is predicted that iron absorption is regulated primarily through the columnar epithelium of the small intestine. In normal iron-replete subjects the mucosal cells may contain a variable amount of iron supplied from the body store. This deposit regulates (within limits) the quantity of iron which can enter the cell from the gut lumen. After the iron has entered the cell, it may proceed into the body to fulfil a requirement. Alternatively a portion of the iron may become fixed in the epithelial cytoplasm to be lost when the cell is sloughed at the end of its life span. Iron deficient subjects apparently possess little or no mechanism to inhibit entrance of iron into the villous epithelial cells or to retain it. Thus dietary iron readily proceeds into the body. In iron-loaded subjects, the body iron incorporated in the epithelial cells is eventually lost, but during the lifespan of the cells its presence inhibits the entrance of iron into the cells. (From Conrad and Crosby[260], by courtesy of *Blood* and Grune and Stratton)

a carrier mechanism that responds adaptively to iron deficiency but not to iron overload[197]. Two interesting genetic defects of iron absorption have been recently described in mice, one involving an inability to transfer iron from the intestinal mucosal cell to the plasma[198], and the other involving an inability to transfer it from the intestinal lumen to the mucosa[199]. The first defect was found in x-linked anaemia of mice (gene symbol SLA). This anaemia is microcytic and hypochromic; stainable iron stores are reduced in these animals. The genetically determined defect in the intestinal mucosa of these mice is probably due to deficiency of an enzyme or a carrier substance necessary for the normal transfer of iron from the intestinal mucosal cell to the plasma[198]. Impaired iron transfer from the intestinal lumen to the mucosa occurs in mice with hereditary microcytic anaemia (gene symbol MK)[199]. Interestingly, the same mice also have difficulty transferring iron from the plasma into the erythroblast. These two genetic defects in iron transport from and into the mucosal cell suggest that one carrier or enzyme is necessary for iron to enter the cell, and another for iron to leave.

The route by which iron passes via the duodenal mucosa while moving from lumen to blood has been studied using high-resolution autoradiography with ^{55}Fe as the tracer[200]. During the first 24 h after instillation of ^{55}Fe into the stomach of normal mice, two phases of iron absorption are seen: (1) iron is taken up quickly by the brush border of the absorptive cell and the terminal web, and (2) it localises in areas rich in rough endoplasmic reticulum and free ribosomes, whereupon iron is rapidly transferred to the vessels of the lamina propria without evidence of any specific cell acting as a 'carrier'. The second phase occurs 3–24 h after iron installation. The uptake of iron by the absorptive cell and its transfer to the lamina propria appear minimal during this period. The iron is found mainly close to rough endoplasmic reticulum and free ribosomes; only a small amount is seen over ferritin granules and lysosomes[200]. Radioiron is not observed in significant amounts over mitochrondria, nuclei, of Golgi zones[200], but is localised over close to the lateral cell membrane. These studies seem to indicate that mitochrondria are not directly involved in the process of transfer or storage of absorbed iron. Moreover goblet, Paneth, argentaffin, and undifferentiated cells of the duodenum apparently take no part in the process of iron absorption. The presence of iron in the region of rough endoplasmic reticulum and areas rich in free ribosomes but poor in ferritin, at all times during the study, suggests that another pool of iron exists besides ferritin, and that it plays a part in iron absorption. This could represent an iron-binding protein[200]. Other studies also cast serious doubt upon the importance of ferritin as a regulator of iron absorption[201]. Thus, although the duodenum of the iron-deficient rat contains little ferritin, the intraduodenal administration of iron rapidly induces the synthesis of ferritin protein. In addition, ferritin synthesis by the duodenum of the iron-deficient rat equals that by the duodenum of the iron-replete control after iron administration[201]. When the ferritin content of the duodenum of iron-deficient rats is raised to a level beyond that of iron-replete rats by previous intraluminal administration of iron, iron absorption is not reduced to the level of control animals (as one would expect if ferritin were the sole regulator of iron absorption). The function of ferritin is unclear, but it may be related to a protective mechanism for detoxification of iron that is not transported to the plasma from the cell for eventual loss by desquamation of mucosal cells, as proposed by Crosby[202].

The relationship between cobalt and iron absorption has been studied by several groups of investigators[203-205]. Both elements are absorbed in the proximal intestine of the rat and seem to share a common absorptive pathway. Cobalt does not decrease iron absorption by a non-specific toxic effect upon the gut or by competing for intraluminal compounds that enhance iron absorption[203]. Cobalt is not incorporated into ferritin, suggesting that ferritin is not involved in any absorptive mechanism common to iron and cobalt. The capability of ferritin to hold absorbed iron in intestinal cells and prevent the transfer of unneeded iron into the body, diminishes iron but not cobalt absorption[203]. The absorption of cobalt and iron in the rat seems to be mediated by a transport system in which two processes occur simultaneously; one is limited by the concentration of the metal in the intestinal lumen, and the second depends on the activity of a mchanism which displays saturation kinetics[205]. The first process prevails when iron stores are replete and the second predominates in the presence of iron deficiency[205]. Cobalt absorption is high in patients with idiopathic haemochromatosis and portal cirrhosis complicated by other endogenous iron overload or iron deficiency; presumably this increase is due to disturbed iron metabolism[204]. In chronic renal disease, alterations in iron absorption are related to disturbances in iron balance and not the presence of renal disease or azotaemia[196]

Administration of phenobarbital, an enzyme inducer, to rats enhances the absorption of inorganic iron and haemoglobin iron *in vivo* and *in vitro*[206]. This phenobarbital-mediated increase in absorption is probably related to an increased synthesis of carrier substance that influences iron transport. Phenobarbital also produces partial reversal of the defect in iron absorption that was previously induced by either iron-loading or treatment with cycloheximide. Phenobarbital would seem to primarily affect the mucosal exit step of iron from the intestinal mucosa[206].

9.11 CALCIUM ABSORPTION

Calcium absorption from the small intestine, studied extensively in animals, involves an active transport mechanism[207-208]. Wensel *et al.*[209], using triple-lumen tube perfusion, measured calcium absorption at various sites along the small intestine and found that the proximal small bowel took up more calcium than the distal small bowel. Basically their studies agreed with previous animal experiments[208]. Calcium flux from the intestinal lumen to the blood was two to three times higher in the duodenojejunal area of the intestine than in the ileal area. Calcium could be absorbed against a concentration gradient and the proportion of absorption varied with intraluminal concentration to a point where the absorption mechanism appeared saturated. Birge and co-workers[210], using radioisotope dilution, found that half the isotopic calcium was absorbed when instilled proximal to the duodenum, compared with 32% absorption when the labelled calcium was injected 4 cm distal to the ligament of Treitz. While the duodenum showed superior absorptive ability, however, it was least sensitive to the enhancing effects of parathyroid hormone on intestinal calcium absorption. The gut distal to the duodenum was most responsive. The effect of parathyroid hormone on intestinal calcium was delayed until 3–5 h after its administration, when one normally sees the peak effect of parathyroid hormone on phosphate transport in the kidney. Calcium-loading, even in amounts as small as 100 mg caused a significant decrease in the uptake of isotopic calcium.

Schachter and Rosen[211] using everted sacs of guinea-pig, rabbit, and rat intestine showed that calcium is actively transported against a concentration gradient. They noted that oxidative metabolism is necessary for the active transport of calcium, and that an agent capable of uncoupling aerobic phosphorylation (2,4-dinitrophenol) inhibits calcium transport. This led them to conclude that such transport depended specifically upon the generation of phosphate-bond energy. In addition, they found that Mg^{2+} and Co^{2+} appeared to compete for calcium by consistently causing a decrease in the mucosal-to-serosal flux of Ca^{2+}. A dependence of intestinal calcium absorption upon dietary vitamin D was observed when calcium uptake rose significantly in animals given supplemental vitamin D in addition to a rachitic diet.

Wasserman[212] and others indicated that the percentage of absorbed intraluminal calcium declined as the intraluminal calcium concentration increased from 1–5 mM, with a plateau response existing between 5 and 125 mM. Absorption rate dropped even more dramatically above that concentration. Analysis of observed curves suggests that an intestinal calcium pump exists that becomes saturated when intraluminal Ca^{2+} exceeds 2–5 mM. Work by Schachter and co-workers[211,213,214] indicates that calcium is absorbed in two steps, one involving uptake from the lumen into the mucosa, and the second involving uptake from the mucosa to the underlying layers. The first step depends only partially upon oxidative metabolism[214], a conclusion by the work of Wasserman[215], who found that calcium uptake by mucosa of everted chick duodenum was enhanced by vitamin D and was not significantly affected by NaCN anerobiosis or 2,4-dinitrophenol.

Studies by Rasmussen et al.[216] studying isolated intestinal villi, produced somewhat different results. Some metabolic inhibitors (dicumarol, 2,4-dinitrophenol and NaCN) suppressed calcium accumulation, while others had no effect. In addition, villi obtained from vitamin-D-deficient rats were able to accumulate and release calcium nearly as efficiently as villi obtained from animals with normal vitamin D levels. Wasserman[217] explained these differences by assuming that in isolated villi the major route of calcium entry is across the serosal and lateral aspects of the tissue (as opposed to transport across the brush border membrane in intact tissue). This, to him, indicated that calcium entry into the cell across non-luminal surfaces depends upon metabolism but is unaffected by vitamin D

Table 9.3   Steps in absorption of calcium from the gut

   I. *Flux from lumen to mucosal cell*
     A. Not dependent on oxidative metabolism
     B. Vitamin-D-dependent
     C. Not regularly saturated by Ca^{2+}

  II. *Flux from mucosal cell to plasma*
     A. Active transport by pump probably located on or near basal and/or lateral surfaces
       1. Functionally significant at low intraluminal levels of calcium
       2. Energy-dependent
       3. Vitamin-D-dependent
     B. Non-active mechanism at high intraluminal calcium levels
       1. Vitamin-D-dependent

 III. *Flux from plasma to mucosal cell*
     A. Not affected by vitamin D
     B. Possibly involves energy-dependent and heat-sensitive components

 IV. *Flux from mucosal cell to lumen*
     A. Vitamin-D-dependent
     B. Dependent on transconcentration

Wasserman[217] has summarised the steps that may involved in intestinal calcium absorption, as shown in Table 9.3.

The lag period required before vitamin D stimulates calcium absorption suggests that the response may be due to the synthesis of a protein involved in calcium transport. The formation of such a protein has been described in several different animals in the past[218-220]. In the chick intestine, Wasserman and Taylor[221] reported some correlation between the amount of calcium binding protein present and the capacity of the intestine to absorb calcium.

Two calcium-binding proteins have been described in the human duodenum[222]. In size, one of them (mol. wt. 20 000) resembles the calcium-binding protein sensitive to vitamin D described in the chick and monkey.

Several studies have indicated that glucocorticoids may affect the intestinal absorption of calcium[223-225]. The action of cortisone on intestinal calcium transport appears to be that of an antivitamin D effect, although the exact mechanisms have not been described. The work of Kimberg et al.[226] suggests that the antivitamin D effect follows the metabolism of vitamin D to 25-hydroxycholecalciferol, since the administration of this compound does not reverse or inhibit the inhibitory effects of cortisone on calcium transport in the rat duodenum in vitro.

9.12 COLONIC ABSORPTION

In man, the colon performs several important tasks, but life is possible without this organ. Excreta are stored in the colon until they can be conveniently eliminated. Colonic absorption is limited primarily to salt and water. Sodium is actively absorbed and water follows passively. As a result, the liquid ileal contents are converted to semisolid faeces in the large intestine. The storage and absorptive abilities of the colon vary greatly from person to person, a fact that may be at least partly explained by the large differences in colonic volume and surface area. Thus, the human colon varies in length from 90 to 150 cm, and its surface area varies from 636 to 1613 cm^2. The estimated colonic pore size in man is 2.1 Å[227]. Thus colon is a much 'tighter' membrane than the jejunum or ileum. The mucosal potential difference (p.d.) is 30–40 mV, much larger than that found in the small bowel.

In the past, the amount of water and solutes absorbed from the colon in healthy humans was indirectly estimated by comparing the volume and contents of ileal effluent in patients with total colectomies to the amount of water and electrolytes lost in the faeces of healthy subjects[228]. Such estimates of colonic function were indirect at best and assumed that ileostomy effluent of patients after total colectomy equalled colonic inflow in health. Because this assumption is probably invalid (colectomy may alter small bowel function), ileal flow in to the healthy colon was estimated by sampling ileal contents after an infusion of markers[229]. The experiments suggested that the amount of ileal effluent entering the healthy colon is about three times larger than the volume estimated from studies done in patients with ileostomies. In normal humans, about 1.5 l of water, 200 mequiv. of sodium, 100 mequiv. of chloride, and 10 mequiv. of potassium enter the healthy colon daily, and 90% of the entering water and salt is absorbed in 24 h by the large intestine[229] (Figure 9.12).

Under physiological conditions, most water and sodium are absorbed in the ascending and transverse colon while the sodium concentration in these regions remains high. In the descending colon and sigmoid colon, the amounts of salt and water absorbed are smaller, but sodium is absorbed against greater concentration gradient so that the colonic sodium concentration is sharply reduced.

Colonic perfusion by peroral intubation with a water-soluble non-absorbable marker permits direct quantitative measurement of absorption of water and solutes from the large intestine in conscious humans[230]. Under steady-state conditions, quantitative measurements of water and solute

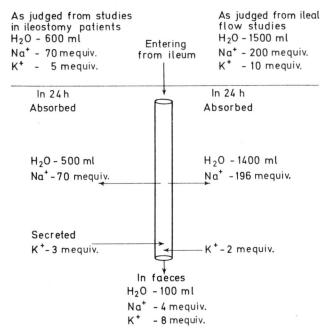

Figure 9.12 Quantitative indirect estimates of colonic absorptive capacity

absorption are obtained. This technique is tedious and certainly uncomfortable and it actually measures absorption under conditions of an artificially induced diarrhoea. However, the data are reproducible from hour to hour and from day to day in the same subjects[231]. The marker usually used in such experiments is polyethylene glycol (PEG), with a mean molecular weight of 4000; it is almost totally recovered in rectal effluent after traversing the entire colon[232]. When the colon is perfused with normal saline at 10 ml min^{-1}, the organ absorbs 0.24 mequiv. min^{-1} of sodium, 1.7 ml min^{-1} of water, and 0.39 mequiv. min^{-1} of chloride; it secretes 0.031 mequiv. min^{-1} of potassium and 0.18 mequiv. min^{-1} of bicarbonate[230]. If this rate of absorption were maintained for 24 h, the colon would have absorbed 2.45 l of water, 403 mequiv. of sodium, and 562 mequiv. of chloride; it would have secreted 45 mequiv. of potassium, and 259 mequiv. of bicarbonate[230] (Figure 9.13).

Both from isotonic and hypertonic solutions, water absorption from perfusates decreases with declining Na^+ concentrations. Also, bile salts decrease absorption from the colon[233]. While the precise colonic absorptive reserve may be debatable, it certainly exists and is extremely useful to compensate for the decreased absorptive ability of the small bowel in disease states. When the colonic absorptive ability is overloaded, diarrhoea results, and mainly small bowel contents are lost from the body. However, in addition, potassium is added to this fluid while it traverses the overtaxed colon, and K^+ loss is substantial. These pathophysiological factors must be considered when one plans fluid replacement in diarrhoeal states. Most of the water and solute absorption occurs in the right side of the colon[230]. These findings may be explained either by great permeability of the right side than the left, or by the presence or a larger mucosal area[227] on the right. In contrast to the right side of the colon, the rectum is relatively impermeable to water and salt[234-235]. This may be due either to a smaller pore radius than in other parts of the colon or because of a reduced pore density.

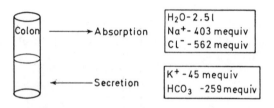

Figure 9.13 Capacity of colon in 24 h as judged from perfusion experiments

Hormones influence colonic absorption. For example, the colonic absorption of water and salt is influenced by pharmacological doses of mineralocorticoids[231, 236-237]. Increased absorption of sodium and salt are invariably induced by mineralocorticoid administration. Mineralocorticoids have also been found to modify the transmural p.d. in the direction of increased absorption[238]. Interestingly, the p.d. increases a few hours after the hormone is given, persisting as long as the mineralocorticoids are administered. Other authors, however, claim that potassium secretion is predominantly affected by the administration of exogenous mineralocorticoids[239] and that aldosterone-producing tumours increase K^+ losses into the colonic lumen[240]. These conflicting observations during colonic perfusion experiments may be accounted for by differences in experimental technics. Clearly, however, all studies show an effect of exogenous mineralcoritcoids on absorption from the colon. The unresolved question is whether mineralocorticoids play a physiological role in regulating salt and water absorption from the colon. We were unable to decrease salt and water absorption from the normal colon by giving spironolactone, an aldosterone antagonist, for periods up to 7 days in healthy volunteers[241]. These experiments suggest either that aldosterone plays no significant role in the normal regulation of colonic salt and water absorption or that spironolactone as given could not block the effect of aldosterone at the colonic level.

Angiotensin is another hormone affecting salt and water transport from the colon. Some of the data on the action of angiotensin conflict. Thus, some authors found stimulated transport of water and solutes in the rat colon[242], while no such effect was documented in the toad colon. Some of these different results can be explained by the presence of a biphasic dose-dependent effect of angiotensin, as shown by Parsons and Munday[243]. They used open-ended, everted, stripped colonic sacs from adrenalectomised and nephrectorised rats. Angiotensin at a concentation of 10^{-10} g ml^{-1} had no effect on transport. At higher concentrations, solute and water transport was inhibited, and at lower concentrations the transport rate was stimulated. Interestingly, at low concentrations angiotensin stimulates transport not only from the rat small bowel and colon, but also across frog skin. Studies using inhibitors suggest that the angiotensin-induced stimulation of fluid transport is secondary to an effect on protein synthesis at the ribosome level and that this results in the translation of precoded RNA to yield a protein associated with fluid transport[243]. In contrast to mineralocorticoids, antidiuretic hormone (ADH) was found to consistently decrease sodium, chloride, and water absorption from the human colon[244]. This effect may be due to a more rapid transit time of the test solution from caecum to rectum during ADH administration. Bile salts and glycine and tuarine conjugates also lower salt and water absorption in man[233]. Hydroxy fatty acids (OHFA) can produce colonic secretion of water and electrolytes. Ricinoleic acid produced such effects on the rat colon. Possibly OHFA contributes to the production of diarrhoea in patients with steatorrhoea[245].

Recent experiments have shown that certain diuretics, such as chlorothiazide decrease salt and water absorption from the intact healthy human colon[246]. While the precise mechanism of the action of diuretics on the colon remains to be established, the effect seems to take place at the cellular level and resembles that in the kidney.

Salt and water absorption is decreased when the colonic mucosa is inflamed[247-248]. In chronic constipation, colonic absorption of salt and water is increased. This change is probably due to a slower transit of colon contents through this organ[249] (Table 9.4).

The following conclusions about colonic absorption summarise much current information.

Table 9.4 Factors influencing water and electrolyte absorption from the intact human colon

Increase absorption	Decrease absorption
Salt depletion	Low Na$^+$ concentration in colonic contents (below 25 mequiv. l^{-1})
Mineralocorticoids	ADH
Angiotensin	Bile salts
Slow transit	Diuretics
	Hydroxy fatty acids (OHFA)
	Inflammatory changes

Sodium absorption from the human colon is an active process. Sodium moves from mucosa to serosa against bulk water flow and against electro-chemical gradients[227,241,250]. On the other hand, potassium movement occurs along electrochemical gradients and can be explained by passive diffusion. The normal colon has a negative mucosal potential difference (30–40 mV), favouring potassium secretion[240]. Sodium absorption seems to be the primary function of colonic absorption in man[227,229-230,239,241,250-252]. The bio-chemical mechanisms for 'active' sodium transport are undefined in man. In the rat colon, however, a Na^+, K^+-activated ATPase is important, and its activity is increased by aldosterone. Water in the colon moves from the mucosa to the serosa passively along osmotic gradients that result from electro-lyte absorption.

Sodium and chloride can be absorbed from the colon against a large concentration gradient. Bicarbonate is secreted into the colonic contents against concentration gradients, against negative mucosal p.d., and against bulk water flow. Chloride absorption is linked to bicarbonate secretion and seems to be an active process. The direction and extent of net water movement influence the movement of chloride, bicarbonate, and potassium[240]. Glucose absorption from the colon and rectum is insignificant[253]. The colon does not possess a sodium non-electrolyte coupling mechanism. Short-chain fatty acids are absorbed from the colon. Thus, the entire colon absorbs as much hexanoic acid as a 30 cm jejunal segment[254]. Quantitative data about the rates of absorption of amino acids and vitamins from the human colon are needed. The human colon is relatively impermeable to urea[227,255].

9.13 CONCLUDING REMARKS

Our understanding of absorptive mechanisms leaves much unsettled. The molecular, biochemical, and physiochemical events during transport in and out of the intestinal cells await deciphering. New knowledge often compli-cates some of our simplistic concepts. For example, a newly recognised factor that influences the kinetics of absorption is the unstirred water layer[256-258], which is a diffusion barrier to actively and passively transported substances in the gut. The unstirred layer causes underestimation of passive permeability, is rate-limiting for passive diffusion, and grossly distorts the kinetics of trans-port. Clearly, all data about transport kinetics accumulated without regard to the unstirred layer need to be corrected; e.g. the previously calculated K_m for certain substances may be six times lower.

References

1. Johnson, F. P. (1910). The development of the mucus membrane of the esophagus, stomach and small intestine in the human embryo. *Amer. J. Anat.*, **10**, 521
2. Olivercrona, H. and Hillarp, N. (1949). Studies on the sub-microscopic structure of the epithelial cells of the intestine, pancreas, and kidney of rats during histogenesis. *Acta Anat.*, **8**, 281
3. Kammaraad, A. (1942). The development of the gastrointestinal tract of the rat. I. Histogenesis of the epithelium of the stomach, small intestine, and pancreas. *J. Morphol.*, **70**, 323

4. Deren, J. J. (1967). Development of intestinal structure and function. *Handbook of Physiology, Section 6, Alimentary Canal, Vol. II. Intestinal Absorption* 1099 (C. F. Code, editor) (Washington, D.C.: Amer. Physiol. Soc.)
5. Koldovsky, O., Heringova, A., Jirsova, V., Jirasek, J. E. and Uher, J. (1965). Transport of glucose against a concentration gradient in everted sacs of jejunum and ileum of human fetuses. *Gastroenterology*, **48**, 185
6. Wilson, T. H. and Lin, E. C. C. (1960): Active transport by intestines of fetal and newborn rabbits. *Amer. J. Physiol.*, **199**, 1030
7. Rosenberg, I. H. (1966). Development of fetal guinea pig small intestine: amino acid transport and sodium potassium-dependent ATPase. *Fed. Proc.*, **25**, 456
8. Moog, F. (1951). The functional differentiation of the small intestine II. The differentiation of alkaline phosphomonoesterase in the duodenum of the mouse. *J. Exp. Zool.*, **118**, 187
9. Auricchio, S., Rubino, A. and Murset, G. (1965). Intestinal glycosidase activities in the human embryo, fetus, and newborn. *Pediatrics*, **35**, 944
10. Auricchio, S., Rubino, A , Tosi, R., Semenza, G., Landolt, M., Kistler, H. and Prader, A. (1963). Disaccharidase activities in human intestinal mucosa. *Enzymol. Biol Clin.*, **3**, 193
11. Dahlqvist, A. and Lindberg, A T. (1966). Development of the intestinal disaccharidase and alkaline phosphatase in the human foetus. *Clin. Sci.*, **30**, 517
12. MacDonald, W. C., Trier, J. S. and Everett, N. B. (1964). Cell proliferation and migration in the stomach, duodenum, and rectum of man: Radioautographic studies. *Gastroenterology*, **46**, 405
13. Shorter, R. G., Moertal, C. G., Titus, J. L. and Reitemeier, R. J. (1964). Cell kinetics in the jejunum and rectum of man. *Amer. J. Dig. Dis.*, **9**, 760
14. Lipkin, M., Sherlock, P. and Bell, B. (1963). Cell proliferation kinetics in the gastrointestinal tract of man. II. Cell renewal in stomach, ileum, colon and rectum. *Gastroenterology*, **45**, 721
15. Brown, A. L. Jr. (1962). Microvilli of the human jejunal epithelial cell. *J. Cell. Biol.*, **12**, 623
16. Ito, S. (1965). The enteric surface coat on cat intestinal microvilli. *J. Cell. Biol.*, **27**, 475
17. Ito, S. and Revel, J. P. (1964). Incorporation of radoactive sulfate and glucose on the surface coat of enteric microvilli. *J. Cell. Biol.*, **23**, 44a
18. Fawcett, D. W. (1965). Surface specilisations of absorbing cells. *J. Histochem. Cytochem.*, **13**, 75
19. Goldfischer, S., Essner, E. and Novikoff, A. B. (1964). The localization of phosphatase activities at the level of the ultrastructure. *J. Histochem. Cytochem.*, **12**, 72
20. Nachlas, M. M., Monis, B., Rosenblatt, D. and Seligman, A. M. (1960). Improvement in the histochemical localization of luecine aminopeptidase with a new substrate L-leucyl-4-methoxy-2-naphthylamide. *J. Biophys. Biochem. Cytol.*, **7**, 261
21. Ashworth, C. T., Luibel, F. J. and Stewart, S. C. (1963). Localization of adenosine triphosphatase in cytomembranes involved in active transport. *Biochemical Problems of Lipids*, 130 (A. C. Frazier, editor) (New York: Elsevier)
22. Miller, D. and Crane, R. K. (1961). The digestive function of the epithelium of the small intestine. II. Localization of disaccharide hydroylsis in the isolated brush border portion of intestinal epithelial cells. *Biochim. Biophys. Acta*, **52**, 293
23. Miller, D. and Crane, R. K. (1961). The digestive function of the epithelium of the small intestine. I. An intracellular locus of disaccharide and sugar phosphate ester hydrolysis. *Biochim. Biophys. Acta*, **52**, 281
24. Overton, J., Eichholz, A. and Crane, R. K. (1965). Studies on the organisation of the brush border in intestinal epithelial cells. II. Fine structure of fractions of Tris-disrupted hamster brush borders. *J. Cell. Biol.*, **26**, 693
25. Rhodes, J. B., Eichholz, A. and Crane, R. K. (1967). Studies on the organization of the brush border in intestinal epithelial cells. IV. Aminopeptidase activity in microvillus membranes of hamster intestinal brush border. *Biochim. Biophys. Acta*, **135**, 959
26. Freeman, J. A. (1962). Fine structure of the goblet cell mucous secretory process. *Anat. Rec.*, **144**, 341
27. Masson, P. (1914). LaGlande endocrine de l'intestin chez l'homme. *Compt. Rend.*, **158**, 59
28. Benditt, E. P. and Wong, R. L. (1957). On the concentration of 5-hydroxytryptamine

in mammalian enterochromaffin cells and its release by reserpine. *J. Exp. Med.*, **105**, 509

29. Oates, J. W., Pettinger, W. A. and Doctor, R. B. (1966). Evidence for the release of bradykinin in carcinoid syndrome. *J. Clin. Invest.*, **45**, 173
30. Mall, F. P. (1908). Development of the human intestine and its position in the adult. *Bull. John Hopkins Hosp.*, **9**, 197
31. Wheeler, E. J. and Wheeler, J. K. (1964). Comparative study of Paneth cell in vertebrates. *Anat. Rec.*, **148**, 350
32. Johnson, F. R. and Kugler, J. H. (1953). The distribution of alkaline phosphatase in the mucosal cells of the small intestine of the rat, cat and dog. *J. Anat.*, **87**, 247
33. McCance, R. A. and Madders, K. (1930). The comparative rates of absorption of sugars from the human intestine. *Biochem. J.*, **24**, 795
34. Althausen, T. L (1939). Test for intestinal absorption. *Amer. J. Dig. Dis.*, **6**, 544
35. Cautrecassas, P., Lockwood, D. H. and Caldwell, J. R. (1965). Lactase deficiency in the adult: a common occurrence. *Lancet*, **1**, 14
36. Thiry, L. (1864). Uber eine neue Methode, den Dunndarm zu isolieren. *Sitzber. Akad. Wiss. Wein. Math. Naturw.*, Kl. I. **50**, 77
37. Mlller, T. G. and Abbott, W. O. (1934). Intestinal intubation; a practical technique. *Amer. J. Med. Sci.*, **187**, 595
38. Abbott, W. O. and Miller, T. G. (1936). Intubation studies of human small intestine; technique for collection of pure intestinal secretion and for study of intestinal absorption *JAMA*, **106**, 16
39. Blankenhorn, D. H., Hirsch, J. and Ahrens, E. H. Jr. (1955). Transintestinal intubation Technique for measurement of gut length and physiologic sampling of known loci. *Proc. Soc. Exp. Biol. Med.*, **88**, 356
40. Cooper, H., Levitan, R., Fordtran, J. S. and Ingelfinger, F. J. (1966). A method for studying absorption of water and solute from the human small intestine. *Gastroenterology*, **50**, 1
41. Fordtran, J. S., Levitan, R., Bikerman, V., Burrows, B. A. and Ingelfinger, F. J. (1961). The kinetics of water absorption in the human intestine. *Trans. Assoc. Amer. Physicians*, **74**, 195
42. Reid, E. W. (1892). Preliminary report of experiments upon intestinal absorption without osmosis. *Brit. Med. J.*, P 1133
43. Wilson, T. H. and Wiseman, G. (1954). The use of sacs of inverted small intestine for the transferance of substances from the mucosal to the serosal surface. *J. Physiol. (London)*, **123**, 116
44. Ussing, H. H. and Zerahn, K. (1951). Active transport of sodium as the source of electric current in the short-circuited isolated frog skin. *Acta Physiol. Scand.*, **23**, 110
45. Dickens, F. and Weil-Malherbe, E. (1941). Metabolism of normal and tumor tissue. 19. The metabolism of intestinal mucous membrane. *Biochem. J.*, **35**, 7
46. Crane, R. K. and Mandelstam, P. (1960). The active transport of sugars by various preparations of hamster intestine. *Biochim. Biophys. Acta*, **45**, 460
47. Hakim, A. A., Lester, R. G. and Lifson, N. (1963). Absorption by an *in vitro* preparation of dog intestinal mucosa. *J. Appl. Physiol.*, **18**, 409
48. Hakim, A. A. and Lifson, N. (1964). Urea transport across dog intestinal mucosa *in vitro*. *Amer. J. Physiol.*, **206**, 1315
49. Kimmich, G. A. (1970). Preparation and properties of mucosal epithelial cells isolated from small intestine of the chicken. *Biochemistry*, **9**, 3659
50. Curran, P. F. (1963). Biophysical nature of biological membranes. *Transfer of Calcium and Strontium across Biological Membranes*, 3 (C. L. Comar and F. Bronner, editors) (New York: Academic Press)
51. Danielli, J. F. (1954). Morphological and molecular aspects of active transport. *Symp. Soc. Exp. Biol.*, **8**, 502
52. Solomon, A. K. (1961). Measurement of the equivalent pore radius in cell membranes. *Membrane Transport and Metabolism*, 94 (A. Kleinzeller and A. Kotyk, editors) (Prague, Czech: Acad Sci.)
53. Crane, R. K., Field, R. A. and Cori, C. F. (1957). Studies of tissue permeability. I. The penetration of sugars into the Ehrlich ascites tumor cells. *J. Biol. Chem.*, **224**, 649
54. Lotspeich, W. D. (1959). *Metabolic Aspects of Renal Function*, (Springfield, Illinois: Thomas)

55. Lotspeich, W. D. and Wheeler, A. H. (1962). Insulin, anaerobiosis, and phlorizin in entry of D-galactose into skeletal muscle. *Amer. J. Physiol.*, **202**, 1065

56. Bihler, I., Hawkins, K. A. and Crane, R. K. (1962). Studies on the mechanism of intestinal absorption of sugars. VI. The specificity and other properties of Na^+-dependent entrance of sugars into intestinal tissue under anaerobic conditions, *in vitro*, *Biochim. Biophys. Acta*, **59**, 94

57. Eichholz, A. and Crane, R. K. (1965). Studies on the organization of the brush border in intestinal epithelial cells. I. Tris-disruption of isolated hamster brush borders and density gradient separation of fractions. *J. Cell. Biol.*, **26**, 687

58. Alvarado, F. and Crane, R. K. (1964). Studies on the mechanism of intestinal absorption of sugars. VII. Phenylglycoside transport and its possible relationship to phlorizin inhibition of the active transport of sugars by the small intestine. *Biochim. Biophys. Acta*, **93**, 116

59. Crane, R. K. and Caspary, W. (1971). Evidence for an intermediate step in sugar translocation across the brush border membrane. *Intestinal Transport of Electrolytes, Amino Acids, and Sugars*, 130 (W. McD. Armstrong and A. S. Nunn, Jr., editors) (Charles C. Thomas)

60. Widdas, W. F. (1968). *Carbohydrate metabolism and its disorders*, 1 (F. Dickens, P. J. Randle and W. J. Whelan, editors) (New York: Academic Press)

61. Riklis, E. and Quastel, J. H. (1958). Effects of cations on sugar absorption by isolated surviving guinea pig intestine. *Can. J. Biochem. Physiol.*, **36**, 347

62. Curran, P. F. (1965). Ion transport in the intestine and its coupling to other transport processes. *Fed. Proc.*, **24**, 993

63. Bihler, I. and Crane, R. K. (1962). Studies on the mechanism of intestinal absorption of sugars. V. The influence of several cations and anions on the active transport of sugars, *in vitro* by various preparations of hamster small intestine. *Biochim. Biophys. Acta*, **59**, 78

64. Bihler, I. (1971). Intestinal sugar transport: Ionic activation and chemical specificity. *Intestinal Transport of Electrolytes, Amino Acids, and Sugars* 144 (W. McD. Armstrong and A. S. Nunn, Jr., editors) (Charles C. Thomas)

65. Bihler, I., Kim, N. D. and Sawh, P. C. (1969). Active transport of L-glucose and D-xylose in Hamster intestine, *in vitro*. *Can. J. Physiol. Pharmacol.*, **47**, 525

66. Crane, R. K. (1965). Na^+-dependent transport in the intestine and other animal tissues. *Fed. Proc.*,, **24**, 1000

67. Caspary, W. F. (1971). Evidence for a sodium-independent transport system for glucose derived from disaccharides. *Na-linked Transport of Organic Solutes* 99, (E. Heinz, editor) (Berlin, Heidelberg, New York: Springer-Verlag)

68. Goldner, A. M., Schultz, S. G. and Curran, P. F. (1969). Sodium and sugar fluxes across the mucosal border of rabbit ileum. *J. Gen. Physiol.*, **53**, 362

69. Parsons, D. S. and Prichard, J. S. (1966). Properties of some model systems for transcellular active transport. *Biochim. Biophys. Acta*, **126**, 471

70. Olsen, W. A. and Ingelfinger, F. J. (1968). The role of sodium in intestinal glucose absorption in man. *J. Clin. Invest.*, **47**, 1133

71. Semenza, G. (1972). Some aspects of intestinal sugar transport. *Transport Across the Intestine*, 78 (W. L. Burland and P. D. Samuel, editors) (Edinburgh and London: Churchill Livingstone)

72. Eichholz, A., Howell, K. E. and Crane, R. K. (1969). Studies on the organization of the brush border in intestinal epithelial cells. VI. Glucose binding to isolated intestinal brush border and their subfractions. *Biochim. Biophys. Acta*, **193**, 179

73. Semenza, G. (1969). In search of molecular mechanisms in intestinal sugar absorption *7th Int. Congr. Clin. Chem. Geneva/Evian. Vol.* **4**: *Digestion and Intestinal Absorption*, 3

74. Semenza, G. (1970). Sucrase and sugar transport in the intestine: A carrier-like sugar binding site in the isolated sucrase-isomaltase complex. *FEBS Symposium*, **20**, 117

75. Fisher, E. H. and Stein E. A. (1960). α-amylases. *The Enzymes*, **4**, 313 (P. Boyer, H. Lardy and K. M. Myrback, editors) (New York: Academic Press)

76. Dahlqvist, A. and Thompson, D. L. (1963). Separation and characterization of two rat-intestinal amylases. *Biochem. J.*, **89**, 272

77. Dahlqvist, A. and Borgstrom, B. (1961). Digestion and absorption of disaccharides in man. *Biochem. J.*, **81**, 411

78. Hoffman, K., Mossel, D. A. A., Korus, W. and Van De Kamer, J. H. (1964). Untersuchungen uber die Wirkungsweise der Lactulose (β-galactosido-fructose) *Darm. Klin. Wochschr.*, **42**, 126
79. Gryboski, J. D., Thayer, W. R. Jr., Gabrielson, I. W. and Spiro, H. M. (1963). Disacchariduria in gastrointestinal disease. *Gastroenterology*, **45**, 633
80. Newcomer, A. D. and McGill, D. B. (1966). Distribution of disaccharidase activity in the small intestine: definition of lactase deficiency (Abstr.) *Gastroenterology*, **50**, 861
81. Welsh, J. D., Rohrer, G. V. and Walker, A. (1966). Human intestinal disaccharidase activity. I. Normal individuals. *Arch. Internal Med.*, **117**, 488
82. Gray, G. M. and Ingelfinger, F. J. (1966). Intestinal absorption of glucose in man: interrelation of hydrolysis and monosaccharide product absorption. *J. Clin. Invest.*, **45**, 388
83. Gray, G. M. and Santiago, N. S. (1966). Disaccharide absorption in normal and diseased human intestine. *Gastroenterology*, **51**, 489
84. Semenza, G., Tosi, R., Vallotton-Delachaux, M. C. and Mulhaupt, E. (1964). Sodium activation of human intestinal sucrase and its possible significance in the enzymic organization of brush borders. *Biochim. Biophys. Acta*, **90**, 109
85. Semenza, G. and Crane, R. K. (1966). Kinetics of Na^+-dependent transport systems. *Int. Congr. Biophys.* (Vienna, Sept 5–9)
86. Eichholz, A. (1967). Structural and functional organization of the brush border of intestinal epithelial cells. III. Enzyme activities and chemical composition of various fractions of tris-disrupted brush borders. *Biochim. Biophys. Acta*, **135**, 475
87. Eggermont, E. and Hers, H. G. (1969). The sedimentation properties of the intestinal α-glucosidases of normal human subjects, and of patients with sucrose intolerance. *Europ. J. Biochem.*, **9**, 488
88. Malathi, P. and Crane, R. K. (1969). Phlorizin hydrolase: a β-glucosidase of hamster intestinal brush border membrane. *Biochim. Biophys. Acta*, **173**, 254
89. Shay, H., Gershon-Cohen, J., Fels, S. S., Munro, F. L. and Siplet, H. (1940). The absorption and dilution of glucose solutions in the human stomach and duodenum. *Amer. J. Dig. Dis.*, **6**, 535
90. Holdsworth, D. C. and Dawson, A. M. (1964). The absorption of monosaccharides in man. *Clin. Sci.*, **27**, 371
91. White, L. W. and Landau, B. R. (1965). Sugar transport and fructose metabolism in human intestine *in vitro. J. Clin. Invest.*, **44**, 1200
92. Andersen, C. M., Kerry, K. R. and Townley, R. R. W. (1965). An inborn defect of intestinal absorption of certain monosaccharides. *Arch. Disease Childhood*, **40**, 1
93. Lindquist, B. and Meeuwisse, G. W. (1962). Chronic diarrhoea caused by monosaccharide malabsorption. *Acta Paediat.*, **51**, 674
94. Lindquist, B., Meeuwisse, G. W. and Melin, K. (1963). Osmotic diarrhoea, in genetically transmitted glucose-galactose malabsorption. *Acta Paediat.*, **52**, 217
95a. Crane, R. K. (1960). Intestinal absorption of sugars. *Physiol. Rev.*, **40**, 789
95b. Holdsworth, R. K. (1966). Enzymes and malabsorption: a concept of brush border membrane disease. *Gastroenterology*, **50**, 254
96. Holdsworth, C. D. and Dawson, A. M. (1965). Glucose and fructose absorption in idiopathic steatorrhea. *Gut*, **6**, 387
97. Gracey, M., Burke, V. and Oshin, A. (1972). Transport of fructose by the intestine. *Transport Across the Intestine*, 99 (W. L. Burland and P. D. Samuel, editors) (Edinburgh and London: Churchill Livingstone)
98. Wilson, T. H. and Landau, B. R. (1960). Specificity of sugar transport by the intestine of the hamster. *Amer. J. Physiol.*, **198**, 99
99. Barnett, J. E. G. and Munday, K. A. (1972). Structural requirements for active intestinal sugar transport in the hamster. *Transport Across the Intestine*, 99 (W. L. Burland and P. D. Samuel, editors) (Edinburgh and London: Churchill Livingstone)
100. Vinnik, I. E., Kern, F. Jr., and Sussman, K. E. (1965). The effect of diabetes mellitus and insulin on glucose absorption by the small intestine in man. *J. Lab. Clin. Med.*, **66**, 131
101. Althausen, T. L., Anderson, E. M. and Stockholm, M. (1939). Effect of adrenalectomy and of NaCl on intestinal absorption of dextrose. *Proc. Soc. Exp. Biol. Med.*, **40**, 432
102. Coupar, I. M. and McColl, I. (1972). Inhibition of glucose absorption by prostaglandin E_1 and F_2a. *J. Pharm. Pharmacol.*, **24**, 254

103. Nasset, E. S. and Ju, J. S. (1961). Mixture of endogenous and exogenous protein in the alimentary tract. *J. Nutr.*, **74**, 461

104. Nasset, E. S., Schwartz, P. and Weiss, H. V. (1955). The digestion of protein *in vivo*. *J. Nutr.*, **56**, 83

105. Cathcart, E. P. and Leathes, J. B. (1906). On the absorption of protein from the intestine. *J. Physiol. (London)*, **33** 462

106. Howell, W. H. (1907). Note upon the presence of amino acids in the blood and lymph as determined by the β-naphthalinsulphochloride reaction. *Amer. J. Physiol.*, **17**, 273

107. Crane, C. W. and Neuberger, A. (1960). The digestion and absorption of protein by normal man. *Biochem. J.*, **74**, 313

108. Prockop, D. J., Keiser, H. R. and Sjoerdsma, A. (1962). Gastrointestinal absorption and renal excretion of hydroxyproline peptides. *Lancet*, **2**, 527

109. Newey, H. and Smyth, D. H. (1959). The intestinal absorption of some dipeptides. *J. Physiol. (London)*, **145**, 48

110. Borgstrom, B., Dahlqvist, A., Lundh, G. and Sjovall, J. (1957). Studies of intestinal digestion and absorption in the human. *J. Clin. Invest.*, **36**, 1521

111. Milne, M. D. (1972). Use of hereditary disorders of amino acid transport in studies of oligopeptide absorption. *Transport Across the Intestine*, 195 (W. L. Burland and P. D. Samuel, editors) (Edinburgh and London: Churchill Livingstone)

112. Tarlow, M. J., Seakins, J. W. T., Lloyd, J. K., Matthews, D. M., Cheng, B. and Thomas A. (1970). Intestinal absorption oand biopsy transport of peptides and amino acids in Hartnup disease. *Clin. Sci.*, **39**, 18

113. Peters, T. J. (1970). The subcellular localization of di- and tripeptide hydrolase activity in guinea pig small intestine. *Biochem. J.*, **120**, 195

114. Peters, T. J., Donlon, J. and Fottrell, P. F. (1972). The subcellular localization and specificity of intestinal peptide hydrolases. *Transport Across the Intestine*, 99 (W. L. Burland and P. D. Samuel, editors) (Edinburgh and London: Churchill Livingstone)

115. Ehrenreich, B. A. and Cohn, Z. A. (1969). The fate of peptides pinocytosed by macrophages *in vitro*. *J. Exp. Med.*, **129**, 227

116. Gibson, Q. H. and Wiseman, G. (1951). Selective absorption of stero-isomers of amino acids from loops of the small intestine of the rat. *Biochem. J.*, **48**, 426

117. Matthews, D. M. and Smyth, D. H. (1954). The intestinal absorption of amino-acid in antiomorphs. *J. Physiol. (London)*, **126**, 96

118. Wiseman, G. (1951). Active sterochemically selective absorption of amino-acids from rat small intestine. *J. Physiol. (London)*, **114**, 7

119. Wiseman, G. (1953). Absorption of amino-acids using an *in vitro* technique. *J. Physiol. (London)*, **120**, 63

120. Jervis, E. L. and Smyth, D. H. (1960). The active transfer of D-methionine by the rat intestine *in vitro*. *J. Physiol. (London)*, **151**, 51

121. Harrison, H. E. and Harrison, H. C. (1963). Sodium, potassium, and intestinal transport of glucose, L-tyrosine, phosphate, and calcium. *Amer. J. Physiol.*, **205**, 107

122. Nathans, D., Tapley, D. F. and Ross, J. E. (1960). Intestinal transport of amino acids studied *in vitro* with L-[131]-I-monoidotyrosine. *Biochim. Biophys. Acta*, **41**, 271

123. Cohen, L. L. and Huang, K. C. (1964). Intestinal transport of tryptophan and its derivatives. *Amer. J. Physiol.*, **206**, 647

124. Saunders, S. J. and Isselbacher, K. J. (1966). Intestinal absorption of amino acids. *Gastroenterology*, **50**, 586

125. Munck, B. G. (1966). Amino acid transport by the small intestine of the rat. The existence and specificity of the transport mechanism of imino acids and its relation to the transport of glycine. *Biochim. Biophys. Acta.*, **120**, 97

126. Reiser, S. (1971). Specificity of pathways of amino acid transport. *Intestinal Transport of Electrolytes, Amino Acids, and Sugars*, 255 (Charles C. Thomas)

127. Wiseman, G. (1964). Absorption from the Intestine. (New York: Academic Press)

128. Wilson, T. H. (1962). *Intestinal Absorption*, 220 (Philadelphia: W. B. Saunders Co.)

129. Newey, H. and Smyth, D. H. (1964). Effect of sugar on intestinal transfer of amino acids. *Nature (London)*, **202**, 401

130. Saunders, S. J. and Isselbacher, K. J. (1965). Inhibition of intestinal amino acid transport by hexoses. *Biochim. Biophys. Acta*, **102**, 397

131. Alvarado, F. (1971). Interrelation of transport systems for sugars and amino acids in small intestine. *Intestinal Transport of Electrolytes, Amino Acids, and Sugars*, 281 (Charles C. Thomas)

132. Thorn, M. B. (1953). Inhibition by malonate of succinic dehydrogenase in heart muscle preparations. *Biochem. J.*, **54**, 540

133. Alvarado, F. (1966). Transport of sugars and amino acids in the intestine: evidence for a common carrier. *Science*, **151**, 1010

134. Munck, B. G. (1972). Effects of galactose on amino acid fluxes in rat jejunum. *Transport Across the Intestine*, 127 (W. L. Burland and P. D. Samuel, editors) (Edinburgh and London: Churchill Livingstone)

135. Riggs, T. R., Walker, L. M. and Christensen, H. N. (1958). Potassium migration and amino acid transport. *J. Biol. Chem.*, **233**, 1479

136. Eddy, A. A. (1972). Neutral amino acids and the ion gradient hypothesis. *Na-linked Transport of Organic Solutes*, 28 (E. Heinz, editor) (Berlin, Heidelberg, and New York: Springer-Verlag)

137. Potashner, S. J. and Johnstone, R. M. (1971). Cation gradients, ATP and amino acid accumulation in Ehrlich ascites cells. *Biochim. Biophys. Acta*, **233**, 91

138. Frizzell, R. A. and Schultz, S. G. (1970). Effects of monovalent cations on the sodium-alanine interaction in rabbit ileum. *J. Gen. Physiol.*, **56**, 462

139. Shimoda, S. S. and Rubin, C. E. (1968). The Zollinger–Ellison syndrome with steatorrhea. *Gastroenterology*, **55**, 695

140. Adibi, S. A., Ruiz, C., Glaser, P. and Fogel, M. (1972). Effect of intraluminal pH on absorption rates of leucine, water and electrolytes in human jejunum. *Gastroenterology*, **63**, 611

141. Visscher, M. B. (1957). Transport of water and electrolytes across intestinal epithelia. *Metabolic Aspects of Transport across Cell Membranes*, (O. R. Murphay, editor) (Univ. Wisconsin Press)

142. Fordtran, J. S. and Dietschy, J. M. (1966). Water and electrolyte movement in the intestine. *Gastroenterology*, **50**, 263

143. Smyth, D. H. (1972). *Introduction to Transport across the Intestine*, 1 (W. L. Burland and P. D. Samuel, editors) (Edinburgh and London: Churchill Livingstone)

144. Whalen, G. E., Harris, J. A., Geenen, J. E. and Soergel, K. (1966). Sodium and water absorption from the human small intestine. The accuracy of the perfusion method. *Gastroenterology*, **51**, 975

145. Fordtran, J. S., Rector, F. C. Jr. and Carter, N. W. (1968). The mechanisms of sodium absorption in the human small bowel. *J. Clin. Invest.*, **47**, 884

146. McHardy, G. J. R. and Parsons, D. S. (1957). The absorption of water and salt from the small intestine of the rat. *Quart. J. Exp. Physiol.*, **42**, 33

147. Fordtran, J. S., Rector, F. C., Locklear, T. W. and Ewton, M. F. (1967). Water and solute movement in the small intestine of patients with sprue. *J. Clin. Invest.*, **46**, 287

148. Fordtran, J. S., Rector, F. C. Jr., Ewton, M. F., Soter, N. and Kinney, J. (1965). Permeability characteristics of the human small intestine. *J. Clin. Invest.*, **44**, 1935

149. Turnberg, L. A., Fordtran, J. S., Carter, N. W. and Rector, F. C. Jr. (1970). Mechanism of bicarbonate absorption and its relationship to sodium transport in the human jejunum. *J. Clin. Invest.*, **49**, 548

150. Bieberdorf, F. A. Gorden, P. and Fordtran, J. S. (1972). Pathogenesis of congenital alkalosis with diarrhoea. Implications for the physiology of normal ileal electrolyte absorption and secretion. *J. Clin. Invest.*, **41**, 1958

151. Torres-Pinedo, R., Rivera, C. L. and Fernandez, S. (1966). Studies on infant diarrhoea. II. Absorption of glucose and net fluxes of water and sodium chloride in a segment of jejunum. *J. Clin. Invest.*, **45**, 1916

152. Pierce, N. F. (1969). Replacement of water and electrolyte losses in cholera by an oral glucose-electrolyte solution. *Ann. Intern. Med.*, **70**, 1173

153. Field, M., Fromm, D., Wallace, C. K. and Greenough, W. B., III (1969). Stimulation of active chloride secretion in small intestine by cholera toxin. *J. Clin. Invest.*, **48**, 24

154. Greenough, W. B., III, Pierce, N. F., Awqati, Q. A. L., Carpenter, C. C. J. (1969). Stimulation of gut electrolyte secretion by prostaglandins, theophylline and cholera exotoxin. *J. Clin. Invest.*, **48**, 32

155. Field, M. (1971). Intestinal secretion: Effect of cyclic AMP and its role in cholera. *New Eng. J. Med.*, **284**, 1137

156. Parkinson, D. K., Ebel, H., Dibona, D. R. and Sharp, G. W. (1972). Localization of the action of cholera toxin on adenyl cyclase in mucosal epithelial cell or rabbit intestine. *J. Clin. Invest.*, **51**, 2292
157. Serebro, H. A., Iber, F. L., Yardley, J. H. and Hendrix T. R. (1969). Inhibition of cholera toxin action in the rabbit by cycloheximide. *Gastroentrology*, **56**, 506
158. Banwell, J. G., Shepherd, R., Thomas, J., Pierce, N. F., Mitra, R. C., Gorbach, S. K., Brigham, K. L. Fedson, D. S. and Mondal, A. (1972). Net and unidirectional transmucosal flux of sodium and water in acute human diarrheal disease. *J. Clin. Lab. Med.*, **80**, 686
159. Hendrix, T. R. and Bayless, T. M. (1970). Intestinal secretion. *Ann. Rev. Physiol.*, **32**, 139
160. Harries, J. T. and Salden, G. E. (1972). The effect of different bile salts on the absorption of fluid, electrolytes and monosaccharides in the small intestine of the rat *in vivo Gut*, **13**, 596
161. Bynum, T. E., Jacobson, E. D. and Johnson, L. R. (1971). Effects of gastrin on intestinal absorption. *Gastroenterology*, **60**, 767
162. Modigliani, R., Mary, J. Y. and Bernier, J. J. (1972). Effects de la pentagastrine sur l'absorption de l'eau des electrolytes et du glucose par l'intestine grele de l'homme. *Biologie et Gastro-Enterologie*, **5**, 635C
163. Ewe, K. and Hoditz, U. (1972). Effect of pentagastrin on water and electrolyte transport in the human jejunum. *Biologie et Gastro-Enterologie*, **5**, 634C
164. Wright, H. K., Hersch, T., Floch, M. H. and Weinstein, L. D. (1970). Impaired intestinal absorption in Zollinger–Ellison syndrome independent of gastric hypersecretion. *Amer. J. Surg.*, **119**, 250
165. Matuchansky, C., Mary, J. Y. and Bernier, J. J. (1972). Effects de la prostaglandine E, sur l'absorption du glucose et les mouvements trans-in-testinaux de l'eau et des electrolytes dans le jejunum human. *Biologie et Gastro-Enterologie*, **5**, 636C
166. Gardner, J. D., Peskin, G. W., Cerda, J. J. and Brooks, F. P. (1967). Alteration of *in vitro* fluid and electrolyte absorption by gastrointestinal hormones. *Amer. J. Surg.*, **113**, 57
167. Soergel, K. H., Whalen, G. E., Harris, J. A. and Geene, J. E. (1968). Effect of antidiuretic hormone on human small intestinal water and solute transport. *J. Clin. Invest.*, **47**, 1071
168. Matthews, D. M. (1965). Absorption of water-soluble vitamins. *Brit. Med. Bull.*, **23**, 258
169. Booth, C. C. (1968). Effect of location along the small intestine on absorption of nutrients. *Handbook of Physiology, Section 6, Alimentary Canal, Vol. III*, 1513 (C. F. Code, editor) (Washington, D.C.: Amer. Physiol. Soc.)
170. Rindi, G. and Ventura, U. (1972). Thiamine intestinal transport. *Physiol. Rev.*, **52**, 821
171. Morrison, A. B. and Campbell, J. A. (1960). Vitamin absorption studies. I. Factors influencing the excretion of oral test dose of thiamine and riboflavin by human subjects. *J. Nutr.*, **72**, 435
172. Ferrari, G., Ventura, U. and Rindi, G. (1971). The Na^+-dependence of thiamine intestinal transport *in vitro*. *Life Sci. (Oxford)*, **10**, 67
173. Kowasaki, T., Miyata, I., Esaki, K. and Nose, Y. (1969). Thiamine uptake in Escherichia coli. I. General properties of thiamine uptake system in Escherichia coli. *Arch. Biochem. Biophys.*, **131**, 223
174. Hatihira, H., Lin, E. C. C., Samiy, A. H. and Wilson, T. H. (1961). Active transport of lysine, ornithine, argine and cystine by the intestine. *Biochem. Biophys. Res. Commun.*, **4**, 478
175. Schanker, L. S. and Tocco, D. J. (1960). Active transport of some pyrimidine across the rat intestinal epithalium. *J. Pharmacol., Exp. Therap.*, **128**, 115
176. Csaky, T. Z. and Lassen, U. V. (1964). Active intestinal transport of d-xylose. *Biochim. Biophys. Acta*, **82**, 215
177. Capraro, V. and Cresseri, A. (1964). Absorption, distribution and excretion of vitamin B_{12}, *Research Progress in Organic-Biologic and Medicinal Chemistry*, 110 (U. Gallo and L. Santamaria, editors) (Amsterdam: North Holland)
178. Sanford, P. and Smyth, D. H. (1971). Intestinal transfer of choline in rat and hamster. *J. Physiol.*, **215**, 769
179. Herbert, V. (1968). Absorption of vitamin B_{12} and folic acid. *Gastroenterology*, **54**, 110

180. Rosenberg, I. H. and Godwin, H. A. (1971). The digestion and absorption of dietary folate. *Gastroenterology*, **60**, 445
181. Chanarin, I. (1969). *Folic Acid-Nutritional Aspects in the Megaloblastic Anemias*, 268 (Philadelphia: F. A. David Co.)
182. Whitehead, V. M. and Cooper, B. A. (1967). Absorption of unaltered folic acid from the gastrointestinal tract in man. *Brit. J. Haemat.*, **13**, 679
183. Herbert, V. (1967). Biochemical and hematological lesions in folic acid deficiency. *Amer. J. Clin. Nutr.*, **20**, 562
184. Burgen, A. S. V. and Goldberg, N. J. (1962). Absorption of folic acid from the small intestine of the rat. *Brit. J. Pharmacol. Chemotherapy*, **19**, 313
185. Kesavan, V. and Nornha, J. M. (1971). Effect of x-radiation on the absorption of naturally-occurring folates. *Int. J. Radiat. Biol.*, **19**, 205
186. Hepner, G. W., Booth, G. H., Cowan, J., Hoffbrand, A. V. and Mollin, D. L. (1968). Absorption of crystalline folic acid in man. *Lancet*, 2: 302
187. Corcino, J. J., Waxman, S. and Herbert, V. (1970). Absorption and malabsorption of vitamin B_{12}. *Amer. J. Med.*, **48**, 562
188. Okuda, K. and Sasayma, K. (1965). Intestinal distribution of intrinsic factor and vitamin B_{12} absorption. *Amer. J. Physiol.*, **208**, 14
189. Okuda, K. and Mito, T. (1965). Absorption of Vitamin B_{12} from the jejunum of man studied with a three-lumen tube. *J. Vitaminol.*, **11**, 28
190. Okuda, K. and Sasayama, K. (1962). Effects of ethylenediariche tetraacetate and metal ions in intestinal absorption of vitamin B_{12} in man and rats. *Proc. Soc. Exp Biol. Med.*, **120**, 17
191. Myberg, W. (1960). The influence of diphyllobothrium latum on the vitamin B_{12} intrinsic factor complex. II. *In vitro* studies. *Acta Med. Scand.*, **167**, 189
192. Peters, T. J., Quinlan, A. and Hoffbrand, A. V. (1970). Absorption of vitamin B_{12} by the guinea pig. I. Subcellular localization of vitamin B_{12} in the ileal enterocyte during absorption. *Brit. J. Haemat.*, **19**, 369
193. Toske, P., Hansell, J., Cerda, J. and Deren, J. J. (1971). Vitamin B_{12} malabsorption in chronic pancreatic insufficiency. Studies suggesting the presence of pancreatic 'intrinsic factor', *New Eng. J. Med.*, **284**, 622
194. Crosby, W. H. (1968). Iron Absorption. *Handbook of Physiology, Alimentary Canal, Section 6, Vol. III*, 1553 (C. F. Code, editor) (Washington, D.C.: Amer. Physiol. Soc.)
195. Bothwell, T. H. and Charlton, R. W. (1970). Absorption of iron. *Ann. Rev. Med.*, **21**, 145
196. Dagg, J. H., Cumming, R. L. C. and Goldberg, A. (1971). Disorders of iron metabolism. *Recent Advances in Haematology*, (A. Goldberg and M. C. Brain, editors) (London: Churchill Livingstone)
197. Howard, J. and Jacobs, A. (1972). Iron transport by rat small intestine *in vitro*: Effect of body iron status. *Brit. J. Haematol.*, **23**, 595
198. Pinkerton, P. H., Bannerman, R. M., Doeblin, T. D., Benisch, B. M. and Edwards, J. A. (1970). Iron metabolism and absorption studies in the x-linked anaemia of mice. *Brit. J. Haematol.*, **18**, 211
199. Bannerman, R. M., Edwards, J. A., Kreimer-Birnbaum, M., McFarland, E. and Russell, E. S. (1972). Hereditary microcytic anaemia in the mouse: Studies in iron distribution and metabolism. *Brit. J. Haematol.*, **23**, 235
200. BeDard, Y. C., Pinkerton, P. H. and Simon, G. T. (1971). Radio-autographic observations on iron absorption by the normal mouse duodenum. *Blood*, **38**, 232
201. Brittin, G. M. and Raval, D. (1970). Duodenal ferritin synthesis during iron absorption in the iron deficient-rat. *J. Lab. Clin. Med.*, **75**, 881
202. Crosby, W. H. (1963). The control of iron balance by the intestinal mucosa. *Blood*, **22**, 441
203. Schade, S. F., Felsher, B. F., Bernier, G. M. and Conrad, M. E. (1970). Interrelationship of cobalt and iron absorption. *J. Lab. Clin. Med.*, **75**, 435
204. Olatunbosun, D., Corbett, W. E. N., Ludwig, J. and Valberg, L. S. (1970). Alteration of cobalt absorption in portal cirrhosis and idiopathic hemochromotosis. *J. Lab. Clin. Med.*, **75**, 754
205. Thompson, A. B. R., Valberg, L. A. and Sinclair, D. G. (1971). Competitive nature of the intestinal transport mechanism for cobalt and iron in the rat. *J. Clin. Invest.*, **50**, 2384

206. Thomas, F. B., McCullough, F. S. and Greenberger, N. J. (1972). Effect of pheno-barbital on the absorption of inorganic and hemoglobin iron in the rat. *Gastroenterology*, **62**, 590
207. Wasserman, R. H., Kallfelz, F. A. and Comar, C. L. (1961). Active transport of calcium by rat doudenum *in vivo*. *Science*, **133**, 883
208. Cramer, F. C. (1963). Quantitative studies on the absorption and excretion of calcium from Thiry-Vella intestinal loops in the dog. *The Transfer of Calcium and Strontium Across Biological Membranes*, 75 (R. H. Wasserman, editor) (New York: Academic Press)
209. Wensel, R. H., Rich, C., Brown, A. C. and Volwiler, W. (1969). Absorption of calcium measured by intubation and perfusion of the intact human small intestine. *J. Clin. Invest.*, **48**, 1768
210. Birge, S. J., Peck, W. A., Berman, M. and Whedon, G. D. (1969). Study of calcium absorption in man: a kinetic analysis and physiologic model. *J. Clin. Invest.*, **48**, 1705
211. Schachter, D. and Rosen, S. M. (1959). Active transport of Ca^{45} by the small intestine and its dependence on vitamin D. *Amer. J. Physiol.*, **196**, 357
212. Wasserman, R. H. (1962). Studies on vitamin D_3 and the intestinal absorption of calcium and other ions in the rachitic chick. *J. Nutr.*, **77**, 69
213. Schachter, D., Kimberg, D. V. and Schenker, H. (1961). Active transport of calcium by intestine: action and bio-assay of vitamin D. *Amer. J. Physiol.*, **200**, 1263
214. Schachter, D., Kowarski, S., Finkelstein, J. D. and Ma, R. -I. W. (1966). Tissue concentration differences during active transport of calcium by intestine. *Amer. J. Physiol.*, **211**, 1131
215. Wasserman, R. H. (1963). Vitamin D and the absorption of calcium and strontium *in vivo*. *The Transfer of Calcium and Strontium Across Biological Membranes*, 211 (R. H. Wasserman, editor) (New York: Academic Press)
216. Rasmussen, H., Waldorf, A., Dziewiatkowski, D. D. and DeLuca, H. F. (1963). Calcium exchange in isolated intestinal villi. *Biochim. Biophys. Acta*, **75**, 250
217. Wasserman, R. H. (1968). Calcium transport by the intestine: a model and comment on vitamin D action. *Calc. Tiss. Res.*, **2**, 301
218. Wasserman, R. H. and Taylor, A. N. (1966). Vitamin D_3-induced calcium-binding protein in chick intestinal mucosa. *Science*, **152**, 791
219. Taylor, A. N. and Wasserman, R. H. (1967). Vitamin D_3-induced calcium-binding protein: partial purification, electrophoretic visualization, and tissue distribution. *Arch. Biochem.*, **119**, 536
220. Corradino, R. A., Wasserman, R. H., Pubols, M. H. and Chang, S. I. (1968). Vitamin D_3 induction of a calcium-binding protein in the uterus of the laying hen. *Arch. Biochem.*, **125**, 378
221. Wasserman, R. H. and Taylor, A. N. (1968). Vitamin D-dependent calcium-binding protein: Response to some physiological and nutritional variables. *J. Biol. Chem.*, **243**, 3987
222. Alpers, D. H., Lee, S. W. and Avioli, L. V. (1972). Identification of two calcium-binding proteins in human small intestine. A preliminary report. *Gastroenterology*, **62**, 559
223. Williams, G. A., Bowser, E. N., Henderson, W. J. and Uzgiries, V. (1961). Effects of vitamin D and cortisone on intestinal absorption of calcium in the rat. *Proc. Exp. Biol. Med.*, **106**, 664
224. Sallis, J. D. and Holdsworth, E. S. (1962). Calcium metabolism in relation to vitamin D_3 and adrenal function in the chick. *Amer. J. Physiol.*, **203**, 506
225. Anderson, J., Dent, C. E., Harper, C. and Philpot, G. R. (1954). Effect of cortisone on calcium metabolism in sarcoidosis with hypercalcemia; possibly antagonistic actions of cortisone and vitamin D. *Lancet*, **2**, 720
226. Kimberg, D. V., Baerg, R. D., Gershon, E. and Graudusius, R. T. (1971). Effect of cortisone treatment on the active transport of calcium by the small intestine. *J. Clin. Invest*, **50**, 1309
227. Billich, C. O. and Levitan, R. (1969). Effects of sodium concentration and osmolality on water and electrolyte absorption from the intact colon. *J. Clin. Invest.*, **48**, 1336
228. Kramer, P., Kearney, M. P. and Ingelfinger, J. F. (1962). The effect of specific foods and water loading on the ileal excreta of ileostomised human subjects. *Gastroenterology*, **42**, 535

229. Phillips, S. F. and Giller, J. The contribution of the colon to electrolyte and water conservation in man. *J. Clin. Lab. Med.*, (in the press)
230. Levitan, R., Fortdran, B. A., Burrows, B. A. and Ingelfinger, F. J. (1962). Water and salt absorption in the human colon. *J. Clin. Invest.*, **41**, 1754
231. Levitan, R. and Ingelfinger, F. J. (1965). Effect of d-aldosterone on salt and water absorption from the intact human colon. *J. Clin. Invest.*, **44**, 801
232. Shields, R., Harris, J. and Davies, M. W. (1968). Suitability of polyethylene glycol as a dilution indicator in the human colon. *Gastroenterology*, **54**, 331
233. Mekhjian, H. S., Phillips, D. G. and Hoffman, A. F. (1971). Colonic secretion of water and electrolytes induced by bile acids: Perfusion studies in man. *J. Clin. Invest.*, **50**, 1569
234. Levitan, R. and Brudno, S. (1967). Permeability of the rectosigmoid mucosa to tritiated water in normal subjects and in patients with mild idiopathic ulcerative colitis. *Gut*, **8**, 15
235. Devroede, G. J. and Phillips, S. F. (1970). Failure of the human rectum to absorb electrolytes and water. *Gut*, **11**, 438
236. Levitan, R. (1967). Salt and water absorption from the normal human colon: Effect of 9-alpha-fluorohydrocortisone administration. *J. Clin. Lab. Med.*, **69**, 558
237. Wrong, O. (1968). Aldosterone and electrolyte movements in the colon. *Brit. Med. J.*, **1**, 379
238. Edmonds, C. J. and Godfrey, R. C. (1970). Measurement of electrical potentials of the human rectum and pelvic colon in normal and aldosterone-treated patients. *Gut*, **11**, 330
239. Shields, R. and Miles, J. B. (1965). Absorption and secretion in the large intestine. *Postgrad. Med.*, **41**, 435
240. Giller, J. and Phillips, S. F. (1972). Electrolyte absorption and secretion in the human colon. *Amer. J. Dig. Dis.*, **17**, 1003
241. Levitan, R. (1968). The human colon: Its study and absorptive function. *Israel J. Med. Sci.*, **4**, 140
242. Davies, N. T., Munday, K. A. and Parsons, B. J. (1970). The effect of angiotensin on rat intestinal fluid transfer. *J. Endocronol.*, **48**, 39
243. Parsons, B. J. and Munday, K. A. (1972). The action of angiotensin on sodium and fluid transport. *Transport Across the Intestine. A Glaxo Symposium*, 59 (W. L. Burland and P. D. Samuel, editors) (Edinburgh and London: Churchill Livingstone)
244. Levitan, R. and Mauer, I. (1968). Effect of intravenous antidiuretic hormone administration on salt and water absorption from the human colon. *J. Clin. Lab. Med.*, **72**, 739
245. Bright-Asare, P. and Binder, H. J. (1972). Hydroxy fatty acids (OHFA) stimulate colonic secretion of water and electrolytes. *Gastroenterology*, **62**, 727
246. Levitan, R. (1972). The effects of chlorothiazide on water and electrolyte absorption from the intact human colon. *Biologie et Gastro-Enterologie*, **5**, 637
247. Harris, J. and Shields, R. (1970). Absorption and secretion of water and electrolytes by the intact human colon in diffuse untreated proctocolitis. *Gut*, **11**, 27
248. Head, L. H., Heaton, J. W. and Kivel, R. M. (1969). Absorption of water and electrolytes in Crohn's disease of the colon. *Gastroenterology*, **56**, 571
249. Devroede, G., Soffice, M. and Lamarche, J. (1972). Idiopathic constipation: Mechanisms and management. *Biologie et Gastro-Enterologie*, **5**, 643
250. Phillips, S. F. (1969). Absorption and secretion by the colon. *Gastroenterology*, **56**, 966
251. Grady, G. F., Duhamel, R. C. and Moore, E. W. (1970). Active transport of sodium by human colon *in vitro*. *Gastroenterology*, **59**, 583
252. Devroede, G. J. and Phillips, S. F. (1969). Studies of the perfusion technique for colonic absorption. *Gastroenterology*, **56**, 92
253. Long, C. L., Geiger, J. W. and Kinney, J. M. (1967). Absorption of glucose from the colon and rectum. *Metabolism*, **16**, 413
254. Levitan, R. and Patterson, J. F. (1966). Sodium hexanoate absorption from the human small bowel and colon. *Gastroenterology*, **50**, 856
255. Wolpert, E., Phillips, S. F. and Summerskill, W. H. J. (1971). Transport of urea and ammonia production in the human colon. *Lancet*, **2**, 1387
256. Wilson, F. A., Sallee, V. L. and Dietschy, J. M. (1971). Unstirred water layers in intestine: rat determinant of fatty acid absorption from micellar solutions. *Science*, **174**, 1031

257. Sallee, V. A., Wilson, F. A. and Dietschy, J. M. (1972). Determination of unidirecticnal uptake rates for lipids across the intestinal brush border. *J. Lipid Res.*, **13,** 184

258. Wilson, F. A. and Dietschy, J. M. (1972). Characterization of bile acid absorption across the unstirred water layer and brush border of the rat jejunum. *J. Clin. Invest.*, **51,** 3015

259. Trier, J. S. (1968). Morphology of the small intestine. *Handbook of Physiology. Section 6: Alimentary Canal, Vol III. Intestinal Absorption*, 1127 (Amer. Physiol. Soc.)

260. Conrad, M. E. Jr. and Crosby, W. H. (1963). Intestinal mucosal mechanisms controlling iron absorption. *Blood.*, **22,** 406

261. Conrad, M. E. Jr. (1969). Humoral regulation of iron absorption. *Gastroenterology*, **57,** 225

10
Absorption of Lipids

W. J. SIMMONDS
University of Western Australia, Perth

10.1 INTRODUCTION

Different lipid molecules vary in their interaction with water and with each other. The main purpose of this chapter is to consider how these differences influence successive events in absorption, from chemical digestion to transport away from the absorptive cell. Intraluminal events will be emphasised, including uptake from the lumen because these events are now better understood at a molecular physicochemical level both in health and disease. Other sources[1-3] should be consulted for comprehensive reviews of absorption of particular lipid classes.

10.2 PHYSICOCHEMICAL BACKGROUND

A brief descriptive account follows. For more detailed information, the reader may consult a number of excellent reviews[4-6,37].

10.2.1 Water as a solvent

Water is a highly polar solvent in which electrons are distributed asymmetrically over individual molecules. The strong intermolecular attraction between the electron-sparse regions of the hydrogen atoms of one water molecule and the electron-dense vicinity of oxygen atoms in adjacent water molecules makes hydrogen bonding a major force in the interaction between water molecules. For a component to be water-soluble, it must be ionised or possess enough strongly-polar hydrophilic groups so that the over-all attraction of the molecule for water is not outweighed by the attraction of water molecules for each other. The latter interaction tends to 'squeeze' the component out of solution. The tendency may be augmented by attractive forces between the added component molecules or between their parts. A solute–solute interaction of this type plays a role in liquid crystal formation and in micelle formation (to be discussed later).

10.2.2 Lipid-water interaction

Various interactions between lipid and water molecules are categorised in Table 10.1, after Small's classification[5].

Non-polar lipids and insoluble polar lipids are virtually insoluble in a bulk aqueous phase because their polar hydrophilic groups are too weak relative to the non-polar parts of the molecule. The water–water interaction predominates, extruding lipid from the watery environment to form a separate

Table 10.1 Classification of lipid interactions with water
(By courtesy of J. Amer. Oil Chemists Soc.)

Class	Examples
(A) Non-polar lipids	Long-chain and cyclic hydrocarbons
(B) Polar lipids	
(1) Insoluble non-swelling amphiphiles	Triglycerides, diglycerides, long-chain non-ionised fatty acids, cholesterol
(2) Insoluble swelling amphiphiles	Monoglycerides, 'acid soaps', lecithin
(3) Soluble amphiphiles	(a) Soaps of long-chain fatty acids, lysolecithin
	(b) Bile salts

phase. Short-range attractive forces between non-polar parts of adjacent molecules help maintain lipid aggregation.

Few lipids of importance in mammalian physiology are completely non-polar, i.e., have a symmetrical electron distribution over the molecule and no polar groups. Most have some polar features. Moreover, there is spatial separation of polar, hydrophilic and non-polar, hydrophobic or lipophilic parts of lipid molecules. Thus, lipids have a dual affinity—hence the term 'amphiphile'—and a tendency to orient in relation to water molecules. At an interface, amphiphiles form a film, with polar parts orientated toward the aqueous phase. In the bulk aqueous phase, the molecules aggregate so that non-polar groups are excluded as much as possible from interaction with water.

Insoluble non-swelling amphiphiles have a weak hydrophilic region, e.g. ester bonds in long-chain triglycerides. At body temperature, the mixture of fatty acids in the usual dietary lipids is above its melting point. The fatty acid chains are fluid either as non-ionised fatty acid or as esterified fats. In the bulk aqueous phase, dietary triglycerides aggregate as an oil with no fixed orientation of the molecules. Solid non-swelling amphiphiles, such as cholesterol, dissolve in the oil. Any excess lipid forms solid aggregates held together by short-range forces between non-polar parts of adjacent molecules.

While insoluble non-swelling amphiphiles may exist in a bulk aqueous phase as a liquid oil or as solid crystals, the characteristic state of swelling amphiphiles is that of liquid crystals. The basis of this liquid crystalline structure is a bilayer in which the polar hydrophilic heads are on the outside and the non-polar paraffin groups are arranged tail-to-tail inside the bilayer. Alternating lipid bilayers and layers of water form a lamellar structure.

Three factors promote formation of liquid crystals. The first is molecular configuration, namely, a strong polar, hydrophilic head relative to a non-polar tail. One can grasp the salient features of this molecular configuration by comparing a long-chain non-ionised fatty acid above its melting point (a non-swelling amphiphile with one CO_2H polar group) with its homologous monoglyceride. The monoglyceride is a swelling amphiphile, with two hydroxyl groups and one ester bond at the head end of the molecule and the same paraffin tail as the fatty acid. Secondly, lack of strong repulsion between head groups that would favour small spherical structures or dissolution rather than a bilayer. Thirdly, the paraffin tails in the bilayer are liquid. When water contacts a non-hydrated swelling amphiphile, it penetrates between the hydrophilic head groups and between the hydrophilic surfaces of adjacent lamellae, causing swelling and a sliding of lamellae over one another to generate the myelin figures seen under the microscope.

Swelling amphiphiles, such as phospholipids and long-chain monoglycerides, are not sufficiently polar to exist as free molecules in solution in more than trace concentrations. Lawrence[7] pointed out, however, that water may be considered to dissolve in liquid crystalline aggregates. Swelling amphiphiles are too polar to dissolve readily in oil droplets composed of non-swelling amphiphiles but are orientated at the surface with their hydrophilic heads outwards. However, certain non-swelling amphiphiles are readily incorporated or dissolved in liquid crystalline lamellae of swelling amphiphiles. Important examples are cholesterol and non-ionised long-chain fatty acids;

their polarity and dimensions allow them to interdigitate with swelling amphiphiles, such as phospholipid and long-chain monoglyceride.

10.2.3 Bile acid–water interactions

In soluble amphiphiles (detergents), the interaction of the polar groups with water is strong enough relative to the hydrophobic portion to render the entire molecule soluble in water. For example, lecithin, with a strongly hydrophilic phosphorylcholine head but two hydrophobic paraffin chains, is a swelling amphiphile. Lysolecithin has one paraffin chain less and additional hydrophilic properties (hydroxyl group instead of one of the ester bonds) at the end. It is a soluble amphiphile.

Soluble amphiphiles exist in monomolecular solution in the bulk aqueous phase only up to a certain concentration, the critical micellar concentration. Above this, their amphiphilic nature asserts itself by the spontaneous formation of aggregates. micelles, the polar groups facing out toward the water, and the non-polar portion facing the interior and shielded from water. The aggregates are small enough not to scatter transmitted light, so that a micellar solution appears as clear as water. Such a micellar solution also contains monomers at the critical micellar concentration. Monomers in the surrounding water and aggregated molecules in the micelles are in thermodynamic equilibrium, exchanging rapidly with one another. Thus, a micelle should be looked upon as a 'flickering cluster'[8] or cloud, whose size and structure remains constant although the component molecules are continuously entering and leaving.

Most of the common detergents are 'head-and-tail' linear types of amphiphiles, tending to aggregate in spherical micelles. Bile acids, the major intestinal detergent, are 'two-faced' planar amphiphiles with the fixed polar hydroxyl groups on one side of the sterol nucleus, the other side non-polar, and a short hydrophilic tail. In a simple bile acid micelle, the molecules appear to aggregate with the non-polar sides of the sterol nuclei back-to-back. This proposed configuration helped explain how bile salts interact with lipids in micellar solubilisation.

10.2.4 Bile acid–lipid–water interactions

Like other detergents, bile acids interact below the critical micellar concentration with insoluble oil, composed, for example, of non-swelling amphiphiles such as triglycerides. They coat the oil–water interface with a hydrophilic layer, thereby lowering the interfacial tension and permitting the formation of small droplets by shearing forces. The layer is also negatively charged due to the bile acid anions, creating repulsion between droplets and delaying coalescence into large globules. However, bile acids are inefficient emulsifiers in the absence of swelling amphiphiles[9].

Above the critical micellar concentration, bile acids interact primarily with swelling amphiphiles, such as phospholipid and monoglyceride. These are solubilised in much higher concentrations in mixed bile acid micelles than in the spherical micelles formed by 'head-and-tail' detergents, such as fatty acid anions or lysolecithin. This difference is probably due to the mode of molecular aggregation. Evidence suggests that a micelle composed of bile acid and swelling amphiphile is structured like a disc punched out of a lipid bilayer (analogous to a liquid crystal) and coated around its edge by bile acids, hydrophilic side outwards. The upper and lower surfaces of the disc (as in a liquid crystal) are also hydrophilic, due to the polar heads of the swelling amphiphiles. The whole aggregate is small enough to be in effect, water-soluble.

The mixed bile acid–swelling amphiphile micelle can further interact with certain non-swelling amphiphiles, notably cholesterol and non-ionised long-chain fatty acids. These are solubilised poorly in the simple bile acid micelle but can be solubilised to form a considerable proportion of the mixed micelle. Presumably this occurs (as in the liquid crystal) by interdigitating with swelling amphiphile molecules. Non-polar lipids or bulky, non-swelling amphiphiles, such as triglyceride, are solubilised in small amounts in mixed micelles. They are probably accommodated in the 'liquid' non-polar core formed by fluid paraffin chains of the swelling amphiphiles.

Finally, it must be emphasised that bile acids are detergents only in the anionic form. Non-ionised bile acids are insoluble non-swelling amphiphiles. The significance of the secretion of bile acids in bile as taurine or glycine conjugates is that the conjugates are virtually fully ionised at the slightly acid pH of the contents of the upper small intestinal. This is not true for unconjugated bile acids, which have a pk_a of $ca.$ 6 compared with pk_a values of $ca.$ 2 and 4 for taurine and glycine conjugates respectively.

10.3 DIGESTION

10.3.1 State of luminal lipids before digestion

The dietary lipids in man are primarily insoluble amphiphiles: triglycerides, phospholipid, cholesterol and plant sterols. The lipids are present in the stomach mainly as oil, because the proportion of unsaturated and other low-melting-point fatty acids in the usual dietary glycerides is sufficient to lower the melting point of the lipid mixture below body temperature.

No data are available on the degree of dispersion of oil as an emulsion by the time the lipids leave the stomach. Our food contains some constituents, such as soluble protein, which could assist emulsification, and some lipid is ingested with detergent additives. However, the efficiency of the gastric antrum as an emulsifying chamber, the effect of varying motility or biliary reflux and other factors have not been studied.

In the duodenum, the dietary oil mixes with a micellar solution of endogenous phospholipid and cholesterol secreted in the bile and with smaller amounts of other endogenous lipids. One should note that the micelles in bile are already almost saturated with phospholipid and cholesterol and that the major dietary lipid, triglyceride, is only slightly solubilised even in expanded bile salt–phospholipid–cholesterol micelles. In the absence of digestion, the micellar phase of intestinal contents would consist mainly of biliary lipid, with the possible addition of small amounts of dietary phospholipids, sterol and fat-soluble vitamins.

10.3.2 Pancreatic lipolysis

Pancreatic enzymes are generally accepted to be the most important agents in lipid digestion. Pancreatic juice contains lipolytic activity against the major dietary esterified lipids—triglyceride, glycerophospholipids and cholesterol esters of long-chain fatty acids—as well as against water-soluble carboxylic esters of fat-soluble vitamins. The number of separate enzymes responsible for all these activities is unresolved. At least three have been isolated and purified with relative success: glycerol ester hydrolase or lipase, a carboxylic ester hydrolase and phospholipase

10.3.2.1 Lipase

Lipase, which normally accounts for virtually all digestion of dietary triglyceride, has two properties of outstanding physiological importance: (a) it acts only at an oil–water interface, and (b) the enzyme behaves towards its substrate, triglyceride, as a specific primary ester hydrolase, the products of digestion being free fatty acid (liberated from the 1- and 3-positions) and 2-monoglyceride. With artificial substrates in vitro, the specificity of lipase for glycerol esters or primary alcohol esters is not absolute[10]. It is appropriate here to consider the physicochemical and physiological implications of these two properties of lipase.

As an interfacial enzyme, lipase activity depends upon the area of the oil–water interface and, therefore, on the particle size distribution of the emulsion. More strictly, however, activity depends on the surface concentration of adsorbed enzyme and the surface concentration of sterically-accessible substrate (triglyceride). Thus, the initial velocity of lipolysis depends on factors modifying the physicochemical properties of the interface as well as its surface area[11].

Digestion by lipase converts an insoluble weakly-polar amphiphile, triglyceride, into a mixture of more polar products which behaves together as a swelling amphiphile. The mixture of 2-monoglycerides liberated from dietary fat has the properties already discussed for a swelling amphiphile. The behaviour of the mixed free fatty acids is more complex[12]. For present purposes, the mixture of non-ionised and ionised long-chain fatty acids (acid soap) found at the slightly acid pH of upper small intestinal contents in the presence of bile acids may be included as a swelling amphiphile in addition to 2-monoglyceride.

In the absence of solubilisation, the digestion products would tend to slow hydrolysis. Being more polar, they would displace triglyceride from the interface, thereby reducing the availability of substrate, and they would possibly reduce lipase activity toward the remaining substrate by making the surface of the oil droplet more hydrophilic. These effects might be offset somewhat by a co-operative action of swelling amphiphiles and bile acids, enhancing emulsification and increasing interfacial area. Nevertheless, a 'clean' hydrophobic interface would seem desirable for an optimal rate of lipolysis. The generation of swelling amphiphiles, which are readily solubilised by bile acid micelles, ensures rapid removal of digestion products from the interface.

A physicochemical basis for the interfacial activity of lipase and for its specificity as a primary ester hydrolase for triglycerides has been proposed by Brockerhoff[13]. Lipase behaves as a weak nucleophilic agent in attacking ester bonds. It is, therefore, efficient only in a non-polar environment shielded from water, i.e. at an oil–water interface. Reducing the hydrophobic properties of the interface would decrease activity. The presence of electron-donating groups adjacent to the site of hydrolysis (e.g., the hydroxyl groups on either side of the ester bond in 2-monoglyceride) would inhibit activity. Steric hindrance must be invoked, however, to explain why the 2-ester bond is not split first in triglyceride, i.e., while it has an electron-withdrawing ester group on either side.

10.3.2.2 Interaction of lipase with bile acids: colipase

Bile acids should promote triglyceride digestion by their emulsifying and solubilising action. Nevertheless, bile acids inhibit the activity of highly purified lipase above the critical micellar concentration. It is restored by a heat-stable low-molecular-weighted fraction first described by Baskys et al.[14]. This substance, colipase, has been purified to give an appreciation of its probable significance in intraluminal fat digestion[15-17].

Colipase is an acid polypeptide, with a mol. wt. of ca. 10 000. It is heat-stable, due probably to its five disulphide bridges. In the presence of bile acids, it binds to lipase, maximally at pH 6 with a colipase: lipase molar ratio of 2:1. Parenthetically, colipase has a remarkably low concentration of aromatic residues. Thus, it is undetectable by absorption at 280 nm when one scans column effluent spectrophotometrically for peptides; this created some difficulties in isolating the active material.

The colipase–lipase complex has important physiological properties. Thus, lipase activity is no longer inhibited in the presence of bile acids above the critical micellar concentration, and the optimum pH for activity is shifted from pH 9 to 6. Lipase activity in duodenal contents resists inactivation by proteolytic enzymes much more than lipase activity in pancreatic juice[18]. This may also be due to the formation of the colipase–lipase complex in the presence of bile acids. Thus, colipase seems to confer properties on lipase which adapt it to function optimally under conditions encountered in the duodenum. Apparently, colipase itself does not enhance lipase activity. The maximum activity of a given amount of pure lipase is the same at pH 6 with colipase plus bile acids as at pH 9 with or without colipase in the absence of bile acids[17].

10.3.2.3 Esterase

Activity of an esterase (mol. wt. 70 000) has been separated from lipase activity (mol. wt. 40 000) by Sephadex gel filtration of pancreatic juice[19]. It resembles the esterase separated from lipase in pancreatic homogenates in that it lacks activity against insoluble esters. The enzyme in pancreatic juice, unlike intracellular esterase, requires bile acids for its activity[20]. The pancreatic juice esterase is active, not only against soluble carboxylic esters, but also against insoluble esters when these are solubilised in bile acid micelles. Thus, it can split monoglyceride and even the minute quantities of triglyceride and cholesterol ester which are solubilised in mixed micelles[19]. The purified enzyme[21] may be identical with cholesterol ester hydrolase previously isolated first as a dimer (mol. wt. 136 000)[22] and then as a monomer[23], and considered to be a separate enzyme. A consensus must still be reached on a number of points, e.g. whether cholesterol ester hydrolase activity can be separated from soluble ester hydrolase activity and whether the sterol hydrolase activity has a more specific requirement for trihydroxy bile acids than the esterase[24]. Bile acids appear to have a dual effect on both activities: protecting against proteolytic activity even below the critical micellar concentration and inducing reversible aggregation to higher-molecular-weight species.

Carboxylic ester hydrolase activity is usually measured against soluble esters that are absent from the diet. Its physiological function is obscure. As a cholesterol ester hydrolase, it would be active mainly against the small fraction of cholesterol ester which is solubilised. It may hydrolyse solubilised esters of fat soluble vitamins. Apparently, it plays no important part in triglyceride digestion. The proportions of 2-monoglyceride and free fatty acid in the intestinal contents and data on the mixture entering the absorptive cell are consistent with the predominance of lipase activity.

10.3.2.4 Phospholipase

The phospholipase of pancreatic juice is secreted as an inactive precursor. In the duodenum, the zymogen is activated by trypsin and protected by bile acid from further proteolysis. The pancreatic enzyme is phospholipase A^2, hydrolysing specifically at the 2 (β)-ester position[25] to 1(a)-acyl lysolecithin and one molecule of fatty acid. Studies in humans by Borgström and his colleagues[26] indicated that this pancreatic enzyme is the main agent of phospholipid digestion. Little or no hydrolysis of 1 (a)-ester occurs either in lecithin or 1-lysolecithin. Phospholipase A^2 activity varies in parallel with the other pancreatic enzymes. 1 (a)-Acyl lysolecithin constitutes up to 50–60% of the total choline glycerophosphatides in intestinal contents after a test meal.

10.3.3 Gastric and pregastric lipolysis

Unesterified long-chain fatty acids are present in gastric contents in man after a test meal containing triglyceride[27]. Lipolytic activity has been demonstrated in gastric contents in man when reflux of duodenal contents was shown to be negligible[28] and in rats after pancreatic juice and bile were diverted for several days[29]. Activity is slight against long-chain triglycerides and moderate against medium-chain triglycerides. Activity against milk triglycerides in the stomach is said to be superior to that of pancreatic lipase. Although eluted from Sephadex gel in a mol. wt. fraction of ca. 40 000 (similar to pancreatic lipase), the gastric activity is stable to low pH and is highly susceptible to tryptic inactivation, even in the presence of bile acids. Histochemistry in rats[30] and the reduction of activity with achlorhydria in man[28] are compatible with a gastric origin of the lipase. However, the contribution of a lingual lipase[31] to the activity found in gastric contents has not yet been evaluated fully.

Whatever the source, it seems that the lipolytic activity in gastric juice contributes little to normal triglyceride digestion. A role has been suggested in the suckling animal and in pancreatic insufficiency.

10.3.4 Factors regulating digestion

The previous section dealt with the enzymology of the lipid hydrolases, particularly with the interactions of substrate, enzyme, bile acid and water. Enzymological studies are particularly concerned with initial reaction rates in a closed system, *in vitro*. Lipid digestion *in vivo* in the intestinal contents is an open system. To use Hofmann's simile[32], the upper small intestine may be considered as a reaction vessel to which substrate, enzymes, fluid and detergent are continuously added, in which enzymes catalyse reactions at oil–water interfaces as well as in the bulk aqueous medium, and from which reaction products are continuously removed. The steps are interdependent physiochemically and physiologically. Thus, it is difficult to determine whether a given factor is affecting the rate of digestion directly and when the rate of digestion is a major determinant in the overall process.

10.3.4.1 Addition of substrate: gastric emptying

The regulation of gastric emptying is discussed in the chapter on motility. Under suitable conditions, a fairly precise adjustment of gastric emptying to triglyceride load can be demonstrated, e.g. in rats given a test meal of finely emulsified triglyceride in a fixed volume of saline[33]. Presumably, this is mediated by solubilised fatty acid in the duodenal contents[34], reducing antral motility by neural and hormonal mechanisms. If these observations are generally applicable, they suggest that stomach emptying is regulated to give a fairly steady supply of lipid substrate to the duodenal reaction vessel. In a mixed meal, however, the lipid content is only one of several factors potentially influencing gastric emptying. Moreover, when the lipid is not pre-emulsified, it leaves the stomach after the main fluid bulk of the meal has been emptied. Suitable markers for the oil phase of gastric contents are now available[35], but whether the rate at which lipid leaves the stomach is specifically regulated, independent of the other constituents of the meal, has not been established.

10.3.4.2 Addition of enzyme: pancreatic secretion

Regulatory mechanisms are discussed in the chapters on pancreatic exocrine secretion and gastrointestinal hormones. Although these mechanisms could conceivably adjust secretion of lipolytic enzymes to the composition of the duodenal contents continuously, it is uncertain that secretory control works in this way. The problem is analogous to that for gastric emptying. Thus, enzyme output in man is stimulated by essential amino acids or fatty acids when these materials are perfused steadily through the duodenum[36], but no evidence exists that the output of lipolytic enzymes is regulated independently. Moreover, in patients on a regimen of three formula meals per day, pancreatic secretion is turned on by the first meal and persists throughout the day at a steady near-maximal rate; it decreases to a minimum during the night (Go, Brunner, Hofmann and Summerskill, personal communication). This suggests that secretory control is geared to provide a continuous surplus of enzymes for duodenal digestion rather than to continuously adjust the enzyme supply to the state of digestion.

10.3.4.3 Addition of detergent: bile acid secretion

In man, on a regime of three homogenised formula meals per day, bile acid secretion varies more than enzyme output. Nevertheless, after the initial surge due to gall-bladder emptying, when the first meal of the day is taken, secretion into the duodenum becomes fairly steady, until digestive–absorptive activity ceases overnight[38].

10.3.4.4 Stabilisation of pH

The prevention of excessive duodenal acidity is important for regulation of lipid digestion. The mechanisms are discussed in the chapters on gastro-intestinal hormones and gastric and pancreatic secretion. Continuous measurement of pH in man and animals[39-40] indicates that digestion takes place mainly in a slightly acidic medium, with occasional swings to more-acid values early in the digestive period. The adverse effects of frequent short periods of high intraluminal acidity have been nicely documented in patients with gross hypersecretion of gastric acid due to a gastrin-producing tumour[41]. Lipase is irreversibly inactivated and solubilisation is impaired.

10.3.4.5 Rate-limiting factors

Little is known about the steps limiting the overall processes of digestion, solubilisation and uptake of lipids from the lumen—thereby determining the point at which a steady state is reached. Evidence has been mentioned which indicates that digestion *in vivo* proceeds with an excess of enzyme, in contrast to the excess of substrate usually used for enzymological studies. Borgstöm has suggested that the rates of hydrolysis and regeneration of ester bonds at the oil–water interface are rapid relative to the removal of triglyceride digestion products by absorption[42]. Thus lipolytic products rapidly accumulate until a balance is reached at which no net lipolysis would occur *in vitro*, while, *in vivo*, further generation of lipolytic products is determined by their absorption. However, when intestinal contents are incubated *in vitro*, net liberation of fatty acids continues, e.g. the concentration may rise by

30–60%[43]. These findings suggest that absorption maintains the concentration of lipolytic products *in vivo* below the true equilibrium value for a closed system *in vitro*.

In man, assemblies of fine plastic tubes passed through the nose allow perfusion and concurrent sampling at a number of sites in the lumen of the small intestine. The composition and physical state of the contents can be measured serially for long periods. Unabsorbable markers and absorbable radioactive tracers, added to the meal or by perfusion into an intestinal segment, allow measurement of rates, e.g. enzyme output into duodenum or generation of lipolytic products. Such techniques may help to identify rate-limiting steps. A steady state can be set up by perfusion and then the system can be perturbed, e.g. by adding further enzyme to see whether enzyme supply is limiting the lipolytic rate[44].

10.3.4.6 Anatomical reserve

Normally, digestion and absorption of lipid are almost completed in the upper half of the small intestine. During overload, the digestive–absorptive process extends into the distal half of the small intestine. This reserve capacity must be taken into account when one compares the results of *in vitro* and *in vivo* studies.

10.4 SOLUBILISATION

10.4.1 Redistribution of lipids during digestion

The concentration of solubilised lipid is an important determinant of uptake and absorption rates. Lipid in the intestinal contents is distributed between an oil phase and an aqueous phase consisting of micelles and a monomolecular solution. Before digestion starts, nearly all the dietary lipid is in the oil phase, and the bile acid micelles in the aqueous phase contain mainly biliary phospholipid and cholesterol. Digestion initiates a complex redistribution of lipid between oil and aqueous phases. Lipase generates micellar solutes, i.e. monoglyceride and fatty acid, while phospholipase reduces the load of micellar solutes by converting lecithin, a swelling amphiphile, into lysolecithin. The latter is a soluble amphiphile, some of which leaves the micelles to enter a monomolecular solution. Absorption also continuously removes lipid solute from the micelles while the micellar solvents, conjugated bile acids, are absorbed very little in the upper small intestine. The distribution of lipid between oil phase and micelles during digestion is thus determined by rates of generation and final removal of micellar solute, as well as by factors which would determine the distribution at equilibrium in a closed system.

10.4.2 Equilibrium distribution between micelles and oil

At equilibrium in a closed system, the chemical potential of a non-ionised lipid would be the same in oil, monomolecular aqueous solution and micelles. Consider first pure non-ionised long-chain fatty acid dispersed as oil droplets in water, in the absence of micelles. In this case, the tendency for fatty acid molecules to escape from oil to water would be very small, but maximal, since fatty acid is the only constituent of the oil (mole fraction $= 1$). An exceedingly low concentration of long-chain fatty acid molecules in water would offset the tendency to escape from oil to water. Nevertheless, the monomolecular aqueous concentration (10^{-5} mol l^{-1} of water, 10^{-5} mol/55 mol water, mole fraction 5×10^{-6}) is a maximal value. The monomolecular solution would be fully saturated. If a second component, say triglyceride, were present in the oil, the mole fraction of fatty acid would be less than one, its chemical potential would usually be lowered, and the monomolecular concentration of fatty acid in water would decrease correspondingly below the 100% saturation value.

The addition of bile acid micelles to the system containing only fatty acid would not materially alter the concentration (percentage saturation) of the monomolecular solution of fatty acid, as long as an oil phase remains. In equilibrium with an oil composed of pure fatty acid, both micelles and monomolecular solution would be saturated with fatty acid. Saturation of the micelles is defined by the mole fraction of non-ionised fatty acid in the micelles, which is much higher than the mole fraction in monomolecular solution. It must be emphasised that only bile acid exceeding the critical micellar concentration acts as micellar solvent.

The concentration of micellar lipid per unit volume of water must be distinguished from the concentration (mole fraction) of lipid in the micelles. The former increases with increasing bile acid concentration, as long as undissolved fatty acid remains. The later remains unchanged as long as the concentration (percentage saturation) of the monomolecular lipid solution in water remains unchanged. In our theoretical situation, when all the fatty acid has been solubilised, a further addition of bile acids would reduce the solute: solvent ratio in micelles below saturation value. A new equilibrium would be established with the monomolecular concentration reduced below saturation to an extent determined by the micellar solute: solvent ratio. In this way, addition of micellar solvent (detergent) may reduce the efficiency of a process in which single molecules of lipid participate, but not micellar aggregates. This can be demonstrated in vitro for diffusion through porous membranes impermeable to micelles[45]. The concept may also be relevant to lipid uptake by absorptive cell membranes (to be discussed later).

When the system contains several micellar solutes, provided they are present only in micelles, in monomolecular solution and in the oil mixture, the same argument can be applied. But there are complications. The different lipids cannot usually be treated as if they were independently solubilised in micelles. First, there is a limit to the mole fraction of total swelling amphiphiles which can be solubilised; the presence of one variety limits the solubilising capacity for another. Second, the presence of swelling amphiphiles greatly enhances the solubilising capacity for certain non-swelling amphiphiles, e.g. cholesterol, as already discussed.

Fairly accurate measurements of concentrations in monomolecular solution are needed to substantiate some of the foregoing arguments. For most lipids, such concentrations are very low and data are not yet available for the complex types of system encountered in the intestinal contents.

10.4.3 Analysis of micellar lipid

The lipid concentration in the aqueous phase depends primarily on micellar solubilisation. Analysis of lipid in the aqueous phase, 'micellar lipid', is complicated by several possible artefacts. The aqueous phase is usually isolated by high-speed centrifugation (10^7 g min), to float the emulsified oil droplets to the surface, and by sampling the clear infranatant layer. If the duration of the centrifuged force is too low, finely-emulsified particles may remain in a seemingly clear infranatant[46]. With more intense centrifugation, the infranatant may show a concentration gradient due to partial sedimentation of micelles[43-46]. With prolonged contact, micellar lipid is taken up by the walls of the cellulose nitrate tubes commonly used[46]. Another complication is continued lipolytic activity during and after collection of intestinal contents. A considerable amount of fatty acid may be liberated by lipase, even during heating to inactive the enzyme. Phospholipase is resistant to heat. Moreover, freezing, thawing and heating of the sample before ultracentrifugation may alter the distribution of the lipid. Passage of intestinal contents through a series of filters of decreasing porosity has been shown to effect a quick and fairly clean separation of oil and aqueous phases and to minimise artefacts due to continued lipolysis[43]. Clearly, measurements of the concentration and composition of micellar lipid in the intestinal contents must still be interpreted cautiously.

10.4.4 Steady-state distribution

In a previous part of this section, the distribution of lipid between oil and micelles was treated as an equilibrium in a closed system. In the intestinal contents *in situ*, a continuous net transfer of lipid occurs from oil to micelles and monomolecular solution and out of the aqueous phase into the absorbing cells. The driving force for this net flux of absorbable lipid is a difference in chemical potential so that, by definition, the oil and aqueous phase cannot be in equilibrium. While proof is lacking, it seems highly likely that lipid in the two aqueous states (monomolecular solution and micelles) is virtually in equilibrium. It is uncertain whether transfer of lipid between oil particles and aqueous phase involves no rate-limiting step; this step would lead to considerable divergence between lipid distribution predicted for a closed system and the distribution found for the same total concentration of lipid, detergent, etc., during absorption *in situ*. Higuchi and his colleagues have studied the role of an interfacial resistance in the transfer of lipid from emulsion particles to mixed micellar solutions[47-49]. They have observed differences, e.g. between cholesterol and betasitosterol which may be relevant for absorption *in vivo*.

10.5 UPTAKE FROM THE LUMEN

10.5.1 General features

Over-all, the intraluminal phase of digestion and absorption is an open system in which digestion products are continuously generated and removed, and the lipid in oil and micelles is constantly redistributed. The aim of this discussion is to consider uptake as a passive process driven by the difference in chemical potential between absorbable lipid in the aqueous phase of intestinal contents and in the aqueous phase of the cytoplasm immediately inside the brush border of the absorptive cell. There are at least two major resistances to flux of lipid down this potential gradient—a diffusion barrier due to an unstirred aqueous layer on the luminal side of the brush border and a more complex resistance encountered in translocation of lipid through the cell membrane itself.

10.5.2   The unstirred layer

However vigorously the bulk of a liquid may be stirred, a relatively undisturbed layer remains adjacent to any surface in contact with the liquid. In this layer, mixing with the bulk of the fluid or transport of solute or solvent molecules can occur only by diffusion. The boundary between the unstirred layer and the well-mixed bulk of the liquid is indistinct. In the intermediate zone, the efficiency of mixing increases with increasing distance from the surface. The thickness of the combined unstirred and poorly-stirred layers is defined operationally as the equivalent thickness of a single layer in which transport occurs only by diffusion. This equivalent thickness can be measured by suddenly altering the composition of the bulk fluid and measuring the rate of change of a property limited by diffusion, such as a diffusion potential, when electrolyte concentration is changed, or a streaming potential for a non-penetrating solute such as sucrose[50,51]. The estimated thickness of the unstirred layer varies with experimental conditions and has no fixed anatomical dimension.

10.5.3   The cell membrane

Transport of lipid through the cell membrane involves at least two steps, both of which might contribute a resistance to absorptive flux.

10.5.3.1   Partition

The first step is passage of lipid molecules from the aqueous environment on the luminal side of the cell membrane to the lipid environment just inside the luminal boundary of the cell membrane. A lipid molecule has less free energy in a lipid environment than in an aqueous medium. Roughly, the tendency to escape from lipid to water is less than from water to lipid. In a closed system, with no absorptive flux, an equilibrium would be established with the concentration of the lipid solute molecules (mole fraction) in the membrane much higher than the concentration (mole fraction) in the aqueous medium. By definition, the chemical potential of the solute would be the same in aqueous medium and in a cell membrane; the lower free energy per solute molecule in the membrane is balanced by the higher concentration. One can regard this as a partition between cell membrane lipids and the aqueous medium just exterior to the membrane. Partition of a lipid solute into the membrane lipid ('solvent') would be decreased by hydrophilic attraction, mainly hydrogen bonding, between lipid solute and water. Attractive forces between lipid solute and cell membrane constituents would favour partition into the membrane.

During absorption, the system is open, with continuous flux of lipid from the aqueous medium into and through the cell membrane. The concentration of lipid solute within the cell membrane must therefore be lower than one would predict from partition in a closed system. If the resistance at the interface between luminal water and cell membrane were low, however, the discrepancy would be small. Whether this is the case cannot yet be determined.

10.5.3.2 Translocation

The second step is penetration of the membrane, that is, translocation through the membrane lipid. This step depends on prior partition, since the higher the concentration of lipid solute in the membrane on its luminal side, the greater the flux to the inner side of the membrane tends to be. For a given concentration gradient within the membrane, the flux is determined by resistances dependent on the size of the moving molecule and its interaction with the membrane 'solvent' lipid and other materials.

Passage of lipids into and through a cell membrane differs in important respects from uptake and diffusion through a bulk oil phase *in vitro*. For example, the membrane lipids are mainly amphiphiles and are part of an organised structure including protein. Also, they form a bilayer in which the distance for solute movement is only about twice the longest dimension of the absorbed dietary lipids. Nevertheless, as Diamond and Wright showed, a model based on partition and diffusion in non-aqueous solvents agrees well, quantitatively, with observed membrane selectivity for the different non-electrolytes. Their excellent review[52] should be consulted for detail and for a more rigorous analysis of membrane permeability than that attempted here.

10.5.4 Resistance to diffusion and membrane penetration

The driving force transferring a given lipid between intraluminal fluid and intracellular fluid is the difference in chemical potential of the lipid in these two aqueous media or, as an approximation, the difference in aqueous concentration $C_1 - C_3$, where C_1 = concentration in the bulk aqueous phase and C_3 = concentration in intracellular fluid. The unstirred layer creates a resistance which depends on two factors. The first is the specific resistance met by the lipid in aqueous diffusion, that is $1/D$, where D = aqueous diffusion coefficient in the layer. This is usually assumed to equal the free diffusion coefficient, but may not. The second is the thickness of the unstirred layer, d. The resistance to diffusion through the unstirred layer is thus d/D.

The second resistance is that encountered on passage into and through the cell membrane. More than one process is involved, but the overall resistance may be expressed as $1/P$, where P = permeability coefficient of the membrane to the molecule concerned. This may be treated as a resistance in series with that of the unstirred layer. The total resistance to uptake into the cell is therefore $(d/D + 1/P)$, and the amount transported (flux per unit area) depends on:

$$\frac{C_1 - C_3}{(d/D + 1/P)}$$

The relative importance of the two resistance terms varies with the type of molecule and the experimental conditions. The resistance of the unstirred layer predominates if d/D is large relative to $1/P$, that is, with a thick unstirred layer (d large) and a slowly diffusing molecule or aggregate (D small) or with a high permeability of lipid through the cell membrane (P large). Under such conditions, most of the fall in chemical potential (concentration), $C_1 - C_3$, occurs across the unstirred layer ($C_1 - C_2$) and only a small proportion across the cell membrane ($C_2 - C_3$). The converse is true when the membrane resistance predominates (Figure 10.1).

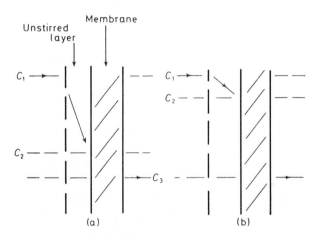

Figure 10.1 Aqueous concentration gradient (A) when diffusion through unstirred layer is the rate-limiting step and (B) when membrane permeability is the rate-limiting step. $C_1 =$ concentration in bulk aqueous phase (well stirred); $C_2 =$ concentration immediately external to cell membrane; and $C_3 =$ concentration in aqueous cytosol. It is assumed that intracellular concentration, C_3, is maintained at a constant low value.

This section has dealt with the restricted case in which diffusion across the unstirred layer and penetration of the cell membrane is monomolecular. When micelles are also present, the aqueous concentration gradient and the resistances to diffusion and membrane penetration must be treated separately for each physical species. This is done in the next section, which also considers the complication introduced when both micelles and monomers diffuse freely across the unstirred layer but only monomers penetrate the cell membrane.

10.6 SOLUBILISATION AND UPTAKE

10.6.1 *In vitro*

Micellar solubilisation unquestionably promotes lipid absorption. The uptake of long-chain fatty acids by everted sacs or rings of small intestine has repeatedly been shown to proceed more rapidly from micellar bile acid solution than from emulsions without bile acids[53,54]. When everted sacs were incubated in media containing a fixed total amount of fatty acid with varying amounts of bile acid, uptake increased *pari passu* with the curve for solubilisation[55]. Uptake varied linearly with the concentration of solubilised fatty acid when this was altered by three methods: (a) by increasing bile acid with a fixed total amount of fatty acid, (b) by varying fatty acid in the presence of a fixed excess of bile acid, so that all the fatty acid was solubilised; and (c) by adding a non-absorbable oil, so that less fatty acid was micellar and more was in the oil with constant amounts of bile acid and total fatty acid. The slope of the line relating uptake to solubilised concentration was much the same, regardless of how solubilisation was altered[56-58].

These observations indicate that micellar solubilisation accelerates uptake by increasing the lipid concentration in aqueous dispersion which provides the driving force for uptake. The amount of insoluble lipid, even in finely dispersed oil droplets, contributes little.

10.6.1.1 *Micellar transport across the unstirred layer*

Although solubilisation increases the effective concentration gradient for uptake, the resistance to aqueous diffusion of solubilised molecules is higher, i.e. the diffusion coefficient is lower. This is due to the greater size of micellar aggregates compared with single molecules in solution. The diffusion coefficient for micellar lipid is lower despite the rapid exchange of individual molecules between micelles and monomolecular solution. Since the ratio of the number of solubilised molecules to the number in monomolecular solution is high at any instant, any given molecule must reside in micelles most of the time, subject to the constraints on movement of the micellar aggregate.

When lipid in micellar solution diffuses across an unstirred layer, the total flux (J_{total}) equals $J_{mic} + J_{mono}$, where J_{mic} and J_{mono} are the fluxes of lipid in micelles and in monomolecular solution, respectively.

$$\text{Flux} = \frac{\text{Driving force}}{\text{Resistance}} - \frac{(C_1 - C_2)}{(d/D)} = (C_1 - C_2) \times D/d$$

where $C_1 - C_2 = $ difference in concentration across the unstirred layer, $d = $ thickness of the layer and $D = $ aqueous diffusion coefficient. Thus,

$$J_{total} = (C_1 - C_2)_{mic} \times \frac{D_{mic}}{d} + (C_1 - C_2)_{mono} \times \frac{D_{mono}}{d}$$

Micellar solubilisation greatly increases the aqueous concentration of certain lipids. For example, in a 10 mM micellar solution of long-chain fatty acids, the ratio $(C_1)_{mic}/(C_1)_{mono} = \dfrac{10^{-2}M}{10^{-5}M} = 1000:1$. The resistance to diffusion $(1/D)$, on the other hand, is (mol. wt.)$^{\frac{1}{2}}$ for molecules of small-to-moderate size and (mol. wt.)$^{\frac{1}{3}}$ for the large micellar aggregate. No reliable measurements of micellar weight are available for mixed micelles in the intestinal contents[6]. Assuming a fairly large value (125 000) the ratio of resistance to diffusion of an 18-carbon fatty acid (micelles: monomolecular solution) $= (125\,000)^{\frac{1}{3}} - (280)^{\frac{1}{2}} = 3:1$. Thus, micellar solubilisation in this example increases the driving force for diffusion ca. 1000-fold, while the resistance increases only ca. threefold.

No great importance should be attached to the number in the example given. It serves merely to emphasise that, for molecules such as long-chain fatty acids which have a low concentration in monomolecular solution but are readily solubilised, diffusion flux is greatly increased by solubilisation and most of the lipid is transported in micelles.

(a) *Rate-limiting effect*—As noted previously, the total resistance to uptake of a lipid may be considered the sum of the resistance to diffusion across the unstirred layer and a resistance term attributable to the cell membrane. That is, total resistance equals $(d/D + 1/P)$, where $d =$ thickness of the unstirred layer and D and $P =$ aqueous diffusion coefficient and membrane permeability coefficient, respectively.

If uptake is unaffected by altering d/D, clearly the resistance to diffusion across the unstirred layer is not a substantial fraction of the total resistance. Wilson, Sallee and Dietschy[59] showed that this was true for a monomolecular solution of short- and medium-chain (6- and 8-carbon) fatty acids. Uptake was unaffected by vigorous stirring, which would reduce the effective thickness of the unstirred layer to a minimum.

Resistance to micellar diffusion of long-chain fatty acid contributed substantially to the resistance to uptake from micellar solution. This was shown by the lower uptake flux per unit concentration in unstirred micellar solution compared with flux from a monomolecular solution of short- and medium-chain fatty acids. It was also demonstrated by a considerable increase in uptake when the micellar medium was stirred. Strictly speaking, these observations do not prove that d/D constitutes a major part of the resistance to uptake from well-stirred micellar solutions (d at its minimum value). However, the conclusions of Wilson et al.[59] are consistent with the data of others[58], who showed that differences in uptake from two types of well-stirred micellar solutions could be correlated with differences in the diffusion coefficients.

Apparently the efficiency of uptake, that is uptake flux per unit concentration in the aqueous phase, is less from micellar solution due to the diffusional resistance of the unstirred layer. The effective thickness of the layer and the size of the micelles, therefore, modifies uptake from micellar solution. However, most lipid digestion products have a very low concentration in a saturated monomolecular solution. This limitation is removed by solubilisation, which greatly increases total uptake, despite the unstirred layer.

10.6.1.2 Micelles and membrane penetration

Enhanced diffusion might not be the only way in which uptake is promoted by solubilisation. Other possibilities are (i) increased membrane permeability; (ii) penetration of the cell membrane by intact micellar aggregates, and (iii) a metabolic effect of bile acids within the absorptive cells. The first two possibilities will be considered here and the third in a later section.

(a) *Permeability*—Evidence exists that bile acids, particularly in high concentration, increase the permeability of the brush border to small water-soluble molecules[60]. No evidence definitely excludes a similar effect on permeability to lipid. Nevertheless, several findings argue against an important permeability effect of bile acids in lipid uptake: (i) solubilised lipid, such as monoglyceride, inhibits the effect of bile acid on permeability to small water-soluble molecules[60]; (ii) the relationship between uptake and solubilised fatty acid concentration is unaffected by bile acid concentration[58]; (iii) damage to cells by unconjugated dihydroxy bile acids is associated with a decrease, not an increase, in fatty acid uptake[53]; (iv) when fatty acid is completely solubilised, a further increase in conjugated bile acids may result in a decreased uptake[61] (see later).

(b) *Micellar or monomolecular penetration*—Presumably, uptake would be promoted if micelles were taken up and penetrated the cell membrane as intact aggregates. Direct evidence from electron microscopy is contradictory[62-64]. It seems unlikely that micellar aggregates passing through the membrane at the time of fixation could survive processing of tissue for electron microscopy. Nor does it seem likely that the labile hydrophilic micellar aggregate would remain intact *in vivo* during passage from an aqueous medium into the lipid environment of the cell membrane.

If the components of micelles were absorbed in the proportions in which they were present in the micelles, this would be strong indirect evidence for micellar penetration. Some results are consistent with this view[59], but evidence favouring independent uptake of micellar components is accumulating. The ratio for uptake of two lipid solutes does not agree consistently with the ratio in the micellar medium[65]. The relation of uptake to concentration solubilised has also been shown to be linear but different for two lipids (fatty acid and glyceryl monoether) when each was the only micellar solute. Furthermore, the proportion in which they were taken up from various micellar mixtures could be predicted from the data for independent uptake[57].

Evidence for independent uptake of different micellar solutes does not, of course, exclude interaction of micelle with membrane before the lipid solutes pass through. If this occurred, the type of micellar solvent might be important for uptake. Cholesterol absorption has been shown to have a specific requirement for bile acid[3] and cholesterol is taken up poorly or not at all when solubilised in other detergents[58]. Apparently, this is not true for fatty acids. Even for cholesterol, the effect of temperature on uptake is consistent with a process of low activation energy, such as diffusion[66], rather than with the higher activation energies of specific types of absorption interaction at surfaces.

(c) *Protein binding*—Most evidence favours uptake of lipid as single molecules. This conclusion is consistent with a process involving partition between water and lipid followed by diffusion in lipid, as in Diamond and Wright's model[52]. In other models, lipid interaction with a mixture of binding sites of low affinity and high affinity has been postulated. The evidence for such models rests rather heavily on data for efflux of labelled lipid after an uptake period[67]. Several difficulties attend the interpretation of such evidence. For example, washout from the unstirred layer could contribute to a 'rapid efflux' component. Also the specific activity of the pools contributing to efflux is unknown. This contrasts with influx from a large 'pool' of incubation medium in which the specific activity changes very little. In addition, it would be difficult to distinguish between the effect of higher affinity sites on efflux curves and the effect of longer mean free path for diffusion. The latter situation might occur if the solution between the lower halves of the villi were less well stirred than that at the tips. In both cases, efflux would be accelerated by increasing the affinity (decreasing the chemical potential) of the medium for lipid, as might occur when albumin was added to bind fatty acid or detergent concentration was raised above the critical micellar concentration.

The concept that protein on or in the cell membrane may influence lipid uptake should not be discarded merely because the evidence is inconclusive. The cell membrane is a highly-organised lipoprotein structure, not simply a lipid film. The high degree of specificity in absorption of steroids, at least *in vivo*, has been ascribed to lipid-binding proteins[68]. Whether these are intracellular or reside in the cell membrane remains undetermined.

One must also remember, however, that apparently small differences in molecular structure may have large effects on lipid:water partition[52] or on penetration of a lipid interface. For example, the plant sterol, β-sitosterol, is transferred much more slowly than cholesterol from oil droplets to water[49], although the plant sterol differs from cholesterol only in addition of a methyl group at C-24 in the side chain. The two sterols have a similar solubility in mixed bile acid-swelling amphiphile micelles. Whether a specificity of uptake or penetration analogous to that for the cell membrane can be obtained with more organised lipid structures, such as liquid crystals or artificial bilayers, needs further study. Detailed information and references on the specificity for absorption of sterols and fat-soluble vitamins may be found in a fine review by Borgström[1].

(d) *Micellar transport and monomolecular gradient*—If micelles do not penetrate the cell membrane and if the resistance to diffusion across the unstirred layer does not limit the uptake from monomolecular solution, it is difficult to explain why uptake is much greater from micellar solution than from saturated monomolecular solution in the absences of micelles. The ultimate driving force for uptake must be the concentration of the penetrating species, i.e. monomers, not micelles. Micellar lipid could, therefore, promote absorption by maintaining a higher monomolecular concentration at the luminal interface of the brush border, after diffusion across the unstirred layer. Since the maximum monomer concentration is that of a saturated monomolecular solution, no enhancement by solubilisation could occur if the unstirred layer contributed no significant resistance to monomer diffusion, relative to the cell membrane resistance. Some mechanism involving lipid loading of the membrane directly from micelles would have to be invoked.

On the other hand, monomolecular penetration would be consistent with decreased uptake found when an excess of micellar solvent is present, e.g. when more bile acid is added to a micellar solution of lipid[61]. In such circumstances, the concentration in monomolecular solution, which is in equilibrium with the micelles, must fall as excess of micellar solvent renders the micelles unsaturated with lipid. The driving force for uptake is thus lower, although the total aqueous concentration of lipid is unchanged.

10.6.2 *In vivo*

In vitro preparations have both limitations and advantages in elucidating mechanisms of lipid absorption[58]. *In vitro* preparations are incomplete models of the *in vivo* process, since they lack the capacity to extrude absorbed lipid from cells as chylomicrons and cannot sustain a steady uptake for long periods. Function starts to deteriorate when the segment is removed, losing its lymph and blood drainage and supply of blood-borne nutrients. Structural disorganisation may be apparent in less than 1 h. Rate-limiting processes may differ from those in the living animal and metabolic handling of absorbed products may be distorted. Selectivity of absorption, e.g. for sterols, may be impaired[1]. The advantage of *in vitro* preparations, particularly in studying transfer from lumen to cell membrane, are that the absorptive area is standardised and the physical state of the absorbate can be closely controlled.

In vivo, quantitative studies comparable to those *in vitro* are difficult to perform. Separation of oil and aqueous phases of human intestinal contents gave the first clear evidence of micellar solubilisation as a key mechanism in lipid absorption[69]. Since then, bile acid deficiency, defective solubilisation and lipid malabsorption have been correlated in a variety of pathological conditions[70-72]. However, a continuous gradation of absorption rates with solubilised concentration, e.g. of long-chain fatty acids, has not been demonstrated in man or animals. Indeed, steady-state lymphatic absorption of long-chain fatty acid in rats with bile fistula was as efficient with duodenal infusions containing a trace of micellar lipid as when all the lipid was solubilised. Absorption was moderately depressed when no micellar lipid was present[73].

Discrepancies between *in vivo* and *in vitro* results may be explained at least partly by differences in the absorptive situation. Normally, lipid is almost completely absorbed before the distal half of the small intestine is reached[27]. Thus, the distal absorptive area remains in reserve. Measures of overall absorption, such as lymphatic output in animals or balance studies in man reveal no absorptive deficit until the reserve area is utilised fully[74]. Similarly, if bile acids are deficient but not absent from the contents of the upper small intestine, progressive absorption of fluid may raise the concentration enough to permit solubilisation before the bile acids are actively absorbed in the distal ileum. Such adaptations have been documented by Knoebel[75].

We have little information on the kinetics of lipid uptake *in vivo* comparable to that obtained *in vitro*. In man, preliminary reports claim that long-chain fatty acid uptake from a perfused intestinal segment is slower in the absence of micelles[76] and that uptake in different patients correlates with the concentration solubilised[77]. Under steady-state conditions, the components of mixed micelles are taken up at different rates by perfused jejunal segments.

Monoglyceride and fatty acid is absorbed faster than cholesterol, and taurine-conjugated bile acids are not absorbed, a finding consistent with uptake of single molecule but not of micellar aggregates[78].

Many animal studies have been reported on absorption from closed segments or continuously perfused segments, *in situ* but usually under anaesthesia. Data suitable for kinetic analysis, however, have come mainly from pharmacological studies of lipid-soluble drugs of low molecular weight[79]. Preliminary reports indicate that uptake of long-chain fatty acid from a closed segment varies with solubilised concentration and that different lipids are taken up at independent rates from the same mixed micelles[58].

Although the evidence is incomplete, apparently when the absorptive area and physiochemical state of the absorbate can be standardised, *in vivo* results are similar to *in vitro* data. They are consistent with the concepts that solubilisation enhances the total delivery of lipid by diffusion to the absorptive surface but that uptake and penetration of the cell membrane occurs ultimately from a monomolecular solution. Nevertheless, the mechanisms of uptake by isolated gut *in vitro* and intact gut *in situ* may not be identical. In particular, an apparently obligatory role of bile acids in cholesterol absorption and a high degree of selectivity for different sterols are more clearly defined *in vivo*. The *in vitro* intracellular events, briefly discussed in the next section, may differ in some respects from those *in vivo*.

10.7 INTRACELLULAR EVENTS

10.7.1 Absorbed lipid mixture

Table 10.2 shows the components of the absorbed lipid mixture and the lipids from which they are derived in the lumen.

Table 10.2

Original lipid	Absorbed components
Long-chain triglyceride	2-Monoglyceride, free fatty acid
Medium-chain triglyceride	Some triglyceride[80], free fatty acid, glycerol
Cholesterol and cholesterol esters	Cholesterol, free fatty acid
Glycerophospholipid	Lysophospholipid, free fatty acid[26, 81]
Sphingomyelin, cerebroside	Undigested[1]
Fat-soluble vitamins: Some as esters or provitamin (A)	Mainly unesterified[1]

The mixture of absorbable components enters the absorptive cell (enterocyte) in a fine dispersion, probably monomolecular. The components leave the enterocyte mainly in particulate form, as chylomicrons and very-low-density lipoprotein, after complex metabolic changes involving re-esterification and incorporation of non-dietary components. This intracellular phase of lipid absorption will be only outlined here. Johnston's fine review contains a detailed discussion[2].

10.7.2 Metabolism

10.7.2.1 Activation of fatty acid

An essential preliminary to incorporation of absorbed free fatty acids into glycerides is the formation of thio-esters with coenzyme A, under the influence of fatty acid thiokinase. The fatty acid–CoA complex is water-soluble and has a detergent structure, with a strongly hydrophilic head group attached to the paraffin chain of the fatty acid[82]. This suggests a role in fatty acid transport from the brush-border membrane to the intracellular membranes, where esterification occurs. However, the thiokinase appears to be located in the microsomal fraction (that is, on the endoplasmic reticulum), whereas for efficient transport one would have expected it to reside on the intracellular side of the brush-border membrane or in the cell sap. There is little activity against short- and medium-chain fatty acids, which pass rapidly, unesterified, through to portal blood (see later for a discussion).

10.7.2.2 Re-esterification of partial glycerides

Both triglycerides and the major phospholipid, lecithin, are incompletely hydrolysed in the lumen and absorbed as the partial glycerides, 2-monoglycerides, and 1-acyl lysolecithin, respectively, together with free fatty acids. In the lumen, incomplete hydrolysis is important for dispersion and uptake, as discussed previously. In the enterocyte, the absorbed partial glycerides provide a potential shortcut for the reconstitution of triglyceride and phospholipid. The demonstration that this biochemical bonus was utilised, by acylation of 2-monoglyceride to triglyceride, was a major advance in research[2]. Evidence suggests that the monoglyceride pathway could account for most of the triglyceride resynthesised in the enterocyte during normal absorption. Less is known about the reconstitution of lecithin from absorbed 1-acyl lysolecithin. Experiments with selectively-labelled phospholipid and analysis of fatty acid distributed in 1- and 2-positions of chylomicron phospholipid in lymph suggest that direct acylation makes a significant contribution[81].

10.7.2.3 Hydrolysis

Partial glycerides may also undergo hydrolysis in the enterocyte. A monoglyceride hydrolase has been demonstrated, but acylation of long-chain monoglycerides normally predominates[2]. Hydrolysis of ester bonds can be a significant factor in the isolated intestine, *in vitro*, and possibly in the normal enterocyte for any medium-chain triglyceride absorbed intact. Sphingomyelins are thought to be taken up intact and split by intracellular or brush-border enzymes[1].

10.7.2.4   Glyceride synthesis

In liver and adipose tissue, triglyceride is synthesised from L-a-glycerophosphate, which is acylated to phosphatidic acid, dephosphorylated to diglyceride and then acylated to triglyceride. The mucosa of the small intestine can also use this pathway. In the enterocyte, L-a-glycerophosphate is generated mainly by glycolysis although, contrary to earlier belief, there is some capacity of glycerokinase to phosphorylate glycerol. The a-glycerophosphate pathway also diverges at phosphatidic acid and diglyceride for phospholipid synthesis.

Thus the enterocyte possesses alternative pathways for the synthesis of both triglyceride and phospholipid. Factors determining the extent of utilisation of the alternative modes of synthesis are not yet understood. The composition of the absorbed lipid mixture may play a part. For example, if fat is absorbed mainly as free fatty acid in animals with bile fistula, as has been suggested[1], the a-glycerophosphate pathway must be used in such circumstances.

10.7.2.5   Cholesterol

Cholesterol esters of long-chain fatty acids are absorbed only after hydrolysis to free cholesterol. Nevertheless, much of the cholesterol recovered in lymph after absorption is esterified. Esterification is thought to occur relatively late in the assembly of the chylomicron, through a small pool of cholesterol ester with a rapid turnover.

10.7.2.6   Non-dietary (endogenous) components

Even at the peak of fat absorption, the absorbed lipid mixture transported in lymph contains a considerable proportion of non-dietary components. The sources of endogenous lipids and the extent to which they participate in lipid turnover by the enterocyte are discussed in detail elsewhere[83]. Biliary cholesterol and phospholipid make a major contribution. Mucosal synthesis is also a significant source of endogenous cholesterol. Endogenous fatty acids are derived mainly from the lumen. In chylomicrons after a fatty meal the proportion of endogenous fatty acid is greater in phospholipid than in cholesterol esters and it is least in triglycerides.

10.7.2.7   Role of bile acids

Metabolism of absorbed lipid in the enterocytes and assembly of transport particles (chylomicrons, very-low-density lipoprotein) is coordinated with intraluminal events, since lymphatic output of absorbed lipid varies *pari passu* with uptake from the lumen, after a time lag of *ca.* 30 min. To a large extent, the coordinating mechanisms could be non-specific, mediated by changing flux of lipid into the enterocyte and by the balance of the absorbed mixture

A more specific role has been claimed for bile acids. Their presence in the lumen inhibits cholesterol synthesis *de novo* by ileal mucosa[84]. In addition, evidence has been advanced for an intracellular effect of bile acids, specific to the trihydroxy acid conjugates, promoting esterification of absorbed cholesterol[3].

A specific effect of conjugated bile acids in promoting triglyceride synthesis has been claimed[53], but the evidence is equivocal[83,85]. In most experiments, non-specific effects have not been excluded. Solubilisation itself could accelerate synthesis by enhancing uptake of fatty acid and ensuring uptake of monoglyceride[58]. Decreased activity of mucosal enzymes, fatty acid thiokinase and monoglyceride acylase, has been demonstrated in animals with bile fistula; it could be partly reversed by returning bile to the lumen[86].

On the other hand, unconjugated dihydroxy bile acids, particularly deoxycholic acid, inhibit many intracellular processes *in vitro*[87], but have less effect *in vivo*[88]. Bacterial deconjugation sufficient to produce an intracellular effect may occur normally in the ileum of some animals, such as rats[87], but not in man. Pathologically, fatty acid malabsorption is associated with bacterial overgrowth, e.g. in the 'blind loop' syndrome. However, the pathogenic mechanisms are complex, including defective micelle formation by unconjugated bile acids[70].

10.7.3 Assembly and extrusion of transport particles

A fairly detailed discussion covering this topic and the remainder of the chapter has recently appeared[83]. Hence, only an outline will be given here, including some more recent findings.

10.7.3.1 Transfer to sites of synthesis

Electron microscopy suggests that lipid is transferred across the cytosol beneath the brush border in fine dispersion, presumably water-miscible[63,64]. As has already been mentioned, fatty acids could be transported as water-soluble coenzyme A complexes. Alternatively, binding to a soluble protein has been suggested. A protein fraction, with a mol. wt. of *ca.* 12 000, has recently been isolated by gel filtration from jejunal mucosa and other tissues. This fraction is present in the organelle-free supernatant of homogenates. It has a high affinity for unsaturated long-chain fatty acids and other properties similar to Z-protein isolated from liver cytosol[89]. Proteins binding sterols[68] and carotenoids[90] have also been described. Much work remains to be done (e.g. competitive binding assays, tests of enzymatic activity) before an intracellular transport function can be ascribed to such protein factors.

10.7.3.2 Assembly of lipid

The metabolic pathways for the lipid components of the intracellular particles have been mentioned. Little is known about how or where in the cell these components are brought together. Most of the enzymes concerned in triglyceride synthesis are microsomal, i.e. in the endoplasmic reticulum. Labelled lipid droplets appear rapidly in the smooth endoplasmic reticulum vesicles and cisterns and labelled fatty acid is incorporated into triglyceride with comparable speed, after exposure of the mucosa to radioactive fatty acids[91]. This suggests assembly within the endoplasmic reticulum.

Location of lipid-synthesising enzymes is not the sole factor determining appearance of lipid transport particles (very-low-density lipoprotein and chylomicrons) within the endoplasmic reticulum spaces. Such particles are scanty, absent, or varied in size when β-lipoprotein synthesis is defective, although some capacity to synthesise triglyceride is retained. Large lipid droplets, some without surrounding membranes, are seen in the cytoplasm in electron micrographs during fat absorption *in vitro*[63] and *in vivo*[92]. They are prominent in α-β lipoproteinaemia in man[93] and in the upper ileum of rats during maximal fat absorption[94]. The composition of these droplets is unknown. Speculatively, triglyceride may be synthesised on the cytoplasmic side of the endoplasmic reticulum but not translocated adequately into the cisterns unless enough apolipoprotein is available.

There is an increase in both the size and number of the chylomicron-sized particles from apical vesicles to lateral and basal exit sites. Whether composition also changes is uncertain, although an increase in the proportion of triglyceride[95] would be likely. The outlying cisterns and vacuoles of the Golgi apparatus contain transport particles during lipid absorption, whereas the medial cisterns and tubules seem to be more concerned with glycoprotein metabolism[96].

10.7.3.3 Protein components and extrusion

Good evidence exists that the protein as well as the lipid components of the transport particles in lymph (very-low-density lipoprotein, VLDL, and chylomicrons) originate in the intestinal epithelium[83,97], although both peptide and lipid components may exchange with soluble lipoproteins to some extent after extrusion from the cell. Lipid particles with the same size distribution as plasma VLDL are seen in the endoplasmic reticulum in fasting animals and man and, mixed with larger chylomicron size particles, after a fatty meal[98]. Particles isolated from the mucosa during fasting have a size and composition like VLDL.

Whether protein is added to the polar lipid surface of chylomicrons inside the cell or after extrusion is more difficult to determine. Analysis of pelleted chylomicron 'membranes' supports an intracellular origin. So does the defect in chylomicron formation in α-β lipoproteinaemia or with inhibitors of mucosal protein synthesis[97]. In the former, a specific apolipoprotein deficiency has now been identified[99]. This is the main apoprotein of β-lipoprotein (normal low-density lipoprotein) and a major consituent of VLDL.

Perhaps, as several workers have suggested, particulate lipid transport from the enterocyte depends primarily on the synthesis of VLDL. This suffices for particulate transport of endogenous lipid during fasting. After a fatty meal, as triglyceride synthesis increases relative to VLDL, chylomicrons form by VLDL aggregation. Similarly, the size of the chymicrons increases with the triglyceride load or with relative deficiency of protein or strongly amphiphilic phospholipid to maintain a fine emulsion. An important technique which may help to test such a concept is the use of isolated enterocytes which retain the capacity to discharge lipid particles into the incubation medium[100].

Transport particles are generally believed to leave the cell by temporary fusion of endoplasmic reticulum vesicles or Golgi vacuoles with indentations (caveolae) in the lateral and basal cell membranes, from where they are discharged into tissue fluid. This has been affirmed by electron microscopic observations made by some investigators[98] but not by others[64]. Experiments with an isolated enterocyte preparation, mentioned above, may offer some clues to the mechanism of extrusion and the factors affecting it.

10.8 LYMPHATIC AND VASCULAR TRANSPORT

After extrusion from enterocytes into tissue fluid, lipid is removed mainly by lymphatics, because most lipid leaves the cells as particles (VLDL and chylomicrons), to which lymphatics are freely permeable but not blood capillaries. The high permeability of lymphatic capillaries in the intestinal mucosa and throughout the body is usually attributed to lack of tight junctions between endothelial cells. A flap-valve action of overlapping cells has been suggested, so that tissue fluid and particles pass in unhindered but do not readily leak out again. This may be an oversimplification. The geometry of intercellular junctions is complex, often making it difficult to tell whether particles are passing between or through cells. Vesicle transport through cells may play a significant role[98,105].

The proportion of absorbed fatty acid and monoglyceride appearing in lymph depends on the extent to which it is incorporated into ester fat, mainly triglyceride. Hence, recovery in lymph is negligible for fatty acids with 8-carbon chains or smaller, low for 10-carbon chains, moderate (*ca.* 50%) for 12-carbon chains, and dominant (80% or more) for 14-carbon chains or longer[83]. Absorbed cholesterol, whether esterified or not, is transported almost exclusively as particles in lymph. Apparently, the same is true for cholesterol synthesised in the intestinal mucosa. Some free cholesterol may be exchanged with soluble lipoproteins in tissue fluid and lymph[101]. Lymph probably transports most of the phospholipid synthesised or reassembled in the enterocytes. However, the complicated metabolism of glycerophosphoryl choline and fatty acid moieties makes it difficult to apportion nascent phospholipid between the transport pathways.

In recent years, advances in lipoprotein analyses have generated an interest in the respective roles of VLDL and chylomicrons as transport particles in lymph. Evidence exists that a large proportion of lipid is transported as VLDL during fasting[102]. After a fatty meal, much of the dietary lipid is transported as chylomicrons. However, the relative importance of VLDL and chylomicron transport may vary with species, with type of lipid, and with composition and size of fatty meal. For example, VLDL transports nearly all absorbed cholesterol in the rabbit[103]. In rats, a high proportion of saturated fatty acid (C 16:0) in the meal promotes triglyceride transport in VLDL[104]. The size of chylomicron increases with increasing load of fat absorbed. The soluble lipoproteins (low-density lipoprotein and high-density lipoprotein) contribute little to lymphatic transport.

The subdivision of transport particles into VLDL and chylomicrons is an operational distinction, whereas the spectrum of particles may be continuous. Nevertheless, the distinction could be important. There seem to be differences in rate of clearance from the circulation and in metabolic fate of transported lipid between VLDL and chylomicrons[104] and between small and large chylomicrons. The rapidly growing body of knowledge concerning interchanges of lipid and apoprotein between particulate and soluble lipoproteins is outside the scope of this chapter.

Increased production of intestinal lymph is a well-known accompaniment of rapid fat absorption. The lymphagogue effect is potent. Evidence suggests that it may be mediated by a humoral agent acting on the microcirculation, but thus far none of the common vasoactive agents has been implicated[83].

Quantitative information is technically difficult to obtain on the proportion of absorbed lipid passing directly into the portal blood capillaries. An upper limit can be set by the discrepancy between amount absorbed and amount recovered in lymph. At one extreme lies cholesterol, which seems to be transported almost entirely in lymph. At the other extreme are short- and medium-chain fatty acids. These appear in lymph only in the small amounts to be expected from bulk drainage of tissue fluid into lymph and, in the case of medium-chain fatty acids, from a minor incorporation into mixed triglycerides. For long-chain fatty acids, as already noted, the discrepancy between absorption and lymphatic recovery is often small (less than 20%). Large differences should arouse suspicion that lymph is by-passing the cannulated duct, either in collateral channels or by lymphatic-venous anastomoses. Recovery of labelled long-chain fatty acid, mainly unesterified, in portal blood of rats with lymph fistula has provided direct evidence of vascular transport. Possibly, if re-esterification of long-chain fatty acids is slow or defective, a larger proportion may be transported in portal blood[83].

10.9 CONCLUSION

The absorption of lipids has been discussed as a physicochemical problem, and some current ideas have been summarised on the way in which interaction of lipid molecules with water and with other lipids influences their fate at each step in absorption.

In the lumen, triglyceride digestion and the entry of bile provide a supply of swelling amphiphiles and of detergents (bile acids), which are particularly well suited for micellar solubilisation of swelling amphiphiles. The latter, in turn, promote solubilisation of other lipid molecules. Thus, triglyceride digestion indirectly promotes absorption of other lipids.

Micellar solubilisation accelerates the delivery of lipid by diffusion across an unstirred layer. The large increase in aqueous lipid concentration with solubilisation outweighs the moderate decrease in diffusibility due to micellar aggregation.

Passage into and through the cell membrane is probably a monomolecular process. Small differences in hydrogen bonding or other hydrophilic properties of the molecule greatly modify the efficiency of transfer into membrane lipid. Small differences in molecular configuration could have a considerable effect on translocation of the molecule through the structured lipoprotein membrane.

The mode of transfer of molecules from lipid membrane to aqueous cytoplasm and the changes in physical state during metabolism are not understood. The binding of lipid by specific proteins may be significant. The end result is mainly a reaggregation of weakly polar lipid, stabilised as small particles (VLDL) or larger ones (chylomicrons) by a swelling amphiphile, phospholipid and a specific apoprotein. Synthesis of this apoprotein by the enterocyte is important for both assembly and extrusion of particles. After leaving the enterocyte, particulate lipid is removed by lymphatics, which are highly permeable. Some of the lipid, usually a small proportion, is removed in water-soluble form by the portal blood stream.

At present, any treatment of lipid absorption as a physicochemical problem will be speculative, incomplete, and—when attempted by a biologist—probably naive. Nevertheless, this account may serve to show how the molecular biophysics of lipids has already illuminated some aspects of absorption and has pointed out problems remaining to be solved.

ACKNOWLEDGEMENTS

The National Health and Medical Research Council of Australia, the Medical Research Grants Committee of Western Australia, and the Raine Foundation provided funds for research support, Dr. N. E. Hoffman and other members of the author's research group made many contributions. The Mayo Foundation offered the author support as a Visiting Scientist during preparation of the manuscript, and Dr. W. H. J. Summerskill generously provided facilities. Finally, Dr. A. F. Hofmann has been a source of stimulus and encouragement for many years, and has offered much constructive criticism.

References

1. Borgström, B. (1973). Intestinal absorption of fats: (1) Digestion and absorption. Gastrointestinal physiology (Smythe, editor)
2. Johnston, J. M. (1968). 'Mechanism of Fat Absorption' in *Handbook of Physiology*, Sec. 6, Vol. 3, 1353 (C. F. Code, editor) (Washington D.C.: Amer. Physiol. Soc.)
3. Treadwell, C. R. and Vahouny, G. V. (1968). 'Cholesterol Absorption' in *Handbook of Physiology*, Sec. 6, Vol. 3, 1407 (C. F. Code, editor) (Washington D.C.: Amer. Physiol. Soc.)
4. Hofmann, A. F. and Small, D. M. (1967). Detergent properties of bile salts: correlation with physiological function. *Annu. Rev. Med.*, **18**, 333

5. Small, D. M. (1968). A classification of biological lipids based upon their interaction in aqueous systems. *J. Amer. Oil Chemists Soc.*, **45**, 108
6. Carey, M. C. and Small, D. M. (1970). The characteristics of mixed micellar solutions with particular reference to bile. *Amer. J. Med.*, **49**, 590
7. Lawrence, A. S. C. (1961). Polar Interaction in Detergency in *Surface Activity and Detergency*, 158 (K. Durham, editor) (London: Macmillan)
8. Hofmann, A. F. (1968). Intraluminal Factors in the Absorption of Glycerides in *Medium Chain Triglycerides*, 9 (J. R. Senior, editor) (Philadelphia: University of Pennsylvania Press)
9. Frazer, A. C., Schulman, J. H. and Stewart, H. C. (1944). Emulsification of fat in the intestine of the rat and its relationship to absorption. *J. Physiol. (London)*, **103**, 306
10. Desnuelle, P. and Savary, P. (1963). Specificity of lipases. *J. Lipid Res.*, **4**, 369
11. Mattson, F. H., Volpenhein, R. A. and Benjamin, L. (1970). Inhibition of lipolysis by normal alcohols. *J. Biol. Chem.*, **245**, 5335
12. Hofmann, A. F. and Mekhjian, H. S. (1973). 'Bile acids and the intestinal absorption of fat and electrolytes in health and disease' in *The Bile Acids*, Vol. 2, (P. P. Nair and D. Kritchevsky, editors) (New York: Plenum Press)
13. Brockerhoff, H. (1968). Substrate specificity of pancreatic lipase. *Biochim. Biophys. Acta*, **159**, 296
14. Baskys, B., Klein, E. and Lever, W. F. (1963). Lipases of blood and tissues: III. Purification and properties of pancreatic lipase. *Archiv. Biochem. Biophys.*, **102**, 201
15. Morgan, R. G. H., Barrowman, J. and Borgström, B. (1969). The effect of sodium taurodesoxycholate and pH on the gel filtration behaviour of rat pancreatic protein and lipases. *Biochim. Biophys. Acta*, **175**, 65
16. Maylié, M. F., Charles, M., Gache, C. and Desnuelle, P. (1971). Isolation and partial identification of a pancreatic colipase. *Biochim. Biophys. Acta*, **229**, 286
17. Borgström, B. and Erlanson, C. (1971). Pancreatic juice co-lipase: physiological importance. *Biochim. Biophys. Acta*, **242**, 509
18. Erlanson, C. and Borgström, B. (1970). Tributyrine as a substrate for determination of lipase activity of pancreatic juice and small intestinal content. *Scand. J. Gastroenterol.*, **5**, 293
19. Morgan, R. G. H., Barrowman, J., Filipek-Wender, H. and Borgström, B. (1967). The lipolytic enzymes of rat pancreatic juice. *Biochim. Biophys. Acta*, **146**, 314
20. Mattson, F. H. and Volpenhein, R. A. (1966). Carboxylic ester hydrolases of rat pancreatic juice. *J. Lipid Res.*, **7**, 536
21. Erlanson, C. (1972). Pancreatic esterase, lipase and co-lipase: purification, characterization and physiological importance. *M.D. Thesis*, 15 (Lund: Rahms Boktryckeri AB)
22. Hyun, J., Kothari, H., Herm, E., Mortenson, J., Treadwell, C. R. and Vahouny, G. V. (1969). Purification and properties of pancreatic juice cholesterol esterase. *J. Biol. Chem.*, **244**, 1937
23. Hyun, J., Steinberg, M., Treadwell, C. R. and Vahouny, G. V. (1971). Cholesterol esterase—a polymeric enzyme. *Biochem. Biophys. Res. Commun.*, **44**, 819
24. Vahouny, C. V., Weersing, S. and Treadwell, C. R. (1965). Function of specific bile acids in cholesterol activity *in vitro*. *Biochim. Biophys. Acta*, **98**, 607
25. de Haas, G. H., Postema, N. M., Nieuwenhuizen, W. and van Deenen, L. L. M. (1968). Purification and properties of phospholipase A from porcine pancreas. *Biochim. Biophys. Acta*, **159**, 103
26. Arnesjö, B., Nilsson, A., Barrowman, J. and Borgström, B. (1969). Intestinal digestion and absorption of cholesterol and lecithin in the human: intubation studies with a fat soluble reference substance. *Scand. J. Gastroenterol.*, **4**, 653
27. Borgström, B., Dahlquist, A., Lundh, G. and Sjövall, J. (1957). Studies of intestinal digestion and absorption in the human. *J. Clin. Invest.*, **36**, 1521
28. Cohen, M., Morgan, R. G. H. and Hofmann, A. F. (1971). Lipolytic activity of human gastric and duodenal juice against medium and long chain triglycerides. *Gastroenterology*, **60**, 1
29. Clark, S. B., Brause, B. and Holt, P. R. (1969). Lipolysis and absorption of fat in the rat stomach. *Gastroenterology*, **56**, 214
30. Barrowman, J. A. and Darnton, S. J. (1970). The lipase of rat gastric mucosa, *Gastroenterology*, **59**, 13

31. Hamosh, M. and Scow, R. O. (1973). Lingual lipase and its role in the digestion of dietary lipids. *J. Clin. Invest.*, in the press
32. Hofmann, A. F. (1968). Functions of bile in the alimentary canal in *Handbook of Physiology*, Sec. 6, Vol. 4, 2507 (C. F. Code, editor) (Washington D.C.: Amer. Physiol. Soc.)
33. Aberdeen, V., Shepherd, P. A. and Simmonds, W. J. (1960). Concurrent measurement in unanesthetized rats of intestinal transport and fat absorption from the lumen. *Quart. J. Exp. Physiol.*, **45**, 265
34. Morgan, R. G. H. (1963). The effect of diverting bile and pancreatic juice on the inhibition of gastric motility by duodenal stimuli in the unanesthetized rat. *Quart. J. Exp. Physiol.*, **48**, 273
35. Morgan, R. G. H. and Hofmann, A. F. (1970). Validity of ^{3}H-labelled triether, a non-absorbable oil-phase marker, in the estimation of fat absorption. *J. Lipid Res.*, **11**, 231
36. Go, V. L. W., Hofmann, A. F. and Summerskill, W. H. J. (1970). Pancreozymin bioassay in man based on pancreatic enzyme secretion: potency of specific amino acids and other digestive products. *J. Clin. Invest.*, **49**, 1558
37. Small, D. M. (1971). 'The physical chemistry of cholanic acids' in *The Bile Acids*, Vol. 1, 249 (P. P. Nair and D. Kritschevsky, editors) (New York: Plenum Press)
38. Northfield, T. C. and Hofmann, A. F. (1972). Relationship between bile acid pool size, bile acid output and production of lithogenic bile in man. *Gastroenterology*, (abst) Amer. Liver Soc. Oct. 1972
39. Brooks, A. M. and Grossman, M. I. (1970). Postprandial pH and neutralising capacity of the proximal duodenum in dogs. *Gastroenterology*, **59**, 85
40. Worning, H. and Mullertz, S. (1966). pH and pancreatic enzymes in the human duodenum during digestion of a standard meal. *Scand. J. Gastroenterol.*, **1**, 268
41. Go, V. L. W., Poley, J. R., Hofmann, A. F. and Summerskill, W. H. J. (1970). The disturbances in fat digestion induced by acid jejunal pH due to gastric hypersecretion in man. *Gastroenterology*, **58**, 638
42. Borgström, B. (1964). Influence of bile salt, pH and time on the action of pancreatic lipase; physiological implications. *J. Lipid Res.*, **5**, 522
43. Porter, H. P. and Saunders, D. R. (1971). Isolation of the aqueous phase of human intestinal contents during the digestion of a fatty meal. *Gastroenterology*, **60**, 997
44. Ricour, C. and Rey, J. (1972). Kinetics of fat hydrolysis and micellar solubilization in children with pancreatic deficiency. *Biol. et Gastroenterol.*, **5**, 36
45. Short, M., and Rhodes, C. T. (1972). Effect of surfactants on diffusion of drugs across membranes. *Nature New Biol.*, **236**, 44
46. Lee, K. Y. (1972). Artifacts in ultracentrifugal estimation of aqueous fatty acid concentration. *J. Lipid Res.*, **13**, 745
47. Bikhazi, A. B. and Higuchi, W. I. (1970). Interfacial barrier limited interphase transport of cholesterol in the aqueous polysorbate 80-hexadecane system. *J. Pharm. Sci.*, **59**, 744
48. Suripurya, V. and Higuchi, W. I. (1972). Interfacially controlled transport of micelle-solubilised sterols across an oil-water interface in two ionic surfactant systems. *J. Pharm. Sci.*, **61**, 375
49. Bikhazi, A. B. and Higuchi, W. I. (1971). Interfacial barriers to the transport of sterols and other organic compounds at the aqueous polysorbate 80-hexadecane interface. *Biochim. Biophys. Acta*, **233**, 676
50. Dainty, J. and House, C. R. (1966). Unstirred layers in frog skin. *J. Physiol.*, **182**, 66
51. Smulders, A. P. and Wright, E. M. (1971). The magnitude of non-electrolyte selectivity in the gall bladder epithelium. *J. Membrane Biol.*, **5**, 297
52. Diamond, J. M. and Wright, E. M. (1969). Biological membranes: the physical basis of ion and nonelectrolyte selectivity. *Annu. Rev. Physiol.*, **31**, 581
53. Dawson, A. M. and Isselbacher, K. J. (1960). Studies in lipid metabolism in the small intestine with observations on the role of bile salts. *J. Clin. Invest.*, **39**, 730
54. Johnston, J. M. and Borgström, B. (1964). The intestinal absorption and metabolism of micellar solutions of lipids. *Biochim. Biophys. Acta*, **84**, 412
55. Hoffman, N. E. (1970). The relationship between uptake *in vitro* of oleic acid and micellar solubilisation. *Biochim. Biophys. Acta*, **196**, 193
56. Lee, K. Y., Hoffman, N. E. and Simmonds, W. J. (1971). The effect of partition of

fatty acid between oil and micelles on its uptake by everted intestinal sacs. *Biochim. Biophys. Acta*, **249**, 548

57. Hoffman, N. E. and Yeoh, V. J. (1971). The relationship between concentration and uptake by rat small intestine, *in vitro*, for two micellar solutes. *Biochim. Biophys.* **233**, 49

58. Simmonds, W. J. (1972). The role of micellar solubilization in lipids absorption. *Aust. J. Exp. Biol. Med. Sci.*, **50**, 403

59. Wilson, F. A., Sallee, V. L. and Dietschy, J. M. (1971). Unstirred water layers in intestine: rate determinant of fatty acid from micellar solutions. *Science*, **174**, 1031

60. Gibaldi, M. and Feldman, S. (1970). Mechanisms of surfactant effects on drug absorption. *J. Pharm. Sci.*, **59**, 579

61. Linscheer, W. G. (1972). Optimal micellar solubilization of oleic acid, an undesirable condition for maximal absorption. *Gastroenterology*, **62**, 777

62. Lacy, D. and Taylor, A. B. (1962). Fat absorption by epithelial cells of the small intestine of the rat. *Amer. J. Anat.*, **110**, 155

63. Strauss, E. W. (1968). Morphological aspects of triglyceride absorption in *Handbook of Physiology*, Sec. 6, Vol. 3, 1377 (C. F. Code, editor) (Washington D.C.: Amer. Physiol. Soc.)

64. Cardell, R. R. Jr., Badenhausen, S. and Porter, K. R. (1967). Intestinal triglyceride absorption in the rat. An electron microscopical study. *J. Cell. Biol.*, **34**, 123

65. Thornton, A. G., Vahouny, G. V. and Treadwell, C. R. (1968). Absorption of lipids from mixed micellar bile salt solutions. *Proc. Soc. Exp. Biol. Med.*, **127**, 629

66. Schultz, S. G. and Strecker, C. K. (1971). Cholesterol and bile salt influxes across brush border of rabbit jejunum. *Amer. J. Physiol.*, **220**, 59

67. Mishkin, S., Yalovsky, M. and Kessler, J. I. (1972). Stages of uptake and incorporation of micellar palmitic acid by hamster proximal intestinal mucosa. *J. Lipid Res.*, **13**, 155

68. Glover, J. and Morton, R. A. (1958). The absorption and metabolism of sterols. *Brit. Med. Bull.*, **14**, 226

69. Hofmann, A. F. and Borgström, B. (1964). The intraluminal phase of fat digestion in man: the lipid content of the micellar and oil phases of intestinal content obtained during fat digestion and absorption. *J. Clin. Invest.*, **43**, 247

70. Krone, C. L., Theodor, E., Sleisenger, M. H. and Jeffries, J. H. (1968). Studies on the pathogenesis of malabsorption: lipid hydrolysis and micelle formation in the intestinal lumen. *Medicine*, **47**, 89

71. Badley, B. W. D., Murphy, G. M., Bouchier, I. A. D. and Sherlock, S. (1970). Diminished micellar phase lipid in patients with chronic nonalcoholic liver disease and steatorrhea. *Gastroenterology*, **58**, 781

72. Porter, H. P., Saunders, D. R., Tytgat, G., Brunser, O. and Rubin, C. E. (1971). Fat absorption in bile fistula man: a morphological and biochemical study. *Gastroenterology*, **60**, 1008

73. Hoffman, N. E., Simmonds, W. J. and Morgan, R. G. H. (1971). A comparison of absorption of free fatty acid and *a*-glyceryl ether in the presence and absence of a micellar phase. *Biochim. Biophys. Acta*, **231**, 487

74. Booth, C. C. (1968). Effects of location along the small intestine on absorption of nutrients, in *Handbook of Physiology*, Sec. 6, Vol. 3, 1513 (C. F. Code, editor) (Washington D. C.: Amer. Physiol. Soc.)

75. Knoebel, L. K. (1972). Intestinal absorption *in vivo* of micellar and non-micellar lipid. *Amer. J. Physiol.*, **223**, 255

76. Hoffman, N. E. and Hofman, A. F. (1972). Absorption rates of micellar versus non-micellar oleic acid: jejunal perfusion studies in man. *Gastroenterology*, **62**, 763

77. Weiss, J. B. and Holt, P. R. (1971). Controlling factors during intestinal fat absorption in man. *J. Clin. Invest.*, **50**, 97a (abst)

78. Simmonds, W. J., Hofmann, A. F. and Theodor, E. (1967). Absorption of cholesterol from a micellar solution: intestinal perfusion studies in man. *J. Clin. Invest.*, **46**, 874

79. Doluisio, J. T., Billups, N. F., Dittert, L. W., Sugita, E. T. and Swintowsky, J. V. (1969). Drug absorption 1: an *in situ* rat gut technique yielding realistic absorption rates. *J. Pharm. Sci.*, **58**, 1196

80. Clark, S. B. and Holt, P. R. (1968). Rate-limiting steps in steady-state intestinal absorption of trioctanoin-1-^{14}C: effect of biliary and pancreatic flow diversion. *J. Clin. Invest.*, **47**, 612

81. Scow, R. O., Stein, Y. and Stein, O. (1967). Incorporation of dietary lecithin and lysolecithin into lymph chylomicrons in the rat. *J. Biol. Chem.*, **242**, 4919
82. Senior, J. R. and Isselbacher, K. J. (1960). Activation of long-chain fatty acids by rat-gut mucosa. *Biochim. Biophys. Acta*, **44**, 399
83. Simmonds, W. J. (1972). Fat absorption and chylomicron formation in *Blood Lipids and Lipoproteins: Quantitation, Composition and Metabolism*, 705 (G. J. Nelson, editor) (New York: John Wiley and Sons)
84. Dietschy, J. M. and Weis, H. J. (1971). Cholesterol synthesis by the gastrointestinal tract. *Amer. J. Clin. Nutr.*, **24**, 70
85. Simmonds, W. J. (1969). Effects of bile salts on the rate of fat absorption. *Amer. J. Clin. Nutr.*, **22**, 266
86. Rodgers, J. B. and Tandon, R. (1971). Effects of infusion of fortified bile and bile salts on jejunal lipid reesterifying enzyme activities of bile diverted rats. *Clin. Res.*, **19**, 401
87. Dietschy, J. M. (1967). Effects of bile salts on intermediate metabolism of the intestinal mucosa. *Fed. Proc. (Fed. Amer. Soc. Exp. Biol.)*, **26**, 1589
88. Cheney, F. E., Burke, V., Clark, M. L. and Senior, J. R. (1971). Intestinal fat absorption and esterification from luminal micellar solutions containing deoxycholic acid. *Proc. Soc. Exp. Biol.*, **133**, 212
89. Ockner, R. K., Manning, J. A., Poppenhausen, R. B. and Ho, W. K. L. (1972). A binding protein for fatty acids in cytosol of intestinal mucosa, liver, myocardium and other tissues. *Science*, **177**, 56
90. Ganguly, J., Krishnamurty, S. and Mahadevan, S. (1959). The transport of carotenoids vitamin A. and cholesterol across the intestines of rats and chickens. *Biochem. J.*, **71**, 756
91. Jersild, R. A., Jr. (1966). A time sequence study of fat absorption in the rat jejunum. *Amer. J. Anat.*, **118**, 135
92. Jersild, R. A., Jr. and Clayton, R. T. (1971). A comparison of the morphology of lipid absorption in the jejunum and ileum of the adult rat. *Amer. J. Anat.*, **131**, 481
93. Dobbins. W. O., Jr. (1966). An ultrastructural study of the intestinal mucosa in congenital β-lipoprotein deficiency with particular emphasis upon the intestinal absorptive cell. *Gastroenterology*, **50**, 195
94. Clark, S. B. (1972). Intestinal absorptive capacity, and regional metabolism and transport of triolein in the unanaesthetized rat. *Gastroenterology*, **62**, 735
95. Sjostrand, F. S. and Borgström, B. (1967). The lipid components of the smooth-surfaced membrane-bounded vesicles of the columnar cells of the rat intestinal epithelium during fat absorption. *J. Ultrastructure Res.*, **20**, 140
96. Sage, J. A. and Jersild, R. A., Jr. (1971). Comparative distribution of carbohydrates and lipid droplets in the Golgi apparatus of intestinal absorptive cells. *J. Cell. Biol.*, **51**, 333
97. Glickman, R. M., Kirsch, K. and Isselbacher, K. J. (1972). Fat absorption during inhibition of protein synthesis: studies of lymph chylomicrons. *J. Clin. Invest.*, **51**, 356
98. Tytgat, G. N., Rubin, C. E. and Saunders, D. R. (1971). Synthesis and transport of lipoprotein particles by intestinal absorptive cells in man. *J. Clin. Invest.*, **50**, 2065
99. Gotto, A. M., Levy, R. I., John, K. and Frederickson, D. S. (1971). On the protein defect in abetalipoproteinemia. *New Engl. J. Med.*, **284**, 813
100. Yousef, I. M. and Kuksis, A. (1972). Release of chylomicrons, by isolated cells of rat mucosa. *Lipids*, **7**, 380
101. Minari, O. Zilversmit, D. B. (1963). Behaviour of dog lymph chylomicron lipid constituents during incubation with serum. *J. Lipid Res.*, **4**, 424
102. Ockner, R. K., Hughes, F. B. and Isselbacher, K. J. (1969). Very low density lipoproteins in intestinal lymph: origin, composition, and role in lipid transport in the fasting state. *J. Clin. Invest.*, **48**, 2079
103. Rudel, L. L., Morris, M. D. and Felts, J. M. (1972). The transport of exogenous cholesterol in the rabbit: 1. Role of cholesterol ester of lymph chylomicra and lymph very low density lipoproteins in absorption. *J. Clin. Invest.*, **51**, 2686
104. Ockner, R. K., Hughes, F. B. and Isselbacher, K. J. (1969). Very low density lipoproteins in the intestinal lymph: role in triglyceride and cholesterol transport during fat absorption. *J. Clin. Invest.*, **48**, 2367
105. Dobbins, W. O. (1971). Intestinal mucosal lacteal in transport of macromolecules and chylomicrons. *Amer. J. Clin. Nutr.*, **24**, 77

Index

377

—,3-*O*-methyl-
  intestinal absorption, 304
Glucosidases in intestines, 294, 303
Glycerides (*see also* Triglycerides)
  absorbed in lymph, 370
  re-esterification, 366
  synthesis, 367
Glycine
  in colonic absorption, 329
  gastrin release by, 13
Glycoamylase in intestines, 302
Glycoproteins in gastric mucus, 242
Goblet cells in intestines, 297
Goldman–Hodgkin–Katz treatment of
  Nernst–Planck equation, 74–77
Golgi apparatus, 369
Golgi complex, digestive enzymes and, 203
Gut (*see also* Intestines)
  blood flow, autoregulation of, 114, 115
  mucosa, colour changes in, 112

Haemoglobin iron, intestinal absorption, 320
Haemorrhage, gastrointestinal circulation
  and, 119, 120
Hartnup disease, intestinal absorption of
  amino acids in, 307
Haustra, 168
Heidenhain pouch, 233
Hemicholinium, acetylcholine synthesis by
  salivary glands and, 212
Hepatic artery autoregulation in, 114
Histamine
  in gastric secretion, 14–17, 235, 244
  gastrin secretion and, 3
  pancreatic blood flow and, 126
  parietal cells in gastric mucosa and, 245
  release from gastric mucosal barrier, 231
L-Histidine
  intestinal absorption, 294
Histidine decarboxylase
  cholecystokinin stimulation of, 21
  gastric secretion and, 14, 15
Hogs—*see* Swine
Hormones (*see also* individual hormones)
  antidiuretic, salivary gland control by, 215
  colonic absorption and, 328
  gastric, interactions, 28–33
  gastrointestinal, 2–43
  in intestinal absorption of sodium, 315
  intestinal absorption of sugars and, 306
  mucosal, mediation, 46–54
  pancreas secretion and, 281–283
  secretion of saliva and, 208
Humans, gastrin, 5
Hydrochloric acid, gastric secretion, 237, 238
Hydrogen bonding in water, 345

Hydrolysis of glycerides, 366
Hyperaemia, gastrointestinal blood flow
  and, 130
Hypercapnia, gastrointestinal blood flow
  and, 130
Hypochlorhydria, gastrin in, 10
Hypothalamus, gastric secretion inhibition
  and, 255
Hypoxia, gastrointestinal blood flow and, 130

Ileocecal sphincter, 168
Ileum
  contraction, 159
  rabbit, shunt pathway across, 97–99
  sodium absorption by, 312
Incretin, insulin secretion and, 8
Inhibition of gastric secretion, 255–259
Injections in gastrointestinal circulation
  studies, 110, 111
Inositol, intestinal absorption, 316
Insulin
  cholecystokinin and, 21
  gastric secretion and, 16, 235
  histidine decarboxylase activity and, 15
  release, secretin and, 26
  secretion, gastrin and, 8
Insulin hypoglycaemia, cephalic stimulation of gastric secretion by, 247
Interaction between gastrointestinal hormones, 283, 284
Intestinal phase of gastric secretion, 253
Intestines (*see also* Gut)
  absorption, methods of study, 298–300
    of water-soluble substances by, 293–341
  arterio-venous anastomoses in, 110
  autoregulation of blood flow in, 115
  blood flow, 128–131
  cholecystokinin in, 19
  electrophysiology and, 82
  epithelium, electrophysiology, 92–99
  gastric secretion and, 234
  gastrin in, 6, 7, 11, 12
  lipid digestion in, 354
  motility, 157–167
    cholecystokinin and, 20
  secretion, cyclic AMP and, 50–54
Intrinsic factor
  in gastric mucosa, 243
  in intestinal absorption of vitamin B_{12}, 318
Ions, movement across membranes, 70–74
Iron, intestinal absorption, 319–324
Isoproterenol
  gastric secretion and, 245
  saliva composition and, 215
Isotopes
  fractionation, in gastrointestinal circula-
    tion studies, 112, 113
  in gastric secretion studies, 232